The Good Vibrations Guide to Sex

The Good Vibrations Guide to Sex

THE MOST COMPLETE SEX MANUAL EVER WRITTEN

Third Edition

Cathy Winks and Anne Semans

Illustrated by Phoebe Gloeckner

CLEIS PRESS

Published in the United States by Cleis Press Inc., P.O. Box 14684, San Francisco, California 94114.

Printed in the United States.
Cover design: Scott Idleman
Text design: Karen Quigg
Cleis Press logo art: Juana Alicia
Third Edition.
10 9 8

LIBRARY OF CONGRESS CATALOGING-IN-PUBLICATION DATA

Winks, Cathy.
The good vibrations guide to sex / Cathy Winks and Anne Semans ; illustrated by Phoebe Gloeckner.
        p. cm.
Rev. ed. of: The new good vibrations guide to sex. 2nd ed. c1997.
Includes bibliographical references and index.
    ISBN 1-57344-158-9 (alk. paper)
    1. Sex. 2. Sex instruction. I. Semans, Anne. II. Winks, Cathy.
New good vibrations guide to sex. III. Title.
    HQ31.W77346 2002
    613.9'6—dc21

                        2002151968

Contents

Illustrations

Acknowledgments

Thanks first and foremost to all our survey respondents, to Joani Blank for creating Good Vibrations, and to all the Good Vibrations employees past and present who shared information, anecdotes, and practical support over the years, particularly Krissy Cababa, Constance Clare, Kate Cunningham, Scout Festa, Staci Haines, Eve Meelan, Laura Miller, Carol Queen, Thomas Roche, Joyce Solano, and Ann Whidden. Thanks also to the many individuals in the sex-positive community who provided resources, referrals, and interviews for the different editions of this book, including Eric Albert, Isadora Alman, Chris Bridges, Ken Dorfman, Gosnell Duncan, M. J. Ecker of Jackinworld.com, Jenne of Clitical.com, Eleanor Hamilton, Chris Mann, Dan Martin, Dr. Marc Nelson, Cory Silverberg, Leonore Tiefer, and Cheri Van Hoover, C.N.M.

We're very grateful to our profile subjects, who were so generous with their time and wisdom: Adrienne Benedicks, Marilyn Bishara, Joani Blank, Susie Bright, Susan Colvin, Betty Dodson, Nina Hartley, Jack Morin, Shar Rednour, Candida Royalle, Russell of sexuality.org, Annie Sprinkle, Jackie Strano, Kat Sunlove, and Tristan Taormino.

Heartfelt thanks to our friends and mentors Susie Bright, Michael Castleman, and Ray Potter for many years of inspiration, encouragement, and advice; to MB Condon for illustrating the first edition of this book; and to Phoebe Gloeckner for illustrating this third edition.

We appreciate the work of our agent, Timothy Seldes, and of Frédérique Delacoste, Felice Newman, and Don Weise at Cleis Press.

Finally, lots of love and thanks to Becky, Jeffrey, Sheila, Trish, and the Semans and Winks families for their support and patience.

Foreword

When Good Vibrations was founded in 1977, it was a very different world than it is now. Founder Joani Blank wanted to establish a clean, comfortable place for women to shop for sex toys.

Since then, we've changed profoundly—but our mission is still founded on the basic principle that accurate sex information and access to sexual pleasure is a birthright for everyone on this planet.

Today, Good Vibrations has grown much larger than its tiny 1977 site in San Francisco's Mission district. We operate two stores (in San Francisco and Berkeley) and a thriving mail order and web business. Our customers are women, men, and transgendered folks from every walk of life and all over the world. We don't just sell erotic products—we manufacture them, with a full line of toys, GV Exclusives, that aren't available anywhere else. We've been publishing erotic and educational sex books since the beginning with our in-house publisher Down There Press; in 2000, we acquired audiobook publisher Passion Press and started our own in-house video department, Sexpositive Productions, which has released four videos to date.

Our sales associates, in the stores and on the phone, are fully trained sex educators, receiving more formal sex education than the vast majority of physicians. They'll answer questions that would get you a blank stare in most college health classrooms, and they'll tell you everything you need to know to use our products safely and effectively. In contrast to other adult businesses, we don't sell our products as "novelties"—they are what they are, *toys*, designed to be fun and life-affirming, to augment your explorations of sexuality.

Similarly, our books, audiobooks, videos, and DVDs are selected with an eye toward accurate sex information that is helpful to the practical user. Erotica and sex instruction videos and books can be hot *and* sex-positive—and, in many cases, can be hot *because* they're sex-positive. Our philosophy is to seek out the best of what's available and, if it's not available, do it ourselves.

The Good Vibrations Guide to Sex has long been one of the cornerstones of that philosophy. It's used in college classrooms and each edition has taken its honored place in many sexuality libraries. This newest revision contains the most up-to-date sexual information available. Authors Anne Semans and Cathy Winks have brought their experiences at Good Vibrations—and the firsthand anecdotes and feedback of our customers—to the task of creating the most comprehensive sex guide ever written. We're proud to present this new volume, and to further our mission every day by offering toys, books, and videos that reflect a positive outlook on sexuality.

Enjoy this newest edition of *The Good Vibrations Guide to Sex*, and let it guide you in your explorations!

The Staff of Good Vibrations

Introduction

People need good sex books. Access to accurate sex information helps us to understand ourselves better and to build more intimate relationships. Not to mention that sex is just good, clean fun—and the more you learn about it, the more fun it becomes.

We were inspired to write the first edition of this book when we worked in a women-run vibrator store. Many customers requested a comprehensive, up-to-date sex manual, but we simply couldn't find one that spoke to a diverse audience, addressed a wide variety of sexual activities, and celebrated sex toy use. So we wrote it ourselves. Since its publication in 1994, *The Good Vibrations Guide to Sex* has made its way onto bedside tables around the world. It is used in health clinics and college sexuality courses, is recommended by sex therapists and medical professionals, and has helped tens of thousands of women and men to enjoy more satisfying sex lives.

What's New?

This is the third edition of *The Good Vibrations Guide to Sex*. We revise this book every few years, which might lead you to wonder, "Is there really anything new to say about sex?" Our answer is, "You'd be surprised." Sure, basic sexual anatomy doesn't change, but cultural attitudes, entertainment technologies, and health information change with every passing year.

Our sex manual offers the most complete guide to sex toys in print, and we consider it a duty (and a pleasure) to bring you up to date on the latest developments in sex toys and technologies. Read on to learn how the microchip is transforming vibrators just as it did computers, making them faster, smaller, and more powerful. Digital video not only makes the latest blockbuster jump off the screen, it's also adding more realism to your porn; and cell phones aren't just for roadside emergencies anymore (at least of the nonsexual kind).

Thanks in part to reader feedback, we've further broadened our scope beyond toys and technique. In a new chapter called Sex Over a Lifetime, we discuss how major life milestones affect your experience of sex, and we offer suggestions for navigating the sexual changes effected by adolescence, pregnancy, parenting, menopause, and aging. Throughout, we have included the most current information regarding sexual health.

Over the past quarter-century, certain sex-positive pioneers have made unique contributions to improving sex in America. We pay tribute to these sex educators, activists, and entrepreneurs with interviews and profiles throughout the book. You'll learn how Candida Royalle, Betty Dodson, Nina Hartley, and many others can enhance your understanding of sexuality, deepen your appreciation for sexual diversity, and show you a good time in the process.

Since this book first appeared in the early nineties, the Web has burst onto the scene, bringing millions of people together to share information, entertainment, and community. Our sexual landscape has been forever altered in the process. We used to lament the fact that people had such limited access to sexual resources, but now, thanks to the Web, you can easily discuss sexual techniques, order a new toy, read some hot erotica, or chat with a sexy cyberpal. We're enthusiastic cheerleaders for the ways in which the Web has advanced our collective sexual literacy, and we've added a new chapter devoted to how the Web can enhance your sex life.

Finally, we've added all new illustrations to give the book a more contemporary feel. When it comes to describing a certain technique or toy, a picture really is worth a thousand words.

In more than fifteen years as sex writers, we've had the privilege of fielding sexual questions, confessions, concerns, and tips from thousands of women and men. Their healthy, candid curiosity dictates what you'll find here—advice, instruction, definitions, illustrations, anecdotes, encouragement, and validation for a variety of sexual interests and activities, courtesy of two women who have been asked a lot of questions about sex. We're convinced that access to good sex information leads to greater health and happiness, and we hope to provide you with all the encouragement you need to explore a whole new world of sexual pleasure. So dive right in and enjoy!

Cathy Winks and Anne Semans
San Francisco
July 2002
www.anneandcathy.com

CHAPTER 1

About Good Vibrations

The Good Vibrations Philosophy

We are two very lucky women. During our decade-long careers at Good Vibrations, San Francisco's women-run sex business, we not only had the opportunity to discuss sex with thousands of customers, but we actually got paid to play with vibrators, read erotica, and review adult videos. Since then, we've written several sex guides, edited an erotic anthology (about sex toys, of course!), and braved numerous media interviews in hopes of sharing the Good Vibrations' philosophy with as many people as possible. We feel fortunate to have found a vocation that fills us with missionary zeal, is consistent with our feminist politics, and is fun to boot.

Good Vibrations was founded on the premise that there's more sexual pleasure available than most people experience, and that achieving this pleasure should not be difficult, dangerous, or expensive. The company mission is to provide access to sexual materials and accurate sex information to combat the fear, ignorance, bias, and insecurity that prevent too many of us from enjoying the sexual pleasure that is our birthright.

Not everyone would agree that selling vibrators and adult videos is consistent with a feminist agenda, but we believe that honest communication about sex is a prerequisite to equal rights both in and out of the bedroom. The adult entertainment industry has traditionally been grounded in male experience and geared toward male consumers—so it's up to feminists to challenge this bias.

Our customers frequently tell us how refreshing it is to shop at a women-owned business, as they feel that our "clean, well-lighted" environment is equally appealing to men and women. Good Vibrations, founded in 1977, is part of a grassroots movement that has been picking up steam ever since: More and more women have stepped forward to name their own sexual desires and to produce their own sexual writings, images, and products, and in the process they've changed the face of the adult industry for men and women alike.

We take a great deal of pride in the revolutionary nature of our work. For one thing, we believe that sex toys are inherently revolutionary. Not only are they self-assertion tools—no dildo is ever going to pressure you into an encounter against your will—but when you plug in a vibrator or cue up an adult video, you're affirming that you deserve to experience pleasure for pleasure's sake. This affirmation is a great leap of faith for many of us. We can experience sexual pleasure in countless ways, yet we tend to rate sexual activities in a hierarchy of best, second best, or better-than-nothing. Whether consciously or not, many of us operate from the belief that sex is okay only if we're motivated by the desire to (a) make babies, (b) express intimacy, or (c) please a partner. The idea that pleasure for pleasure's sake is sufficient motivation for sexual activity, and that no means of experiencing sexual pleasure is morally, aesthetically, or romantically superior to another, is the subversive philosophy behind the enjoyment of sex toys.

When Good Vibrations first opened its doors, the vast majority of manufacturers and retailers in the adult industry dealt in overpriced, shoddy merchandise—many still do. They can count on the fact that their customers are simply too ignorant or embarrassed about sexuality to demand the same quality control from sex toys that they would from household appliances or other products. Good Vibrations revolutionized the marketing of sex toys by taking a consumer-friendly approach. We display samples of all products on the shelves for customers to handle and compare before making their selection. We want our customers to make informed choices, so we acknowledge the drawbacks as well as the advantages of everything we carry.

By holding sex toys to the same standards as any other consumer goods, we've been blessed with an enthusiastic, trusting, and loyal customer base. Good Vibrations' success has had a ripple effect—other retailers and catalogers have adopted the same straightforward approach to selling sexually explicit materials, while manufacturers and distributors have begun improving the quality of their products.

We call the products we sell and love "sex toys," rather than "sexual aids" or "marital aids." A lot of the stigma attached to sexual merchandise seems to result from the misconception that vibrators, dildos, lubricants, and erotica are "aids" for those troubled by sexual "problems." Certainly sex toys are useful tools for individuals and couples who wish to explore and enhance their sexual imaginations and responses, and they can be immensely helpful to preorgasmic women, men with erectile dysfunctions, and couples with desire discrepancies. But identifying sex toys as relevant only to those with special needs, let alone relevant only to married couples, is inaccurate at best.

Our products were created first and foremost for fun, and that's why we call them "toys." You don't need to be experiencing a sexual dysfunction to justify purchasing a sex toy, and you shouldn't feel that purchasing a sex toy exposes you as someone with a "problem." No one would describe a bakery as an establishment that sells "dietary aids"—to us it seems equally illogical to describe Good Vibrations as an establishment that sells "sexual aids." Whether or not you yourself enjoy playing with sex toys, we hope you'll agree that they are among the many "normal" options available in erotic accessories, no more and no less.

Yet the Good Vibrations mission to normalize the purchase of sex toys is just the thin end of the wedge—our ultimate goal is to normalize sex as a vital, life-affirming, primal force in human experience. All of us suffer when the Powers That Be—whether religious, political, or social—ignore, repress, or distort the free expression of sexual energy. This suffering is most disturbingly evident in sexual abuse and most commonly evident in the shame, discomfort, and insecurity many of us feel around sex. Sexual shame is completely unnecessary, and in our work and in this book we strive to bring the subject of sex into the light while encouraging a spirit of fun and adventure.

What's Between These Covers

Good Vibrations customers come from a wide range of cultural, religious, and political backgrounds; they are all ages and all sexual preferences. We supply sexual resources to urban professionals, bikers, suburban newlyweds, mobile-home-dwelling retirees, college-age lesbians, transsexuals, stroller-pushing moms, therapists, and nuns. We hope to reach a similarly wide range of people with this book—gay, straight, bisexual, transgendered, young, old, novices, old-timers, singles, partnered, multipartnered, the physically challenged, and the sexually jaded, to name a few. And we dream that this book will wind up in the hands of folks too shy to enter stores like Good Vibrations. We try, through our language, illustrations, and attitude, to reflect and be respectful of a variety of interests.

It's our experience that people from a wide range of backgrounds share certain traits: They crave accurate, practical, nonjudgmental information about sex, and they relish the opportunity to speak frankly about sexual activities. Furthermore, people of all sexual preferences take pleasure in many of the same toys and activities and have similar questions about what toys to play with and how to play with them. The teen looking for ways to enjoy safer sex and the transsexual looking for alternatives to intercourse may discover identical solutions in one of our chapters.

We've arranged the chapters according to types of sexual activities. For example, whereas many mainstream sex manuals will discuss penetration in a chapter on penis/vagina intercourse—usually billed as the ultimate sexual experience—we describe the variety of ways to penetrate a partner of either sex (vaginally, anally, with toys, fingers, etc.) and as only one of many enjoyable sexual activities.

You won't find chapters entitled "How Monogamous Heterosexuals Can Spice Up Their Love Lives" or "What Lesbians Do in Bed." We like to think that the contents of every chapter are relevant to women and men of all sexualities. To this end, we speak to our readers directly in the second person, as this seems to us the most graceful way to avoid any presumptions about sex or sexuality. You'll notice that we tend to describe sexual activities from the point of view of the active partner. We've done so to keep the descriptions simple and the language clear. We certainly don't mean to imply that the experience of the passive partner is of less worth.

Even the most well-intentioned sex books have a tendency to abuse statistics, and readers can't help but use these statistics to assess whether they're "normal"—are they having the right kind of sex, the right amount of sex? Yet surveys are just as vulnerable to cultural biases and trends as any other popular literature. Whether you're reading survey results claiming that less than 3 percent of the general population is gay, or that 40 percent of women and 30 percent of men suffer from "sexual dysfunction," keep in mind that it's notoriously difficult to compile accurate statistics on a subject as highly charged and as subjective as sexual behaviors and attitudes.

We won't be able to say it enough throughout this book: Everyone's different. This book is not about keeping up with the Joneses or judging the Joneses. It's about finding out what activities strike your own fancy. While we cop to citing a statistic now and then, it's usually to counter a stereotype. No matter how often you ask, we won't tell you how many vibrators it would take to satisfy the staff at the White House.

One of the most exciting aspects of working at a business like Good Vibrations is bearing witness to the breadth and variety of human sexuality and encouraging people to trust their own experiences and respect their own unique responses. The single most frustrating question Good Vibrations clerks field every day is, "What's the best vibrator (or lubricant or massage oil or erotic video)?" The myth that there's one sure-fire sexual silver bullet that will guarantee orgasm for one and all dies hard. Yet, you wouldn't dream of asking the clerk at a record store, "What's the best CD you've got in here?"

We all have the same basic body parts, and our bodies undergo the same basic sexual responses, yet the range in what stimulation people enjoy and how they subjectively experience arousal and orgasm is breathtaking. You'll probably consider some of the activities described in this book old hat. Some activities will strike you as intriguing, some will seem completely unappealing, and some will make you want to rush right out and try them for yourselves. The beautiful and fascinating thing about sexual taste is its diversity.

Our Contributors

When we set out to write this book, we knew it wouldn't be complete without input from the people from whom we've learned so much over the years: our customers. Resources describing sex toys and sexual activities that are somewhat off the beaten track are few and far between. At Good Vibrations, we rely heavily on the pooled knowledge of our entire community—vendors, coworkers, peer educators, and, above all, the customers whose honest, unabridged feedback we disseminate back through the community.

To solicit information we thought would be helpful, we composed and distributed a brief questionnaire, asking our customers to describe their experiences of orgasm, masturbation, partner sex, sex toys, and fantasy. Our goal was not to compile statistics, but simply to get first-person quotes as to what kinds of sexual activities our customers enjoy, and why.

For the first edition of this book, we received more than 150 responses. For the current edition, we posted the survey on Good Vibrations' website and received some 400 responses from women and men ranging in age from 18 to 73. Reading their completed questionnaires was the best part of writing this book. The responses were sincere, enthusiastic, open, funny, poignant, and arousing. We feel privileged to have been entrusted with such honest and forthcoming feedback, and we've included numerous quotes from these questionnaire respondents in the following pages. In some cases, it's impossible to know the sexuality, and even the sex, of the person quoted. How does this affect your reaction to the quote? Perhaps you'll want to read the same quote several times over, imagining a different identity for the subject each time. If this exercise should happen to subvert some of your assumptions about gender and sexuality, so much the better.

We've included a copy of our survey in the Appendix in case you'd like to fill one out yourself—many of our respondents told us they enjoyed having the opportunity to think and write about their sex lives, and you too may find the process enlightening and enjoyable.

Who We Are

In exchange for the intimate personal details our customers shared in their questionnaire responses, it's only fair that we introduce ourselves and tell the stories of how we each came to work in a vibrator store.

Cathy

I wound up working for a vibrator store because vibrators wound up working so well for me. You could say we have a certain affinity, which dates back to my college years. While debates about feminism, pornography, and censorship raged about me, I was in single-minded pursuit of "the big O": the elusive orgasm that always seemed just out of reach. Thorough student that I was, I did extensive research on the subject: reading "The Playboy Advisor" column religiously, combing through *Penthouse Forum* articles for possible techniques, quizzing all my girlfriends about what "it" felt like, and gamely tackling a variety of sexual positions and activities, to no avail.

Finally, after reading the classic texts *For Yourself* and *Becoming Orgasmic*, I decided to buy myself a vibrator and see what would come of it. Off I went to the Pink Pussycat Boutique in Greenwich Village, where I purchased a battery vibrator made of gleaming gold plastic. Sure enough, reliable, consistent stimulation did the trick for me—I still have sentimental memories of the long summer evenings I spent with that vibrator, enjoying the first orgasms of my life.

My first vibrator got quite a workout, and its motor died within a couple of months. The thought of facing the smirking clerks at the Pink Pussycat again was just too intimidating, so from then on I made my vibrator purchases from mail-order catalogs and drugstores. When I moved home to San Francisco and heard about Good Vibrations, a women-run sex toy store, it sounded too good to be true. On my first visit to Good Vibes, I was struck by the low-key, living-room atmosphere of the place—the worn carpet, the homemade bookshelves, and the friendly librarian-type behind the counter stood in sharp contrast to the garish walls of the Pink Pussycat and the sterile aisles of a drugstore. Both the store and the electric vibrator I walked out of there with made a lasting impression.

Over the next couple of years, the image of that cozy, hospitable storefront stayed with me—and so did my fascination with sex. When I decided that I wanted to give up temporary office jobs in favor of retail work, I took a trip to Good Vibrations to see if they were hiring. Lo and behold, they were, and before I had much chance to wonder just what I was getting myself into, I had a new job.

I started out in a part-time sales job, and eventually became store manager and toy buyer. For a period of several years, I worked full time in the store, and there was hardly anyone who came through our doors whom I didn't wait on. Sometimes, I'd have trouble understanding why complete strangers blushed or smiled broadly when they saw me on the street, and then I'd realize they were customers identifying me as "the girl from the vibrator store."

Selling vibrators proved to be both an empowering and entertaining experience. A sex toy salesperson is sort of a cross between a stand-up comic and an advice columnist. My job as a store clerk was to try to make people comfortable with highly charged subject matter and to offer accurate sex information without judgment or personal bias. I learned how to coax people into handling the display vibrators rather than eyeing them nervously from five feet away and how to diplomatically insist that someone buying an anal toy buy some lubricant as well. I negotiated the treacherous shoals of whether our books were "erotica" or "pornography." The fact that I'm the hopelessly respectable, wholesome-looking product of girls' schools finally seemed to serve a purpose—many customers' worst fears about entering a sex store dissolve when they see a "nice girl" like me behind the counter.

I loved the wide variety of people I met, and the way my own preconceptions were constantly challenged. The hippest leftie was likely to walk out of the store in a panic of shyness. The most Republican of military men was likely to display complete familiarity and affection for our product line. I couldn't guess customers' sexualities, and they couldn't guess mine. It was very liberating to be forced to toss out assumptions and start from square one with each new customer.

In the decade I spent at Good Vibrations, the staff expanded from four to sixty people; we launched a nationwide mail-order business, opened a second store, and became a democratically managed, worker-owned cooperative. There's no way the company could have become as successful as it has if there weren't hundreds of thousands of people across the country who appreciate sexual products and yearn for sex information. This gives me hope that one day there really will be shops like Good Vibrations in every urban neighborhood, suburban mall, or small-town square.

Working at Good Vibrations changed my life. For one thing, it "ruined" me for any traditional workplace—once you've had a job that offers a huge amount of fun along with a sense of right livelihood, it's hard to settle for less. I learned that grassroots information-sharing can effect incremental social change, so I dare to dream big (vibrator stores in the Vatican! sex ed in schools!). I gained the training and confidence to write, along with a subject matter that's infinitely fascinating to write about. And I met my partner, Becky, who used to work for one of our vendors. After years in a long-term relationship, I've discovered that it's a lot easier to communicate about sex with strangers than up close and personal—but both are well worth it.

Anne

Vibrators first entered my consciousness in ninth-grade English class. Two girlfriends and I staged a sixties' version of *Romeo and Juliet* that featured Lady Capulet draped over her chaise longue reading *The Sensuous Woman* (on loan, without permission, from my friend's mother). Desperate for any and all sex information,

we devoured this book in which the mysterious "J" extolled the virtues of vibrators, revealing that these devices could help women have orgasms. After eight years of Catholic school and no real sex education, I barely knew what an orgasm was, but I was quite certain I hadn't had one. I knew I simply had to learn how, but turning to this machine seemed so daring and risqué. I traveled to the next town to buy birth control for fear of being discovered, so there was absolutely no way I'd risk being seen purchasing a vibrator!

Somewhere in those high-school years I became best friends with my best friend's shower massager. I experienced long sessions of self-pleasuring in that tiny shower; I would emerge certain that my prunelike skin and rosy glow would be a dead giveaway to her parents and brothers. I know now, of course, that they were none the wiser, but the fear of being caught or discovered acted as a powerful aphrodisiac. While I was busy wasting one of California's precious resources, a friend from English class had gone out and bought herself a vibrator. On a trip we took together, I tried it while she was out shopping. What bliss! I came instantly and powerfully. I paused for a few seconds and then went for broke—three or four more orgasms later, I was a convert. After we got back from our trip, I headed straight for the nearest drugstore. I didn't care who saw me; no one was going to keep me from such intense pleasure! Selecting my little Oster Coil was easy—it was the only one on the shelf—but that little gem lasted me ten years. Not only that, it serviced many of my roommates and lovers along the way.

During college, the teacher in one of my women's classes arranged a field trip to San Francisco to visit the Women's Building, a women's bookstore, and her favorite taqueria. Someone casually mentioned a vibrator store in the neighborhood, but to my disappointment no one suggested we visit. I snuck away from the group that day and crossed the threshold of Good Vibrations for the first time.

I, like so many others before and after, walked through the door, stopped, and just gazed, with equal parts wonder, embarrassment, and terror. I headed straight for the bookshelves, picked up a book of illustrations of women's genitals, and gasped. I picked up a magazine full of images of lesbians having sex and gasped again. I walked over to the vibrator section, started to gasp, and then laughed—sitting next to the modern vibrators were a dozen or so antique vibrators. Everything clicked for me then: People long before me were using these things for more than just massage; there was a historical precedent for my activity. There I was standing in a store devoted to, and not ashamed of, getting people off! My sexual self-esteem soared through the roof.

My euphoria was interrupted by a cheery sales clerk asking if I needed help, which of course rendered me completely mute and sent waves of color up to my roots. I stammered something and stumbled out of the store, only to come back a week later and buy my roommate a vibrator. Since then, I've supplied many of my pals with toys from Good Vibrations—showers, birthdays, and weddings are all perfect excuses to slip that little pleasure box discreetly in with the other gifts with a note saying "open in private."

During my post-college job search, a feminist publisher unexpectedly referred me to the owner of Good Vibrations. Much to my astonishment and delight, I soon found myself answering questions about vibrator speed and dildo size for an adoring and curious bunch of customers. Having been raised believing sex was something you didn't talk about, you just "knew," speaking frankly about it to strangers was awkward at first, but eventually became as effortless as giving directions to lost tourists. I learned an incredible amount from my interactions with people, and the thought that I may have been responsible for a few customers' sexual enlightenment—as they were for mine—made me proud. Sure, we all blushed and stammered, but the payoff was the glee in the eyes of a customer about to purchase a new vibrator, or the hungry anticipation of one who couldn't wait to leave the store and try out new toys.

There are other things I appreciated during my thirteen years working at Good Vibrations—the sight of a store clerk restocking the shelves with a basket overflowing with sex toys conjured up images of a naughty Little Red Riding Hood. It was a joy to visit the warehouse every afternoon, to marvel at the five-foot-high wall of packages being shipped and to imagine each customer opening a box and touching his or her toy for the first time. Working with a bunch of people who talked about sex like other employees talk about the football pool was a perspective I'll never take for granted.

Even though I'm no longer with the company, the Good Vibrations philosophy continues to influence my professional and personal growth. Knowing that we all have an inalienable right to sexual pleasure has inspired me to write additional sex books, work with other women's sex businesses, and improve my public speaking. And now as the mother of two, I am enjoying the challenges of passing on sex-positive attitudes to my own children. It's definitely not as easy as directing lost tourists, but helping my daughters find their way to a life full of ecstatic discovery, good health, and rich sexuality is a journey I'll gladly make any day.

GV Tale: Customer Snapshots

Over the years our customers have brought us great joy. Imagine waiting on two women in their sixties who are sporting corsages and buying each other a vibrator as part of their day on the town. Imagine getting a thank-you letter from a woman who had never had an orgasm before purchasing her vibrator. Or the woman who feared that the trauma from a violent rape might permanently interfere with her ability to feel sensations during sex, but who shared sex toys with her husband as a way of overcoming her fear and inhibition. She told us, "I have shared many triumphs with your products—without your company, I would never be as far along on my path to sexual freedom as I am today."

Imagine a friendly conversation between two lesbians helping a nervous husband decide which dildo to buy his wife. Or our sympathy when a self-described "sex-starving female from a forgotten land" wrote us from Iran asking if we could smuggle some lesbian magazines to her. "Here there is no explicit, and everything about sex is forbidden, especially for female creatures," she confided. We consider ourselves honored to have access to the confidences and concerns of all the curious, courageous folks who come into our store or write to our mail-order department. Several years ago, a rural customer wrote to thank us for rushing her order and to say that she was going to dedicate her next vibrator orgasm to the staff of Good Vibrations. How could we help but feel a vicarious glow of sexual pleasure? We feel extremely privileged to have contributed in our own humble way to so many people's pursuit of happiness.

How to Use This Book

In our fantasies, we dream of this book with its cracked spine and well-thumbed pages lying on your nightstand next to your vibrator, lube, massage oil, and condoms. In reality, we hope you'll use this book to explore your own sexuality in whatever way you see fit. Whether you're interested in one particular practice or searching for fresh ideas, we encourage you to read the entire book—you never know what might spark your imagination!

The other advantage to reading this book in its entirety is that you can increase your comfort level, not only with your own sexuality, but with that of others as well. Our book is about exposing yourself to and exploring a range of sexual activities. We certainly don't expect you to like them all; we don't even expect you to try them all. But if your sex life or your feelings about your sexuality improve even the slightest bit thanks to something you read here, we'll have been successful.

The Good Vibrations Guide to Sex is not a program or an exercise book. For example, we won't promise you twenty-four hours of ecstasy in exchange for using six toys four times a day. This sort of goal-oriented approach only serves to make people more self-conscious about performance at the expense of enjoying themselves in the moment. We merely offer you a menu; it's up to you to sample whatever you please.

We've chosen not to write about subjects we felt were out of our league. While we expect that individuals with sexual dysfunctions will benefit from much of the information in this book, we're not qualified to explore medical or psychotherapeutic issues in depth, and we direct you to the resource listings for referrals. Whether you're looking for the sex toy outlet nearest you, a good sex-information line, or a sex therapist, our resource listings should be helpful. We've also compiled a bibliography and videography with recommendations of self-help, informational, and fantasy material.

Most of the activities and toys we describe can be enjoyed at any age and whether you're partnered or not. We hope that teenagers will be able to get their hands on this book, since we feel that information and encouragement are critical to becoming a sexually healthy, responsible adult. Similarly, while society tends to label older adults as sexless, we've tried to make this book equally relevant to both the old and the young. If you're experiencing some physical constraints, sex toys and fantasies are among the many options at your disposal—all it takes is the time and desire.

More than anything, this book celebrates each person's unique sexual nature. A healthy sex life is your birthright, and no one should be deprived of either the information or the tools to pursue it. By reading this book, you're acknowledging and taking responsibility for your sexual self—welcome to the celebration! It is not only possible, it's exciting to have great sex safely. We'll offer our suggestions throughout the book—but it's up to you to put them into practice.

Joani Blank

"There's a great deal more sexual pleasure available than most of us now experience, and getting it need not be difficult, expensive, or dangerous."

You wouldn't be holding this book in your hands if it weren't for the pioneering work of Good Vibrations' founder, Joani Blank. As a publisher, entrepreneur, and consultant, Joani epitomizes the Good Vibrations motto, "If you want something done right, do it yourself." Whether publishing the first (and still the only) *Complete Guide to Vibrators*, launching the nation's most successful women-run sex business, or supporting other sex-positive entrepreneurs, Joani puts her time, money, and considerable energy where her mouth is.

Joani worked as a public health educator when she moved to the San Francisco Bay Area in the early seventies—the heyday of women's self-help clinics and consciousness-raising groups. She was trained by Lonnie Barbach to lead preorgasmic women's groups, participated in the very first training group for SFSI (San Francisco Sex Information), the peer education hot line, and self-published her *Playbook for Women About Sex* and *Playbook for Men About Sex*. These experiences inspired Joani's philosophy that "There's a great deal more sexual pleasure available than most of us now experience, and getting it need not be difficult, expensive, or dangerous." After hearing from numerous women who yearned for "a clean, well-lighted place" to shop for vibrators and books, Joani opened Good Vibrations in March of 1977; the first store was only two hundred square feet of retail space dominated by her collection of antique vibrators.

Joani always followed open business practices, putting principles before profits. She kept prices low, maintained open financial records, allowed customers to test-drive vibrators (through their clothing), and prioritized accurate information-sharing about sex. She encouraged a democratic business structure and initiated the sale of the company to her employees, who formed a worker-owned cooperative in 1992. It has always been her dream to see Good Vibration's mission spread throughout the country, and she's been unfailingly generous toward fellow entrepreneurs, offering advice, consultation, or business loans to numerous sex-positive companies over the past two decades.

As a sexuality publisher and entrepreneur, Joani has had plenty of first-hand experience with censorship and discrimination. She has had to battle printers to publish ground-breaking Down There Press books such as *Anal Pleasure and Health* and *Femalia*, negotiate with banks to obtain basic credit card services, and confront magazine publishers who refused to allow the words "vibrator" or "sex" to appear in ad copy. Despite these ongoing challenges, she remains positive about our overall progress toward "making sex a regular part of life." She hopes that sexuality will come even further out of the closet over the next quarter century, noting: "We still have almost no good data about what people do in bed or how they feel about it." Joani continues her grassroots work to obtain this kind of data, publishing what she calls "field notes": collections of first-person narratives about subjects such as masturbation (*First Person Sexual*) or sex and aging (*Still Doing It*). Her video production projects include *Faces of Ecstasy*, close-up images of individual faces during orgasm.

When asked about her own contribution to America's sexual evolution, Joani says, "It comes easily and naturally to me to be open around sexuality, and people who hear me talk or who read my books realize that they can probably do it too without all that much difficulty. I'm still saying the same things I said twenty-five years ago. And I still would love to see a store like Good Vibrations in every major metropolitan area in this country. Hey, why not all over the world!"

To read more about Joani Blank's latest projects, visit her website at www.joaniblank.com.

Sexual Self-Image

A healthy sense of self-esteem can improve your sex life, just as a healthy sex life can improve your self-esteem. Allow us to illustrate this maxim with a few examples. If you feel good enough about your body and your sexual desires to masturbate, the act of masturbating will make you feel even better about your body and your desires. Or try this one on for size: Asserting your chosen approach to safer sex will contribute to an erotic, safe sexual encounter with a new partner, resulting in increased self-confidence.

Clearly, self-esteem is an integral part of your sexuality. Self-acceptance is a prerequisite for any intimate relationship—especially the one with yourself. Whether you're gathering the nerve to try a new sex toy or preparing to negotiate a sexual scene with a partner, the more confidence you bring to a sexual encounter the more likely you are to meet with success. At Good Vibrations, we've been able to witness first-hand how access to basic sex information and tools can benefit self-esteem:

> I was nonorgasmic for years, but with a little advice/assistance from your store and a vibrator, I am now orgasmic. I can't tell you how happy this has made me. Tapping into this sexual energy has vitalized me and improved my life in every way!

This book describes a myriad of sexual activities you can try alone or with others. We recognize, however, that nothing is ever as easy as it sounds on paper. Experimentation requires that you assert yourself and take a few risks. Above all, it requires that you feel entitled to sexual pleasure.

In this chapter, we invite you to explore some common challenges to claiming pleasure. The more familiar you are with your own sexual profile (including past and current attitudes, roadblocks, battles won and those being waged), the more confident you'll be in your approach to sex. Everyone suffers from poor sexual self-esteem occasionally—there are times when we simply don't feel attractive, loved, or satisfied with ourselves. It's normal! But being in a perpetual state of dissatisfaction might indicate some more-ingrained problems. We hope what you read here will help you identify any problem areas, uncover many reasons to love yourself, and ultimately emerge with a happier, healthier self-image.

Body Image

Physical Appearance

You're probably familiar with the statistics revealing that only a very small number of people in the United States are satisfied with their bodies. While most of us continue to have sex despite wishing we had better hair or thinner thighs, the extent to which these anxieties about appearance erode our sexual self-esteem is painfully disproportionate and can be enough to sabotage a sexual encounter:

> My biggest fear is that I will take my clothes off and he will not be aroused anymore. Now this has never happened, but it doesn't mean that the first time I am with someone I am not still thinking about it. Fear gets in the way of my being relaxed, and so it takes me longer to actually achieve an orgasm. Then I am worried about how my partner might feel if I don't have one.

Almost everyone has experienced, in some form, the effects that a negative body image can have on one's sex life, whether you're feeling unattractive and plan to put more energy into your sex life after you've lost ten pounds or you're having trouble enjoying sex because you're embarrassed by a specific physical attribute.

Even though we may know better, it's not easy to steel ourselves against the (often sexualized) media images of perfect body-types that bombard us daily. Whether you're a woman trying not to envy the curves on the latest *Cosmopolitan* models or a man who notices he doesn't fill out his briefs like the athletes do in the underwear ads, the images can be depressing at best and damaging at worst (as when taken to extremes in the case of eating disorders).

You can't very well close your eyes to the media, but you *can* keep a few things in perspective. Remember, these images reflect a small segment of the population, the young and thin; there are folks of all ages, sizes, physical abilities, ethnicities, and proclivities enjoying sex. Real diversity is visible right outside your door—take a walk or ride the bus; what you see is far more representative of America's sexual jigsaw puzzle than what's plastered up on a billboard. All kinds of bodies enjoy all kinds of sex with all kinds of other bodies. Maybe you prefer burying your nose in soft flesh to bouncing off hard muscle. Maybe that bald head heats you up at night whereas those golden locks

leave you cold. Maybe you're the only one who even cares about the size of your feet. The point is, trying to live up to a glorified ideal in hopes that it will bring you better sex is a waste of time and energy because sexual chemistry is not that formulaic. What's more, society's definition of beauty changes with the wind—by the time you've lost twenty pounds, thin might be out and Rubenesque in. We encourage you to scoff at the societal ideal and celebrate your body's uniqueness.

> I've been a chunky female my entire life, and while society may not celebrate it, finding hot men who worship chubby women was amazing for my ego.

> When I realized that I was attracted to other women, I became less concerned about my own imperfections. I realized that the girls I found most attractive were not super-skinny, huge-boob types, but a variety of body types: real-looking girls with small boobs and large stomachs and stretch marks and the whole shebang— sexy girls!

While we wish we could tell you to "accept your body unconditionally," and you'd do it, we know that's not very realistic. Some of us have been harboring visions of self-transformation for our entire lives and can't just wish them away. But questioning whether your vision is necessary, productive, and realistic might alleviate the pressure. Here are a few suggestions for improving your self-esteem:

- Start a list of all the attributes you like about your body. Keep it somewhere and add to it. Share it with a partner.
- Strip down to your birthday suit, stand in front of the mirror and get used to looking at your body. Tell yourself what you like—appreciate your body's uniqueness. If you get good at this, you may end up with some hot erotica!
- Listen to compliments that people give you and try to accept and believe them.
- Seek out sexual images that show a greater variety of body types—you can find erotica that reflects diversity at large newsstands, libraries, and the Web.
- Talk to a close friend—share your anxieties as well as what you admire about yourselves and each other. Try exploring where some of your attitudes originated.
- Change something about your physical appearance that will boost self-esteem—new clothes, fresh

hairstyle, designer glasses. If you're bound and determined to diet, be realistic. Set reasonable goals, eat nutritiously and get plenty of exercise.

- Learn how to give and receive massage. This can enhance your appreciation and enjoyment of your body and of others' as well.
- Read some self-help books about body image and self-esteem.
- Visit a nude beach or a spa to surround yourself with ordinary people comfortable in their nudity.

Our survey respondents shared some of the ways in which they've successfully overcome negative body image:

I pose nude for a couple of local photographers. This helps me love my body and see my body as a beautiful thing.

The two most positive influences on my sexual self-esteem have been the Internet and science fiction fandom. In fandom, all different sorts of body shapes are valued. It was really amazing to me that in this community, people actually really liked looking at short, round men.

I have always felt that I wasn't sexy because I'm a little overweight. I've found that I have to focus on the things that I like about myself instead of those I dislike. I wear clothes that my husband thinks I look sexy in because it makes me feel good about myself, and then I feel sexy.

When I was 18 and 19 I worked as an erotic dancer and that gave me more self-esteem than anything. This was an unusual job for me to take on because I had grown up in an upper-class family and had attended private boarding school. But I always had this fantasy about being a stripper— and I had also tended to suffer from low body image and occasional bouts with anorexia. Being a stripper was marvelous! Men loved all kinds of body types, and that was amazing. That experience taught me to get in touch with my body—literally and figuratively.

I think that maturity has had the biggest influence on my sexual self-esteem. I am no longer afraid to be myself, and I realize that it doesn't matter if my body isn't perfect. It's what's inside that counts.

Genitals

Few of us have ever been given permission, let alone encouraged, to familiarize ourselves with our genitals. Any childhood self-discovery was usually accidental and nearly always secretive. Particularly for women, this ignorance can manifest itself in adulthood as a tendency either to ignore our genitals, or to consider them off limits, dirty, and shameful. We simply aren't exposed to a broad enough range of vulva imagery— you can find realistic images of penises in any art museum, but vulva lovers have to make do with Georgia O'Keefe paintings. As a result, women with labia that aren't precisely symmetrical may worry that they are somehow deformed, and those who chance upon pictures of shaved and "prettied-up" labia in men's magazines may fear that their own genitals are ugly and abnormal:

Thanks to those stupid girlie-mags my dad hid around the house, I discovered that my pussy did not look like the girls' in the photos! I was gifted with more of an iris than a clam. That inhibited me in ways I am only now coming to grips with. It hurt me in a very deep, well-hidden way, and robbed me of a lot of self-esteem that I deserved to enjoy.

Despite the fact that we're well into the twenty-first century, and decades have passed since the feminist women's health movement inspired a generation of women to switch on the lights, haul out the hand mirrors, and take a long, loving look between their legs, vulva shame remains rampant. And certain unscrupulous medical professionals are more than willing to take advantage of this sad state of affairs by offering surgery to "aesthetically modify" women's genitalia. The best way to fight shame is with information, and we encourage you to seek out authentic visual representations of vulvas in all their glorious variety: *A New View of a Woman's Body* and *Femalia* feature full-color photographs, and Betty Dodson's *Sex for One* includes black-and-white illustrations.

It turns out my plump, full-lipped vulva is not only normal, it is hereditary, and it is beautiful! The book Femalia *went a long way in helping me come to grips with what I have "down there." The final dismantling of all my negative fantasies about my body came when I found myself with a lover who totally reveled in my pussy, who loved and praised it in every aspect. He kept asking me to open my legs so he could admire me. A thousand and one ugly lies shattered, and I have since become a proud priestess of the pussy! If I could ever add one thing to human sexuality books for adolescents, it would be photos or illustrations of lots of vulvas. There are snake-oil doctors out there performing labia reductions on countless emotionally suffering women, and it is an outrage! Not only is my vulva, and all its components, beautiful, it works like a souped-up BMW!*

Men can also harbor less than enthusiastic feelings about their genitals, with anxiety over penis size being most common. Yet the idea that sexual satisfaction is directly related to penis size is a ridiculous myth. For one thing, everybody has a different preference when it comes to penetration, which minimizes the likelihood of a "perfect fit." For another, sexual satisfaction depends on communication, generosity, and a whole-body approach to pleasure—not on genital anatomy.

My sex life improved the day I realized that size wasn't the only thing that a partner was interested in and that it could be forgotten in place of getting her to the bliss that was possible from so many other things.

If you feel negative or ambivalent about your genitals, perhaps you too just need to familiarize yourself with your own anatomy. Sit down in the nude with a mirror and the following chapter on anatomy, and explore. Masturbate—this is an excellent way to appreciate your genitals; it feels great and can have a direct impact on self-esteem!

I think that my most memorable masturbation experience was when I was learning about how I looked and what made me feel good. I watched myself masturbating while looking in a mirror I had near my bed.

Attitudes about Sex and Pleasure

Just as we should question media messages about body type, so too should we question the messages we receive about sex and pleasure. Whether it's a politician telling you to "just say no" to sex, a support group urging you to admit that you're a "sex addict," or a teacher warning that "boys are only after one thing," you've got to stay on your toes to keep your sexual self-esteem intact. We're exposed to negative messages at

every turn—from parents, religious institutions, friends, media, sex "experts," medical professionals, lovers. Internalizing these messages can leave you feeling—depending on the script—inadequate, oversexed, presumptuous, promiscuous, or ignorant.

Early on, young men would always express shock that was half excited and half scornful of my powerful desire and aggressive sexuality. It has taken me a long time to get over feeling like my passion is bad, and I still fight it with my whole being.

My mother and my old religion, Mormonism, really affected my sexual development. My mom always had a sort of negative outlook on sex. She never actually said, "Sex is bad. Avoid it, because that's all they want from you," but I felt it from her, and I never heard her say the reverse, "Sex is beautiful."

I've been sexually active since I was 15, so a huge change for me has been just claiming my own desire, learning to communicate what my needs are, what I require of a partner, etc. Our culture doesn't always allow this of women, and especially as a woman growing up under a Republican administration, in the deep South, with conservative parents, sexuality and sexual freedom weren't exactly subjects of household conversation.

Thanks to Puritan and Victorian ancestors, many of us have inherited the belief that abstinence and self-control are the highest virtues. As a result, we sometimes question whether we even deserve sexual pleasure. If we answer yes, the next question becomes: How much do we deserve? Won't too much lead to dependency? Disease? A bad reputation? This fear can play itself out in our sex lives in many ways—perhaps we don't masturbate as often as we like, or we feel selfish having more than one orgasm, or we don't ask for what we really want to avoid the risk of sounding greedy. Even if you are well-informed about sex, you may still find it a bit overwhelming to confront the sheer amount of pleasure you're capable of having. You may unconsciously find an abundance of pleasure intimidating and wonder if there must not be something wrong with feeling so good.

We can't wave a magic wand and erase centuries of social conditioning, but we would urge you to be conscious of these underlying influences. A lot of our customers are so accustomed to the notion of sexual deprivation that they become alarmed at how easy it is to feel good with sex toys. A common concern is, "If I buy this vibrator, won't it ruin me for regular sex?" What an interesting concern! After all, no one refuses to bake a chocolate mousse cake on the grounds that it might "ruin" them for apple pie—more likely, you'd leap at the chance to expand your dessert repertoire. Our experience suggests that increased sexual pleasure doesn't lead to anarchy, the destruction of your relationship, or the degradation of family values. Instead, the more pleasure you have, the more pleasure you're capable of having.

Confidence Boosters

Nothing boosts your self-image like confidence. How do you gain sexual self-confidence? The same way you gain anything else worth having—practice, determination, feedback, study, and some risk-taking. You've got to want good sex badly enough to work for it. Here are a few suggestions.

Sexual Agency

Identifying as a sexual person who deserves a life full of rich, glorious, and endlessly satisfying sexual encounters is vital to your sexual self-image. If you believe you're not worthy of good sex, others will sense this too. If you wait around for others to bestow great sex upon you, it may never happen. Be active, articulate, and selfish when it comes to your sexual desires.

I feel lucky that I grew up during the reign of Madonna. I truly credit that woman for helping me be the sexually aggressive and sexually unashamed woman I've become. I was about 8 years old when Madonna first appeared on the scene and I've been a fan since then. She made it perfectly clear that her sexuality was important and that it should be respected. I really took that to heart. I don't expect a partner to be solely responsible for my sexual pleasure. I've been using vibrators since I was 18. I know how to please myself.

I'm mature enough to understand that I shouldn't settle for less than what I want, or expect others to settle for less than what they want. And I stick with people who accept me for who I am.

When my partner is sexually aggressive and her desire to touch me is evident—that makes me feel sexy and beautiful.

Resources

Remember those teachers who told you, "no question is too stupid"? Take this to heart when it comes to satisfying your sexual curiosity. Sexual ignorance is nothing to be ashamed or embarrassed of; it's not as though you flunked a standardized test somewhere along the way. Most of us receive a negligible amount of sex information in our youth, yet suddenly when we reach "the age of consent" we're supposed to know how to please ourselves and our partners. Where are we supposed to have gained this expertise? Certainly not from our peers, who are fumbling around in the dark as much as we are. Use resources. Many books, videos, and websites today offer excellent sex information. Or you may find that an approachable relative, older sibling, friend, therapist, or knowledgeable sex partner can provide enlightening advice.

I always feel more sexually confident when I feel knowledgeable. So if I've just read a book or talked to a friend and learned about a new technique, it makes me feel more excited about trying it.

I have for years gone in search of positive images and words that have helped me raise my sexual self-esteem. On Our Backs and movies like Hard Love and How to Fuck in High Heels helped me realize the beauty and eros of my body and my desire, as well as books such as Stone Butch Blues, Doing It for Daddy, and The Good Vibrations Guide to Sex. Also, my experience and conversations with a few caring lovers have provided opportunities to explore my sexuality and push my edges.

Practice

This is obvious! The more sexual experience you gain, the more confident you'll be when it comes to pleasing yourself or a lover.

After doing it alone so much, I now have the confidence to masturbate in front of my partners, and I get off seeing them become aroused by this. I've learned how to satisfy a man and I enjoy being told that I give the "best sex he's ever had." I am not prudish so am willing to act out fantasies.

When I changed from being a "get on, get in, get off, get out, get gone" kind of a guy, to one who allowed his partner to use every tool and every inch I had, I forgot about how small I was and started enjoying the journey rather than the destination. I became a woman's dream, because all the focus was on her climaxes, her self-esteem, her fulfillment—that lead to her fulfilling my desires.

Older people often comment that age has given them experience and perspective that allows them to more fully enjoy their sexuality.

Age has had a significant impact on how I feel about myself. While I am less svelte than I used to be when I was younger, as an older woman, I feel sexier than I ever did as a young woman.

I'm not a "hardbody." I'm older and out of shape, but I devote all my energies to making love-making extremely enjoyable for my partners. I've learned that even an older guy that's far from a "10" can seriously satisfy women if he puts his partner's enjoyment first.

Age to some people is a bad thing, but it brought me a new sense of freedom. My self-esteem is better these days for a lot of reasons, and yes my sex life is one of them. I am less afraid to try new things.

Communication

Learn to be a vocal lover. Give your partner specific compliments—on technique, appearance, or attitude—and enjoy the results. His or her self-esteem will blossom, and you'll undoubtedly have a more eager lover on your hands. And remember, the more you give, the more you get!

My partners' reactions have had a lot of influence on me. When he went down on me, my first lover said, "You smell funny and taste funny." It's taken me a long, long time to get over that one. In contrast, my second lover boosted my sexual self-esteem a lot by telling me enthusiastically how much he liked the way I smelled and tasted, the sounds I made, everything.

Little comments are good for me. People telling me I'm a good kisser, that I give good head. A "wow" now and again. Just this morning my boyfriend was rubbing his hands all over me, saying how soft my skin is. It's also good to be recognized as a sexual person outside the bed. My boyfriend whispering, "You're so sexy" in my ear when I'm washing dishes.

Nonverbal communication is often just as effective:

I get a boost listening to the sounds my girlfriend makes as I am pleasuring her. Or the way she touches me as I touch her. The look on her face as her eyes glaze over when it's getting intense. Watching her does it for me.

Adventure

Sexual risk-taking can get you out of a rut and help you discover new facets of your sexuality, which will ultimately boost your self-esteem.

Learning what I like through masturbation, coming out as (mostly) lesbian, and having sex with women—these have given me more confidence about my body and helped me be more assertive about what I like and what I don't.

I have been into BDSM for several years and the experience has opened me up to so many new things. I am soooo much more free now and I love myself… even though I am not perfect. I look in the mirror and say, "Wow, what a sex goddess!!"

Self-Acceptance

When it comes to sex, we're all vulnerable to the temptation to whip out a ruler or a stopwatch and calculate how we measure up: Is everybody else having more fun, more excitement, more orgasms? All too often, curiosity about what the neighbors are doing in bed generates performance anxiety and a lurking sense of inadequacy. But cultivating curiosity about your own unique sexuality can set you on the path to pleasure.

Sex is fun, and it's serious when you're really intimate with someone. What it shouldn't be (in my view) is a competitive performance where you are rated X out of ten. And you don't have to have vast numbers of orgasms a week for it to be brilliant.

Folks need to know that whatever their preferences are, they needn't feel guilty or inadequate. Over the course of my life, I've had less adventurous friends, or lately, vanilla friends, who felt that celebrations of brazenness, leathersex, etc., were somehow indictments of their quieter sex lives.

Life Changes

Dealing with physical changes can provide an opportunity to expand your experience or definition of sex.

I lost my inhibitions and self-consciousness after childbirth. Once the world has seen your private bits, why not show a new partner as well?!

My inability to maintain an erection definitely created a serious dent in my sexual self-esteem. Fortunately I spent time learning to be more oral with my partners, something that I now excel in. That is a good ego booster.

On the Road to a Soaring Self-Image

Obviously, not everyone struggles with self-esteem issues. Some of us were raised by loving and understanding parents who modeled healthy attitudes:

My mother's attitude that sexuality was natural and wonderful and an expression of love laid the groundwork for a healthy self-esteem. Also my sister's passion and love of sexuality encouraged me to be open and natural.

Others have had their sexual development challenged by specific life experiences:

Memories of a rape damaged my self-image, and my partner and I had to work through my triggers. We have been together for almost fifteen years and we are doing well sexually.

Whether you're recovering from sexual trauma, are coming out as queer to conservative parents, or have questions about gender identity, you are taking a huge step toward sexual self-assertion simply by seeking information. We're not qualified to address all these issues in depth, but we refer you to our resource listings and bibliography, and we hope that, like this survey respondent, you will benefit from the honesty, acceptance, and encouragement you find within these pages:

As a survivor actively healing from childhood sexual abuse, I want to tell you what an important place your products, catalog, and philosophy hold in my life. It is incredibly validating to me as I continue my healing journey to realize that sexuality chosen and desired by consenting adults is not only okay but fun. Thanks for being a part of my healthy and whole sexuality in a powerful way.

Finally, we suspect that all of you have a fairly positive sexual self-image, or you wouldn't be reading this book! We applaud your initiative and hope to provide you with the tools and motivation to pursue your sexual dreams.

Annie Sprinkle

"I may not have children, but I've birthed a lot of bliss."

Public Cervix Announcement. Bosom Ballet. Intervaginal Superhighway. You've got to admit, Annie Sprinkle has a knack for coming up with unforgettable and utterly enticing ways of teaching people about sex. Take a tour of her website, known as the Intervaginal Superhighway, and you'll be invited to view her cervix, appreciate the breast choreography of the Bosom Ballet, and learn a thing or two about full-body orgasms.

If you're looking for someone who projects a strong sexual self-image, Annie's your woman. Throughout her life she's used her art—primarily performance art and photography—to expand both her own and her audience's experience of sex. Because Annie's work is so accessible, she makes a great flesh-and-blood role model. She publicly celebrates her own body and sexuality in books such as *Post Porn Modernist* and videos such as *Sluts and Goddesses*. Her performance piece *Ellen/Annie*, which documents her transformation from shy, small-town girl to sexually empowered sex goddess, will resonate with every woman who's ever dreamed of being sexually desirable.

As a former sex worker and porn star turned sex guru with a Ph.D. in human sexuality, Annie's reinvented herself more times than Madonna. Yet each incarnation marks an important milestone on her quest for sexual enlightenment. Says Annie, "Sex has been my spiritual path. Sure, it's been a hobby and business, but ultimately it's a form of worship, a path to understanding the universe and life."

Annie's journey is unique in its impact. Over fifty thousand people have viewed Annie's cervix as part of her performance art, and thousands more have seen it on the Web. Her contribution to women's understanding of their genital anatomy, and subsequent sexual confidence, cannot be underestimated. "Lots of folks, both women and men, know very little about female anatomy and so are ashamed or afraid of the cervix. I do my best to lift that veil of ignorance." Of her many performances, the show Annie found most satisfying was "The Sacred Prostitute and Masturbation Ritual." Annie demonstrated full-body orgasms to thousands of people around the world, many of whom came along with her. "I may not have children, but I've birthed a lot of bliss," she says of the experience.

Annie's sexual activism ignited during the seventies, when she discovered a small, sex-positive feminist community. "It was so different then. Women didn't know about their bodies, there was no sex education, and women weren't supposed to like sex. Now women are asking for what they want, and demanding their orgasms. Back then people weren't sure women really could have orgasms, and if they could, so what!"

She's certainly done her share to change that; today she works on projects ranging from empowerment courses for sex workers to sexuality workshops on college campuses, from designing erotic tarot decks to creating videos on tantric breathing.

Visit Annie's website at www.gatesofheck.com/annie.

CHAPTER 3

Sexual Anatomy 101

Although there's a lot more involved in sexual pleasure than what's "down there" between your legs, it's also true that many men and women could be experiencing more sexual pleasure if they were better informed about their own and each other's genitals:

I'm always shocked at how few of my partners—women or men—know anything about female anatomy. I've had girlfriends who thought their urethras were in their vaginas. People act like it's all just blurred together "down there."

I wish I had a dollar for every time I've asked a woman to grab hold of my penis more firmly. They always act like it's so delicate and they're afraid they might hurt me if they take off the kid gloves.

So before we go any further, we'd like to offer you a brief tour of human genital anatomy. Why not get undressed, get comfortable, grab a hand mirror, and follow along on this guided tour of your own genital landscape?

On the surface, women's and men's genitals don't seem to have a whole lot in common. But a closer look reveals that they are two very similar structures. Every part of the vulva has its corresponding counterpart in the penis—and vice versa.

Female Anatomy

The female external genitals are generally referred to as the *vulva*. Your vulva includes the outer lips, or *labia majora*; the inner lips, or *labia minora*; the tip of the clitoris; the urethral opening; and the vaginal opening. The two long fleshy folds of the outer lips are composed of fat and erectile tissue and covered with pubic hair. The smooth, hairless inner lips enclose the urethral and vaginal openings. The inner lips tend to be the most distinctive feature of the vulva, and they rarely come as a matched pair. Women's labia vary greatly in size, shape, and coloration. Similarly, the clitoral tip, or glans, of the clitoris varies in size, shape, color, and the extent to which it protrudes from under the clitoral hood.

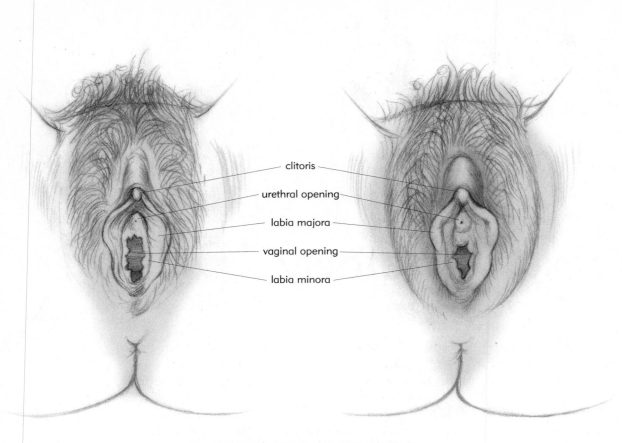

clitoris

urethral opening

labia majora

vaginal opening

labia minora

Unaroused vulva (left) and aroused vulva (right)

When I took Betty Dodson's Bodysex workshop, my favorite part was the genital show-and-tell. We each took turns sitting in front of a hand mirror and displayed our vulvas to each other, while Betty extolled their virtues and variety. It was amazing to hear the sighs of awe as we each unveiled ourselves. One woman had a blue clitoris; another, black feathered lips contrasted against a rosy interior; another, rich layers of folds; and another had labia that folded right up like a heart-shaped Ziploc.

The Clitoris

You can easily locate your clitoris, the most sensitive spot in your pubic area, tucked under the folds of skin where the top of your labia meet. Pull back the hood of skin over the clitoris to reveal the clitoral glans. You may be surprised at how much it resembles a miniature penis—or how much a penis resembles a large clitoris.

If you press your fingers down on the skin above your glans, you should be able to locate something that feels like a short rod of cartilage directly beneath

the skin and extending up to your pubic bone. This is the clitoral shaft. Beneath the skin the clitoral shaft separates into two legs (or *crura*), which extend in a wishbone fashion for about three inches on either side of the vaginal opening. The entire clitoris consists of erectile tissue made up of blood vessels, spongy tissue, and nerves, just like the erectile tissue of the penis. During sexual stimulation this tissue fills with blood, and the clitoral glans, shaft, and legs swell and become firmer. Since the clitoral legs extend beneath the labia, when you stimulate the urethra, vagina, or anus, you indirectly stimulate the clitoris as well.

The clitoris is the only organ in the human body whose sole function is to transmit sexual sensation. It is made up of approximately eight thousand nerve fibers, a higher concentration than in any other body part, and twice as many as in the penis. Despite the constant outpouring of sex "information" in popular culture, thousands of men and women still have no idea that the clitoris exists or how to locate it. At the same time, many women who know all about the clitoris and who regularly enjoy orgasms from clitoral stimulation are convinced that "vaginal orgasms" are somehow superior. Freud's dictum that clitoral pleasure is an "immature" substitute for vaginal pleasure cast a long shadow over the twentieth century, even though medical writers down through the ages have always identified the clitoris as the main site of female sexual pleasure.

In truth, the majority of women require direct clitoral stimulation to reach orgasm. However, some women do report that clitoral and vaginal stimulation result in what they identify as different types of orgasm:

> *In my experience, there are clitoral orgasms and G-spot orgasms. Clitoral orgasms feel like a roller-coaster ride. G-spot orgasms feel deeper and somehow more intense, like my whole body is involved.*

Researchers have proposed that different nerve pathways between the genitals and the brain account for variances in orgasmic experience. John Perry and Beverly Whipple, two of the authors of *The G-Spot and Other Recent Discoveries about Human Sexuality*, theorize that subjective perceptions of orgasm are based on which of two primary nerve pathways is involved. The pudendal nerve is connected to the clitoral glans and the PC muscle (see below), while the pelvic nerve is connected to the clitoral shaft, clitoral legs, G-spot, bladder, uterus, and deepest part of the PC muscle. Perry and Whipple suggest that the ways in which nerve signals travel on one or both of the pathways can create a variety of different or blended sensations. That the pelvic nerve connects to internal organs and inner muscles could explain why many women describe orgasms resulting from vaginal or G-spot stimulation as "deep" and "full-bodied."

If reading about these distinctions makes you worry that you're missing out on some "better" type of orgasm, remember that orgasm is a subjective experience that can't really be neatly categorized. After all, the clitoris and vagina don't inhabit separate postal codes, and the sexual pleasure each provides is completely interconnected.

The Urethral Sponge and Female Ejaculation

As you move your attention down from your clitoris toward your vaginal opening, you should be able to locate the opening of the urethra, the tube that conducts urine from the bladder out of the body. The urethral opening is more visible in some women than others. You may have to spread your labia and bear down with your pelvic muscles to get a good look at this area. The spongy, acorn-shaped protrusion around the urethral opening is loaded with nerve endings and is an erogenous zone for many women. For others, stimulation of this area may be irritating and unpleasant.

Inside your body, the urethra runs parallel to and above the vagina, so that the ceiling of the vagina is closest to the floor of the urethra. The urethra is surrounded by spongy tissue dense with blood vessels and containing glands similar in their makeup and in the fluids they produce to the male prostate gland. These glands are most densely concentrated in an area equivalent to the outer third of the vagina. This urethral sponge is what has come to be called the *G-spot*, or female prostate, named after Ernst Grafenberg, a gynecologist who first published research on the erotic pleasure potential of the urethra in the 1940s and 1950s. Some women greatly enjoy stimulating the urethral sponge, and some women experience an ejaculation of fluids through the urethra as a result.

SO YOU WANT TO FIND YOUR G-SPOT
We've chosen to use the somewhat arbitrary term *G-spot* throughout this book because it's made its way into popular usage, thanks to the publication of a book by the same name in 1982. Unfortunately, this terminology plays into a common sexual misconception that specific physiological buttons need only be located and pressed to produce mind-blowing pleasure. The G-spot has variously been described as a dime-sized, quarter-sized, or half-dollar-sized raised area located in the front wall of the vagina. Many women are understandably confused by this notion of the vagina as piggy bank and fret that they "don't have" or "can't find" their own G-spot.

> *It took me a while to realize that the G-spot wasn't just a button you press to cause orgasm (from all the talk…well, it was a bit exaggerated), but with a little patience, it's fantastic. For me it creates a totally different experience than clitoral orgasm—equally pleasurable, but more involved…a whole-body thing.*

The G-spot is not a vaginal ecstasy button—rather, it's simply a cushion of tissue wrapped around the urethra. The reason this cushion can aptly be

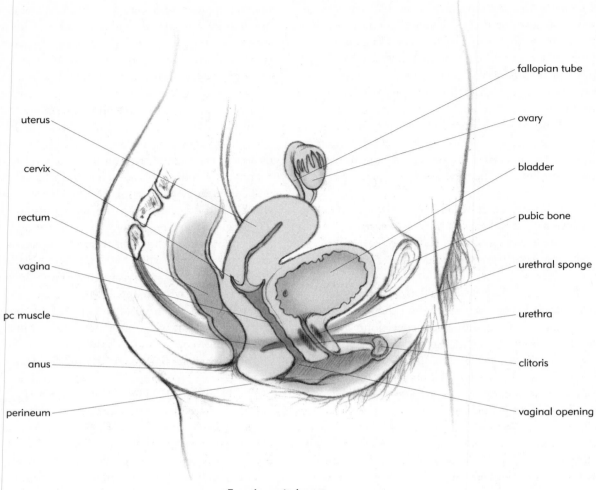

uterus

cervix

rectum

vagina

pc muscle

anus

perineum

fallopian tube

ovary

bladder

pubic bone

urethral sponge

urethra

clitoris

vaginal opening

Female genital anatomy

described as a "spot" is that the urethra is only about one and a half to two inches long. Your urethral sponge can be stimulated through the front wall of your vagina in the same way that a man's prostate gland can be stimulated through the front wall of his rectum. While every woman has a urethral sponge, not everyone has the same response to its stimulation—your reaction could range from pleasure to indifference to irritation:

I've never had an orgasm through intercourse or stimulation of the G-spot. I can't seem to find it!

The only orgasm I have ever experienced was elicited by intense penetration and stimulation of my G-spot by my partner, using her fingers.

G-spot stimulation to me simply feels good; it does not generate an orgasm.

If you'd like to explore G-spot stimulation, warm up first with other types of sexual stimulation. If you are tense or insufficiently aroused, prodding your urethral sponge will probably only irritate your bladder. Once you're aroused and your erectile tissues are swollen with blood, the urethral sponge will be easier to locate. You may find that G-spot stimulation initially makes you feel like you need to pee—this is a natural response to pressure on the urethra, and the sensation should subside in a few moments.

Choose the position that best enables you or your partner to reach the front wall of your vagina—squatting, lying on your stomach, or rear-entry intercourse are all good bets. Dildos are also particularly handy helpers, as they can reach farther than most people's fingers. The G-spot is not responsive to light touch, so you'll need to press firmly into the vaginal wall—the G-spot can't be felt *on* the vaginal wall, but only *through* it. If you explore with your fingers, you should encounter a slightly ridged area just behind the pubic bone that feels distinct from the smoother vaginal walls around it. Press down on this area—experiment with rocking, massaging, and rhythmic touch to discover what you like best. Some women find it helpful to place one hand above the pubic hair line and press down through the belly to feel the urethral sponge swelling between their hands. Others only become aware of the G-spot if they're being penetrated by something larger than fingers.

I have experienced G-spot stimulation more on my own than with a partner. I can take the intensity longer by myself than with someone else.

Doggy-style sex seems to provide a highly pleasurable form of G-spot stimulation.

I found my G-spot with a vibrator. I have to angle it toward my belly and put it on high. Intense.

There are numerous G-spot vibrators and vibrator attachments, curved to hit the front wall of the vagina. You may or may not find these long enough or curved just right to hit your individual G-spot.

FEMALE EJACULATION

With continuous stimulation of the urethral sponge, the paraurethral glands fill up with a clear, odorless fluid. This fluid can seep, flow, or spurt out of the urethra during ejaculation. While all women have a urethral sponge, not all ejaculate. Of those who do, some ejaculate during orgasm and some during arousal. Ejaculation and orgasm are two distinct physiological phenomena in both women and men.

Female ejaculation has been around as long as females have been around, and was recognized in folk wisdom and medical literature from classical antiquity through the Renaissance. Until the eighteenth century, the prevailing theory in the Western world was that successful conception depends on the mingled sexual fluids and sexual enjoyment of both men and women. When the invention of the microscope revealed that only male fluids contribute to conception, female fluids (and the value of female orgasm) disappeared from medical literature. For centuries thereafter, doctors dismissed anecdotal reports of female ejaculation as evidence of urinary incontinence:

I had never experienced ejaculation before I was with a woman. I have always had orgasms, but never like those I have now. At first I would love the wet sensations but seconds later feel guilty, thinking maybe it was pee. It smells like pee, and there aren't too many documents supporting the female ejaculation theory. I wish I wasn't so uptight, because it is a very enjoyable experience.

In fact, research shows that female ejaculate is chemically distinct from urine. If you've ever felt embarrassed or intimidated by the fear that you're peeing in bed, we hope the following quotes will inspire you to go ahead and do what comes naturally:

I've found that ejaculation happens when I've been slowly aroused and teased maximally (clitorally speaking) by a patient partner, as this can take one to two hours. It's wonderful and very intense! At first I thought I peed, but then I thought, "Who cares?"

I've ejaculated many times, especially during pregnancy when I'm particularly juicy anyway. Has made me nervous (partner reaction-wise), but it feels goo-oo-ood.

I ejaculated the first time when I was 25 and was on top during intercourse with a man. The next time I ejaculated was recently during G-spot stimulation by my girlfriend's hand. I just realized that urination anxiety was holding back my ejaculate, so I let it go, and I did ejaculate!

When I was younger, I thought ejaculation during masturbation was wrong, sorta like peeing the bed. I'd feel great, but guilty, because I'd left a huge wet stain on my mattress (of course having the urge to masturbate just before leaving for church might have had something to do with that). Now that I've read a bit more, I realize that ejaculate is a natural and normal occurrence, even if it doesn't happen all the time. Now I plan ahead by bringing in towels.

While sitting on top of my lover with his lovely curved cock inside me, he said, "Look at you, baby," and when I looked down, I was coming and it was gushing! The G-spot exists and he really hit it. It was a glorious release!

If you've never experienced ejaculation and would like to, try incorporating G-spot stimulation into your usual masturbation techniques. As your urethral sponge grows more swollen and sensitive, bear down with your pelvic muscles. Women's experiences of ejaculation can range from simply feeling more wet than usual to shooting jets of fluid. Of course, plenty of women may never ejaculate and may never want to. We are pleased that female ejaculation is now acknowledged as a genuine sexual response, but we don't like to see it promoted as a new goal that every woman should strive to achieve. Ideally, you'll undertake your explorations in a spirit of fun and curiosity, rather than one of grim determination. Whether or not you "find" your G-spot or hit the ceiling with your fluids, you're certain to learn new things about your sexual responses:

Discovering my G-spot, actually seeking it out rather than just having occasional, accidental stimulation of it, has totally increased my sexual pleasure—whether alone with a dildo or with a partner. I never knew what was producing the giant wet spot underneath me until then. I love the feeling that I might be about to pee.

I still haven't found the G-spot yet, but I'm enjoying the search. The longest, most intense multiorgasm I had was with a man stimulating my clit while thrusting my new G-spot vibrator in. Whoa. I didn't realize how much fun that G-spot vibrator was until I put someone else behind the wheel.

I was so blown away the one time I climaxed with G-spot stimulation that I didn't notice if I ejaculated, though I wouldn't be surprised if it happened. I definitely ejaculated verbally!

The Vagina

You'll notice that the vaginal opening appears as folds of skin, rather than as an open space. The vagina is extremely expandable—think childbirth—yet most of the time the vaginal walls rest companionably against each other. The vagina is about four inches long. After the initial bulge over the urethral sponge, the vaginal canal curves back to the cervix, the neck of the uterus. The outer third of the vaginal walls consists of ridges and folds of tissue, has more nerve endings, and is more sensitive than the rest of the vagina. The inner two-thirds of the vaginal walls are smoother and contain fewer nerve endings—therefore, the inner part of the vagina is more responsive to pressure than to light touch, friction, or vibration. Like the inner vagina, the cervix can be quite sensitive to pressure. During sexual arousal, the uterus elevates and the inner vagina balloons, creating a sort of cul-de-sac behind the cervix—some women find pressure on this spot particularly pleasurable.

Every woman's vaginal geography is unique, and we encourage you to explore your own to discover any "hot spots" or particularly pleasurable areas inside your vagina. Some women have no interest in pursuing vaginal stimulation during sex, while others find that penetration enhances a sexual experience:

I've definitely noticed a difference between coming with penetration and coming without. With penetration, there's more of a total body sensation, whereas without (i.e., with finger, tongue, or vibrator on my clitoris), sensation is more localized. Both are great.

I differentiate between the intense clit-centered climaxes I have during oral sex or manual stimulation and the wave of full-body climaxes I experience during vaginal penetration. They are both equally desirable, and I usually experience both.

Male Anatomy
External Organs

While most of us are familiar with what the penis and the scrotum look like externally, there's a surprising amount of mystification around what's beneath the surface. There are no bones and no muscles inside the penis. Instead, two long cylinders containing erectile tissue run down the length of the penis. These cylinders are called the *corpora cavernosa* and correspond to the clitoral legs in women. The urethra runs along the bottom of the penis, surrounded by a third cylinder of spongy tissue, the *corpus spongiosum*, which is connected to the glans, or head of the penis. The urethral opening is in the glans. The head of the penis is

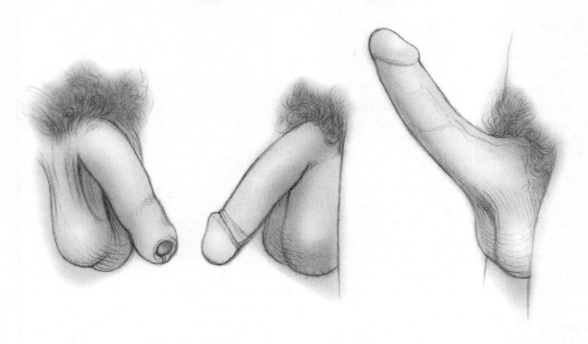

Uncircumcised, circumcised, and erect penis

generally the most sensitive part, particularly around the coronal ridge at the base of the glans, and corresponds to the tip of the clitoris. However, nerve endings are not as densely concentrated on the head of the penis as they are on the clitoral tip, so the glans of the penis is considerably less sensitive than the clitoral glans.

If you hold your penis in your hand, you'll notice that the skin covering the penis slides easily over the shaft. All men are born with a foreskin, a retractable extension of the skin of the penis, which covers the glans. When boys or men are circumcised, this loose skin is cut off. Since the glans of an uncircumcised man is protected by his foreskin, it is usually more sensitive when exposed than the glans of a circumcised man. Try stroking all around your glans and coronal ridge to see what spots feel particularly pleasurable. Some men find stimulation of the urethral opening pleasant, while others find it irritating. The frenulum, the piece of skin on the underside of the coronal ridge between the shaft of the penis and the glans, is another area rich in nerve endings. As you move your hand down the shaft of your penis, pay attention to the hump of skin running along the underside of your penis—you are feeling the *corpus*

spongiosum, which lies just beneath the skin. This ridge, known as the raphe, runs from the frenulum all the way down the shaft of the penis, along the middle of the scrotum, to the anus and is particularly sensitive to touch.

The scrotum is the loose sac of skin hanging below the penis that contains the two testicles. Testicles are the glands involved in the production of both testosterone and sperm. They can vary from grape-sized to egg-sized. The scrotum serves to protect the testicles from injury and from extremes of temperature, which would inhibit sperm production. You've probably noticed that when you're cold, physically active, or sexually excited, the muscles in your scrotum contract, thereby pulling your testicles protectively closer to your body. It's common that one testicle will hang lower than the other.

As we're sure you're aware, most men's testicles are extremely sensitive to pain and require gentle treatment. Although even light tapping on the testicles can be painful, firm pressure or steady pulling on the scrotum can feel good. Many men enjoy having their scrotums stroked, squeezed, and tugged on. This is one principle behind the numerous cock-and-ball toys on the market. Cock-and-ball toys, which resemble

A Word about Circumcision

The foreskin, nature's way of keeping the glans of the penis protected and lubricated, is a sheath of skin lined with mucous membrane. Not only is the foreskin itself packed with sensory tissue, rich with blood vessels and nerve endings, but it serves to enhance the sensitivity of the glans of the penis and to provide natural lubrication.

Nothing feels quite as good as my lover's uncut penis. I must emphasize that my favorite form of penetration is from an uncircumcised penis. As for circumcised, bleah! Once you've felt the amazing feeling of a foreskin sliding back and forth over the penis inside you, you'll never want a cut man again. Believe me.

In recent years, many men and women have begun to question the American social norm of circumcising infant boys. While circumcision is a religious ritual in both Judaism and Islam, it's a purely secular, medical tradition for the majority of American families, one that is arguably outmoded and unnecessary. Circumcision became widespread in twentieth-century America owing to a legacy from the Victorian age, when circumcision was promoted as a method of controlling masturbation, and owing to post–World War II standards of hygiene. By the sixties, doctors routinely circumcised between 80 and 90 percent of American boys, as it was widely believed that circumcision

would reduce chances of infant urinary tract infections (UTIs), penile cancer, cervical cancer, and the transmission of STDs.

Recent research has shown that good hygiene and safer sex practices are the key to avoiding infections (including genital warts, which are linked to cervical cancer). Penile cancer is very rare, and while circumcised infants are at lower risk for UTIs, the risk for uncircumcised boys is at most 1 percent. In 1999, the American Academy of Pediatrics reversed its former position, stating that circumcision does not have enough benefits to warrant routine recommendation. If you're an expectant parent, we strongly advise you to research and come to your own decision before the birth of your child, so that you'll be prepared to communicate your wishes to doctors after delivery.

The majority of circumcised men in America experience the penis as a great source of pleasure. There are, however, men who experience desensitization of the glans and mourn the loss of the foreskin to such an extent that they seek "uncircumcision" or "foreskin restoration." If you're interested in pursuing the nonsurgical methods of restoration, all of which involve gradually stretching the skin of the penile shaft until it covers the glans, more power to you. However, we'd strongly advise against surgical intervention, which frequently results in scarring and other problems.

---

harnesses for the male genitals, are variously designed to snap around the base of the penis and scrotum, lift and separate the testicles, or stretch the scrotum. Some men enjoy hanging light weights off their scrotums to create a sensation of steady pulling. And some men crave more vigorous treatment:

I like lots of strong stimulation of my balls. Squeeze them, smack them, twist them, pull them apart from side to side, slap them on the steering wheel of my car—I don't care. I love it all!!!

Internal Organs

There's more to the male genitals than what's visible outside your body. The base of the penis extends into the body—in fact, there's enough room in the pelvic cavity that the entire penis and testicles can be tucked inside the body when soft. If you press your fingers against your perineum—the area between your testicles and anus—you can feel this root, or bulb, of your penis. The root of the penis is sensitive and can be stimulated through the perineum or the rectum—one reason anal penetration feels pleasurable to many men.

The urethra passes into the body and through the prostate gland to the bladder. The prostate gland, an

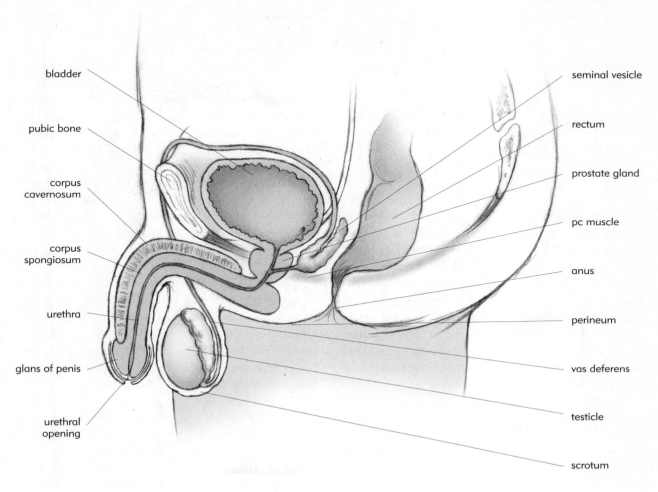

bladder

pubic bone

corpus
cavernosum

corpus
spongiosum

urethra

glans of penis

urethral
opening

seminal vesicle

rectum

prostate gland

pc muscle

anus

perineum

vas deferens

testicle

scrotum

Male genital anatomy

internal organ that produces ejaculatory fluid, is situated behind the pubic bone and just below the bladder. The prostate is a source of sexual pleasure for many men. Tucked close to the root of the penis, the prostate lies along nerve pathways between the penis and the brain, and is exceptionally well situated to pick up pleasurable signals both coming and going. Many men can have orgasms purely from prostate stimulation. Prostate massage also enhances genital stimulation, as it produces pressure against the root of the penis that feels like an internal erotic massage. The prostate corresponds to the G-spot in women—like the G-spot, it is connected to the pelvic nerve, rather than the pudendal nerve, which may explain why prostate-triggered orgasms are often described as particularly "deep."

You can massage your prostate by inserting a finger about three inches into your rectum and stroking toward the front of your body. You'll feel the prostate as a firm bulge about the size of a walnut (it may be larger in men over 40). Given the angles you're working with, you may find it difficult to reach your prostate with your own fingers, but a partner's fingers, an insertable vibrator, or a dildo can come in handy. As with G-spot stimulation in women, men are more likely to enjoy prostate stimulation once they're already aroused, and responses to prostate stimulation can range from extreme pleasure to irritation:

Too much prostate stimulation makes me lose the desire to orgasm. Is this common, I wonder? Perhaps it "oversatisfies" me.

The most intense orgasms I've ever had in my life have come through prostate stimulation. I have a particularly delicious memory of a threesome in which I was fucking a friend of mine while my wife pushed her fingers into me and touched my prostate. The orgasm that resulted was truly shattering.

Since my wife turned me on to the "male G-spot," I have had orgasms that far surpassed anything I had previously experienced.

Erection

The penis would be blood-engorged all the time were it not for smooth muscle cells that constrict local arteries, minimizing blood flow into the corpora cavernosa. In response to sexual stimulation, your brain signals the nerve cells around the penis to release a neurotransmitter that causes these smooth-muscle cells to relax, and voilà: Arteries widen and the erectile tissues fill with blood. The corpora cavernosa expand against their surrounding membrane, thereby squeezing shut the veins that would normally carry blood back out of the penis and creating a firm erection.

An erect penis can hold eight times as much blood as a nonerect penis. Erect penises don't, however, expand in direct proportion to their nonerect size. Some penises increase in size more during erection than others; there's actually a smaller range of sizes among erect penises than among nonerect penises.

ERECTILE DYSFUNCTION: More commonly referred to by the loaded term *impotence*, the inability to sustain an erection is something that all men experience at one point or another in their lives, whether as a result of a few too many drinks, physical fatigue, or lack of desire. Recurring erectile dysfunction is another matter, and is generally the result of ongoing physical conditions, rather than temporary, situational problems.

A number of neurological and/or circulatory problems can short-circuit the physical process of erection. Pelvic surgery, spinal cord injuries, multiple sclerosis, or diabetes can all cause nerve damage, while certain drugs—such as antidepressants or high-blood-pressure medications—can interfere with signals to the smooth muscle cells. Circulatory problems, such as hardening of the arteries, can interfere with blood flow into the penis. Diabetes, smoking, pelvic injury, and aging can

all reduce the elasticity of the erectile tissues, resulting in blood leaking out of the erection.

If you have had recurrent episodes in which you couldn't sustain an erection, the first thing to do is determine whether this failure has physical or psychological causes. All men who are physically capable of having erections have several throughout the course of a night's sleep, and most wake up with an erection at least one morning a week. If you haven't woken with an erection in a few weeks, you can try a low-tech diagnostic test by attaching a ring of postage stamps around the base of your flaccid penis before going to bed—check to see if the ring is broken when you awake. Or, a doctor can set you up with a device like a mechanized cock ring, which will measure the quantity and firmness of the erections you have throughout the night.

If you are having erections while you sleep, presumably your difficulties with erection during waking hours are psychological, not physiological in origin. Maybe you are forcing yourself into sexual situations you don't want to be in; or your sex life has become oppressively goal-oriented; or you're experiencing stress that is affecting your sexual responsiveness.

At 27, I assumed I was too young to have to worry about sexual problems, but during a stressful separation and divorce, I found myself unable to get or maintain an erection. This not only was a problem in itself, but it also proved to be somewhat of a self-fulfilling prophecy. The more I thought about it, the more depressed I got, and the less responsive my body became to sexual stimulation. Then I started deep reflection, and relaxing exercises…this was all the help I needed. While I'm not back to 100 percent, things are definitely "looking up."

Consider taking a sabbatical from partner sex; restricting your partner interactions to nondemand touching, such as massage; or adopting a less performance-based approach to genital sex. Many couples have discovered that erections aren't necessary for pleasurable sexual encounters. You can focus on alternatives to intercourse or experiment with "soft entry" penetration. You'll find soft entry easiest if you are on top, so that gravity is on your side, and if you clasp the base of your penis to create a cock ring effect. Bear in mind that your penis can be an erotic tool regardless of how firm it is:

My husband has erection problems at times, so we spend more time with creative foreplay and pleasuring each other in a variety of ways, which we both really enjoy when he is not able to enter me in the usual manner. I especially love it when he takes the soft head of his penis and strokes it against my thighs or rubs it against my clit.

Sex therapy and/or talk therapy can help you address the emotional components that may be complicating your erection difficulties. Even when erectile dysfunction has a physiological cause, it can create intimacy and relationship issues that benefit from open discussion.

If you do find that there are physiological causes for your erectile dysfunction, you don't lack for treatment options. Over the years, treatments have included vacuum pumps; injections to produce temporary, involuntary erections; and surgical implants. Viagra is the first oral pill to hit the market, and its convenience (you take it approximately one hour prior to intercourse) and effectiveness (it's been found to work for seven in ten men, with the exception of diabetics and those recovering from prostate surgery) have led to skyrocketing sales. The active ingredient in Viagra is sildenafil, which aids in relaxing smooth muscle cells, thereby improving blood flow to the penis.

Things have definitely slowed down with age, but Viagra is the best thing since sliced bread! Timing and dependability of my erections started to fade a few years ago. With Viagra, it's like borrowing a younger penis for three hours.

I rarely orgasm as strongly as I used to when I was younger. I now use Viagra to help me get and keep an erection, and I am satisfied with the results.

While Viagra is a useful sex enhancer for many men, it's no magic bullet. It doesn't necessarily create firmer or longer-lasting erections than you would otherwise have. It won't inspire desire, boost a flagging libido, or bridge the emotional distance created by insufficient intimacy or communication. Before running to your doctor for a prescription, we'd encourage you to take the time to evaluate how crucial erections are to your sex life. Many men find that as they get older and are less able to have erections on demand, they expand their sexual activities to include more nongenital touch, oral sex, playing with vibrators, and penetrating their partners with either a dildo or a soft penis. It may be that your partner is less attached to intercourse than you might think and would be happy to build a sex life based on any one of the numerous pleasurable alternatives.

At the age of 64, the sensitivity of my penis diminished markedly, and erection and orgasm became much more difficult to achieve. This has not been a difficult adjustment for me as sex can now be much more relaxed and less goal-oriented. When I do achieve orgasm, the sensation is definitely still there.

Ejaculation

Although they tend to be inseparably linked in many folks' minds, ejaculation and orgasm are two distinct physiological phenomena, controlled by different nerve groups in the spine. Ejaculation is the result of a build-up of sexual tension that causes muscles near the prostate gland to contract, sending fluids from the prostate gland and seminal vesicles into the urethra. This produces the sensation referred to medically as "ejaculatory inevitability" and popularly as "ohmigod, I'm about to come!" Seconds later, intricately timed signals from the brain close off the valve between the bladder and the urethra and propel the ejaculate down the urethra and out the penis. Generally, ejaculation is accompanied by the involuntary, rhythmic contraction of the pelvic muscles, which is experienced as orgasm. However, it's possible to pass over the neurological point of no return and ejaculate without having yet reached orgasm:

I don't remember having an orgasm without ejaculation, but I have ejaculated without an orgasm—a disappointing experience!

It's also possible for a man to reach orgasm without ever ejaculating. Orgasm without ejaculation can be the result of retrograde ejaculation, which occurs when the valve between your bladder and urethra doesn't close and ejaculate is forced back into the bladder, rather than out the urethra. Retrograde ejaculation sometimes happens in men with spinal injuries or in men who have had prostate or bladder surgery—it should not adversely affect the pleasure you experience during orgasm.

After surgery to reduce an enlarged prostate, ejaculation no longer happens as usual—it's retrograde ejaculation with the semen being voided with the urine. It's been an adjustment but no problem. Also, no mess!

Orgasm without ejaculation can also be a conscious technique in men who train themselves to bypass the expulsion of semen and to experience the pleasurable full-body sensations and muscular contractions of orgasm without ejaculating. We'll discuss the phenomenon of orgasm without ejaculation in the Multiple Orgasm section below.

PREMATURE EJACULATION: Whether you are ejaculating "prematurely" or not is, of course, in the eye of the beholder. There are no absolutes when it comes to how long intercourse "should" take place before a man ejaculates. Whether the time involved is a minute or an hour, ejaculation is only premature if either partner wishes it had been delayed. It's worth noting that very few gay men report problems with premature ejaculation—presumably since they're not worrying about whether or not a female partner will reach orgasm, they don't feel pressure around how long they do or don't take to ejaculate. As men age, the rate at which they reach orgasm slows down naturally.

Popular remedies for premature ejaculation tend to focus on trying to counteract sexual arousal or to deaden sensation in the penis. You're probably familiar with the stereotype of a man reciting baseball statistics to himself during intercourse so that he can "last longer," and the adult industry does a booming business in numbing gels sold as "erection prolongers" (these contain anesthetic ingredients).

Actually, the best way to gain control over one's physical responses is to increase rather than decrease awareness of sensation. Common and highly effective treatments for premature ejaculation involve learning to identify the moment of "ejaculatory inevitability" right before orgasm. If you feel that you're reaching orgasm sooner than you'd like, practice the following stop–start exercises. Start by masturbating. Pay attention to your level of arousal, and when you feel you're about to reach orgasm, stop moving, stop touching yourself for a moment, and let the arousal ebb slightly before starting up again. Repeat this a few times and see how long you can stimulate yourself each time before you have to back off again. After fifteen minutes or so, consciously allow yourself to come. The

fact that you've built up to orgasm slowly and deliberately could well result in a particularly enjoyable orgasm.

The next step is to incorporate this stop–start technique into partner sex. Gradually intensify the stimulation you're receiving in each session, so that you gain confidence that you can control your responses under increasingly arousing circumstances. It's usually recommended that a man learning to control ejaculation progress from masturbating with no lubricant, to masturbating with lubricant, to intercourse with his partner on top of him while he lies still, to intercourse with him on top and moving. Some men utilize a variation of the stop–start method known as the squeeze technique. With this technique, you forestall an imminent orgasm by grasping the area right below your glans between your thumb and forefingers, and squeezing. After a few seconds of squeezing, you can resume stimulation and build yourself up to the point of ejaculatory inevitability again.

You may also find it helpful to use your PC muscle to delay ejaculation. See the Multiple Orgasm section below for tips on how you can modulate your level of arousal by consciously contracting and relaxing your PC muscle.

Bear in mind that you're not going to gain control over your body by denying yourself sensation. Instead, let yourself take conscious pleasure in the different levels of arousal you're capable of experiencing. As you learn to postpone the immediate gratification of orgasm, you may well discover a subtle range of sensation that is infinitely more gratifying.

Male and Female Anatomy
Anal Eroticism

The anus is an erogenous zone that doesn't always receive the acknowledgment it so richly deserves. For many people, the anus is the seat of a lot of physical tension and is associated with uncleanliness, discomfort, and pain. Anal eroticism is all too frequently dismissed as "unnatural." Yet if you can get past societal taboos and personal fears, you may be pleasantly surprised by the erotic possibilities of anal play.

After all, the anus is not only loaded with blood vessels and nerve endings, it also shares in the genital engorgement of arousal and the muscular contractions of orgasm. Many women and men find that direct stimulation of the anal opening enhances sex. The perineum, the area between the vaginal opening and the anus in women and between the base of the scrotum and the anus in men, is another potential erogenous zone.

> When my fiancé is masturbating me, I just about come right away when he slips one of his fingers to the spot in between my vagina and my anus and rubs that while rubbing my clitoris with another finger—sexual heaven! My orgasm is definitely far more earth-moving and intense.

The anal opening is controlled by two sphincter muscles, which you can learn to relax and contract at will. The anus is only about one inch long and leads into the rectum, a five to nine inches long, highly expandable canal lined with smooth tissue. Many men and women enjoy the feeling of fullness and pressure in the rectum resulting from anal penetration. Since rectal tissue is not as sturdy as vaginal tissue, and since the rectum takes a sort of S-shaped curve, you should take care not to insert anything rectally that isn't smooth, flexible, and well-lubricated. The rectum leads into the colon, so you shouldn't insert anything anally that doesn't have a flared base, to prevent its slipping into your body.

Pelvic Muscles

The pelvic organs are supported by a complex muscle system that lies just beneath the surface of the pelvic floor. The pubococcygeus muscle group—known as the PC muscle, for short—runs from the pubic bone to the coccyx or tailbone and surrounds the genitals in a figure eight. The PC muscle contracts involuntarily during arousal and orgasm. Learning to contract it voluntarily can be a great sexual enhancer.

The easiest way to locate your PC muscle is to practice stopping the flow of urine—the muscle you use to do this is your PC. Once you've found it, you can exercise your PC muscle in a variety of ways. It's helpful to try to coordinate your breathing with these exercises. For example, inhale and contract your PC at the same time. Hold both your breath and your contraction for a few seconds, then exhale and relax your muscle. Or try inhaling slowly while rapidly tightening and releasing your PC as many times as you can before exhaling and relaxing the muscle. Another

exercise that involves abdominal muscles as well as pelvic muscles is to inhale and pull up your pelvic muscles as though you were sucking water into your anus and/or vagina, then exhale and bear down as though you were pushing the water out.

These exercises are sometimes referred to as Kegel exercises, in honor of the gynecologist who first popularized them. The benefits of "doing your Kegels" are numerous. You'll gain greater awareness of sensation in your pelvic region. Exercise increases blood flow to the area, which is pleasurable in and of itself. Toned muscles are more flexible and better able to transmit sensation. You may well experience increased vaginal lubrication or easier, stronger erections thanks to a well-toned PC muscle. Techniques of controlling ejaculation and experiencing male multiple orgasm are based on learning voluntary control of pelvic muscles. Many people report increased sexual sensitivity and stronger orgasms as a result of exercising the PC. And, of course, there are no expensive gym memberships to worry about—you can do your Kegels anytime and anywhere.

> For a long time, I thought that feeling a penis inside my vagina would make my otherwise "superficial" orgasms feel more intense and deep. But I was wrong. I started exercising my PC muscle, and from then on whenever I was close to orgasm, I would squeeze my PC muscle, and the orgasm would go straight to my core.

The Sexual Response Cycle

The *sexual response cycle* is the term used to refer to the physiological changes our bodies go through during arousal and orgasm. Masters and Johnson can be credited with popularizing this phrase in the sixties. Their laboratory studies of thousands of men and women engaging in a variety of sexual activities led them to develop the concept of a four-stage cycle of sexual response. These four stages are: excitement, plateau, orgasm, and resolution.

According to the Masters and Johnson model, the excitement phase in both men and women is characterized by an increase in heart rate, muscle tension, and blood flow. Increased blood flow results in engorgement of the genitals, lips, and breasts; general body warmth; and flushed skin. Women's responses include vaginal lubrication, swelling of the clitoris and vaginal lips, and a lifting up or ballooning of the inner vagina and the uterus. Men's responses include erection, contraction of the scrotum, and elevation of the testicles. Many men and women also experience nipple erection. The entire body experiences muscular tension and warmth. Arousal frequently produces increased sensitivity to stimulation as well as reduced sensitivity to pain.

The plateau phase is a continuation and heightening of the excitement phase. In women, the clitoris retracts under the clitoral hood; the outer third of the vagina becomes even more congested with blood; and the uterus becomes fully elevated, creating a tenting effect in the inner vagina. Men often secrete a clear glandular fluid that may contain some stray sperm. Often referred to as "pre-come," this fluid is the reason withdrawal before ejaculation is an ineffective method of birth control.

Orgasm is the discharge of sexual tension through involuntary muscular contractions. These contractions take place in the outer third of the vagina and the uterus in women and in muscles throughout the pelvic region in both men and women. Anywhere from three to fifteen contractions occur, at intervals of eight-tenths of a second. Orgasm releases the blood from engorged genital tissue.

During resolution, the body returns to an unaroused state. Heart rate, breathing, and blood pressure return to normal; the body flush subsides; and genitals return to their usual size, shape, and color. If you've been aroused but haven't had an orgasm, it will take somewhat longer for the blood to ebb out of your congested genitals and for resolution to be completed.

Your body undergoes certain distinct physiological changes regardless of what kind of stimulation you are receiving or how subjectively different your arousal and orgasm may feel. Please don't despair, however, if you've never noticed your skin flush during arousal, if you find it hard to conceive of eight-tenths of a second, or if you're not sure if you've ever experienced "the plateau phase." Masters and Johnson's sexual response cycle is a fairly arbitrary construct. They interpreted their data selectively, to create a model that could be applied to men and women alike. In fact, few of us experience sexual arousal as though our bodies were spaceships moving inexorably from one discrete launching phase to another as we lift off toward a guaranteed orgasm.

Masters and Johnson's emphasis on the physiology of sexual response has influenced sex therapy and the treatment of people's sexual dysfunctions since the sixties. The idea that sexual response is not only natural, but quantifiable, is appealing. Who wouldn't be tempted by the notion that if we're just taught to push the right physiological buttons, sexual pleasure will automatically follow? The trouble with this mechanical approach to sex is that it doesn't take into account the huge influence that subjective conditions, social factors, and psychological readiness have on our experience of sex. Furthermore, physiological arousal doesn't necessarily indicate a readiness to have sex. Just because a woman is lubricating or a man has an erection doesn't mean she or he feels like being sexual. People need to *desire* sex to enjoy *having* sex.

In the seventies, sex therapist Helen Singer Kaplan amended the Masters and Johnson sexual response cycle to include desire as a prerequisite to excitement and orgasm, and this model (desire, excitement, and orgasm) has been widely followed since then. Yet, as the lesbian sex therapist JoAnn Loulan points out, even desire isn't necessarily required to initiate a satisfying sexual experience. If you enter into sex with willingness, desire may follow. Desire doesn't necessarily begin with sexual stimulation or come to an end upon orgasm. Perhaps the only absolute truth about sexual response is how fundamentally fluid it is. One can move from arousal to desire, from excitement to indifference, from boredom to passion, from orgasm to arousal and back again.

Desire

Sex therapists had only just begun to explore the powerful, subjective complexities of sexual desire when Viagra burst on the scene (and the stock market) in the late nineties. The resulting avalanche of interest in the *physiology* of sexual response has all but buried any more nuanced discussions of desire. In recent years, the concept of sexual desire has become so medicalized that so-called "desire disorders" are now clinically categorized in the DSM (*Diagnostic and Statistical Manual of Mental Disorders*). "Female sexual dysfunction" is a particularly broad category—never mind that fifty years ago, women were pathologized for having "too much" desire, now they're pathologized for having "too little." If you are experiencing difficulty with arousal or orgasm, or admit to having "low interest" in sex, you have a medically treatable condition. And you'd better believe that pharmaceutical companies are ready and willing to treat you.

A breathtaking array of products is being developed to relax smooth muscle cells (thereby facilitating erection), enhance genital blood flow, and increase vaginal lubrication: Prostaglandin creams, androgens such as testosterone and DHEA, and the amino acid L-arginine are all being touted as modern-day aphrodisiacs. The prevailing medical models put such focus on constructing firm erections and supple, lubed vaginas that they almost seem to lose sight of the men and women attached to those high-functioning genitals.

Sure, some of these products may ultimately prove to be useful sexual enhancers. However, we question the motives of snake oil salespeople such as the doctor who promotes his vaginal cream with the promise that it "basically eliminates the need for foreplay." Do we really need gels marketed to "increase clitoral sensitivity" that cost thirty times more than any water-based lubricant? Our culture has a knee-jerk affinity for quick-fix solutions: We'd rather pop a pill, apply a lotion, or switch on a medically approved vacuum device than take the time and energy to cultivate sexual self-awareness.

As we'll discuss in the next chapter, sexual desire fluctuates over the course of our lives, for numerous situational, emotional, cultural, and hormonal reasons. We hope that everything you read in this book will inspire you to take the long view and let your own authentic desires be your guide through a lifetime of sexual flux.

Know Yourself: Hormones and Desire

You've probably heard or read that hormones affect sexual desire. Growing interest in the physiology of arousal have put the spotlight on the role hormones play in sexual desire and response.

Hormones are chemical messengers produced in one part of the body that stimulate activity in another part. While there are many types of hormones, those that get the most press belong to the category of so-called "sex" or "steroid" hormones: estrogen, testosterone, and progesterone. Progesterone is present only in women, but estrogen and testosterone are present in both women and men. As women have up to ten times more estrogen than men during their reproductive years, and men have over ten times more testosterone than women, it's often claimed that differences between these two hormones "explain" the differences between the sexes.

We encourage you to be skeptical when you read popular articles naming testosterone as the source of all lust and aggression or explaining that postmenopausal women feel less "womanly" because of declining estrogen levels. The study of hormones is a young science, and new research is constantly overturning previous theories. There is so much more to sexual desire than chemistry—body image, self-esteem, health, relationship status, and access to resources such as information, time, space, and privacy all play a far bigger role in your enjoyment of sex than hormones alone.

That said, estrogen, progesterone, and testosterone do have physiological effects that will impact your sex life and that are well worth learning to identify. If you have never noticed these effects, don't be alarmed; some people are simply more responsive to hormonal fluctuations than others.

ESTROGEN AND PROGESTERONE: The most influential form of estrogen is estrodiol, which a woman produces in her ovaries during the first half of the menstrual cycle throughout her reproductive years. Estrogen promotes blood flow throughout the body (including the genitals), vaginal lubrication, a general sense of well-being and energy, and greater physical and emotional sensitivity. Progesterone, which a woman produces in her ovaries during the second half of the menstrual cycle, blocks the effects of estrogen, suppresses the immune system, and sedates the central nervous system. Some women experience progesterone as soothing and relaxing, others as fatiguing and depressing.

If you're not on birth control pills, you may have noticed an increase in libido midcycle (right before ovulation) when your estrogen levels are highest, or right before menstruation, when progesterone levels drop.

Desire has definitely changed for me! I've noticed as I've gotten older, my level of horniness rises in response to ovulation. Some months, I'm ready to jump on anyone!

I'm finding that in the last year or so, I have marked monthly fluctuations in desire and responsiveness. Ten days of the month, I think of little but sex, and have incredible orgasms. The rest of the month is more ordinary.

If you are on birth control pills, you may have noticed that your libido sags for most of the month, but rebounds during the week you're off hormones. Birth control pills contain just enough estrogen to prevent breakthrough bleeding, along with the high quantities of progesterone necessary to short-circuit ovulation and implantation. Progesterone is responsible for most of the Pill's negative side effects: bloating, headaches, depression, and reduced desire.

Most of my lifetime I have been on birth control or other medications that altered my ability to "want" to have intercourse. Seems like I'm most aroused during my periods and while pregnant.

I found that birth control pills really did a number on arousal for me. And of course, if I couldn't get aroused, I didn't want sex as often…it was a nasty cycle.

The Pill killed my sex drive. Who knew? I went on it when I was 17 because of a broken condom and stayed on it till I was 25, when I went off it because I was no longer in a monogamous heterosexual relationship and kind of wondered what my hormones would be like without it. Best damn decision I ever made. I'm not suicidally depressed anymore. I have a libido! For a few months after I went off the Pill things became ridiculous: I'd have one day a month where I wouldn't get any work done because I'd just sit and clutch the arms of my chair and fantasize. I'd know my period was coming because I'd find myself looking at people I normally didn't find at all attractive and becoming mesmerized by the way the little hairs on their cheek caught the light.

Other progesterone-based birth control methods, such as Norplant implants and Depo-Provera shots, can be equally hard on your libido. However, individual responses to hormones vary greatly. Plenty of women experience no negative effects from progesterone, while others report increased desire while on birth control. Certainly, freedom from the fear of unwanted pregnancy can be highly arousing in and of itself.

I got a Norplant shortly after starting to have sex, and it affected my sexual response in ways I didn't notice until I got it removed. For me, those few extra hormones kicked me up from what appears to be a more or less average libido to a hair-trigger orgasm girl who wanted sex three times a day.

TESTOSTERONE: Women produce testosterone in their ovaries and adrenal glands. Men produce ten to twenty times as much in their testicles. Testosterone appears to play a significant role in sexual sensation for both men and women—from boosting libido to enhancing genital sensitivity to heightening orgasm.

Researchers have proposed that variations in sex drive are influenced by variations in testosterone levels: that some of us are naturally "high-T" individuals, while others are "low-T." (To avoid charges of sexism, some researchers hasten to add that even though women have much lower levels of naturally occurring testosterone than men, they might compensate by having a higher sensitivity to testosterone.) On the other hand, most of us have had the experience of feeling "high-T" at some point in our lives (usually in the first flush of a new relationship) and decidedly "low-T" at others. Context can often trump chemistry.

Ebb and Flow

We all take for granted that "women have their cycles," but desire and energy fluctuate for men and women alike—in daily, monthly, seasonal, and situational cycles. Some research suggests that testosterone levels in men peak in the morning and dip in the evening; they've also been found to increase in the autumn, and decrease during times of stress. We'd encourage you to explore your unique personal patterns and body rhythms so that you can make the most hay when your own sexual sun is shining:

I want sex more in the spring, summer, and fall, we're at the nadir of my sex drive right now (late March). I also find I want sex more when I am happy or angry. When I am anxious or depressed, nope. No need for sex here. Not even masturbation. I really think, overall, each sexual relationship I have had has resulted in changes in my experience of desire and arousal. With each new person, new things turn me on and get me off.

Being pregnant allowed me to realize just how much hormones do play a part in my body, and how strongly they affected me…. It helped both me and my husband in later years when I had to take pain meds after I was in a car accident. We could realize what the drugs were doing to me, and that it was not anything personal going on when my libido went on strike!

Gender versus Anatomy

Sexual identity involves so much more than anatomy, and sexual expression is not controlled by biology alone—after all, we aren't uniformly hard-wired to insert tab A in slot B and call that satisfying sex. Each individual's sexuality is shaped and mediated by cultural values and expectations. And the social construct that has the greatest influence on our experience of sex is gender. Gender identity becomes the prism through which we perceive and relate to our anatomy.

We all have experience with our culture's rigid gender categories, the arbitrary rules that dictate appropriate "masculine" or "feminine" ways of moving, dressing, and speaking, as well as appropriate professions and pastimes. According to these rules, each biological sex has its own accompanying gender, and no swapping is allowed! Sure, we're making progress in overturning certain gender stereotypes, but as any boy ballet-dancer or girl football-player can testify, we've got a very long way to go.

The truth is that our binary view of gender is not only absurdly restrictive, it's woefully inadequate to represent reality. Gender is a human construct, and as such, it exists on a continuum that reflects the variety of human experience. For one thing, gender identity doesn't necessarily "match" biological sex: A butch woman can assert a masculine identity and appearance without having the slightest interest in adopting a male body. For some people, gender is a toy; for others it's an integral, immutable part of their identity; and for still others it's a nonissue.

Think about the influence of gender in your own sex life: Are you attracted by certain feminine or masculine styles? Or does gender ambiguity makes your pulse race? Do you feel sexually confident when you slip into spiked heels, biker boots, or both? Are there ways in which gender stereotypes are restricting your sexual pleasure? Perhaps you're ashamed of your own lust because you were raised to believe that "women prefer cuddling to sex." Perhaps you're not sure how to express your desire for anal penetration because you're convinced that "only gay men take it up the ass." Self-awareness is the first step toward cultivating your gender identity in ways that enhance your sexuality rather than repress it.

The good news is that the increased visibility of transgendered people and gender-bending trends in popular culture seem to be bringing about a greater acceptance of gender playfulness in bedrooms around the country. There's no question that feminine and masculine role-playing are loaded with erotic possibilities, especially if you approach your gender play with a spirit of generosity. Too often, people allow gender roles to limit, rather than expand, their sexual horizons. We encourage you to experiment with gender play as a way of adding options, not subtracting them—whether you slip into some silk, strap on a dildo, or try out a new way of walking and talking. Gender isn't static, and you can expect your relationship to your own gender identity to evolve in new and unexpected ways throughout your life.

I've gone from very femme to genderqueer and almost androgynous to being comfortable having a number of different gender identities that live in a thoroughly female body.

Transsexuals

Transsexuals are people who are assigned a gender at birth that doesn't fit their sense of self. Most transsexuals alter their bodies in some way, through either hormone treatment or sex-reassignment surgery or both, to bring their physical self into better alignment with their gender identity. Others simply live as the gender that feels right to them, without making any physical changes.

Hormone treatment—in which male-to-female transsexuals (MTFs) take estrogen and antiandrogens and female-to-male transsexuals (FTMs) take testosterone—is more common than surgery. Hormones alter secondary sex characteristics such as fat-to-muscle ratio, body hair, facial hair, and vocal pitch—all of which are among the primary cues we use in reading gender. Naturally, these hormones also affect sexual anatomy and responsiveness: MTFs taking estrogen often report that their penises can no longer become erect and that they must explore other paths to arousal and orgasm, while FTMs taking testosterone often report clitoral enlargement and an increased libido.

Genital surgery is more common for MTFs than FTMs. It's been argued that the medical establishment finds it less threatening to surgically create a vagina than a penis, and this may well be true—it's also true

While most of us take for granted that there are two, and only two, biological sexes, anatomical sex actually exists on a continuum. In fact, there are a wide range of intersex conditions, in which individuals are born with sex chromosomes, hormonal patterns, genitals, or reproductive organs that don't fit into tidy categories of male or female.

Intersex conditions have many causes—including genetic abnormalities or prenatal exposure to hormones—and manifest in a variety of ways. In some cases, intersexed individuals are clearly male or female in appearance, and their condition is not identified until puberty or adulthood. Some men with Klinefelter's syndrome, a genetic variation in which men are born with an extra X chromosome in addition to the standard XY, may not become aware of the syndrome until they discover their infertility in adulthood. Individuals with androgen insensitivity syndrome (AIS) are genetically male (they have XY chromosomes and testes), but their androgen receptors are not responsive to male hormones, and they develop female bodies. Sometimes AIS isn't identified until a young women reaches the age of puberty without menstruating. Women with MRKH syndrome are genetically female (they have XX chromosomes), but are born without a vagina, uterus, and fallopian tubes, a fact they may not discover until becoming sexually active.

Other intersexed individuals are identified at birth. An estimated one in two thousand babies is born with ambiguous genitals—estimates are imprecise in part because most of these infants are surgically altered at birth to be "assigned" one sex (usually female). An even higher number of babies are born with unambiguous genitals that doctors nonetheless consider medically "unacceptable," for example girls with large clitorises or boys with hypospadias, a condition in which the urethral opening is not located at the tip of the penis. The sad truth is that an infant girl born with a clitoris deemed "too long" (longer than three-eighths of an inch) will probably be subjected to clitoral reduction surgery—regardless of the resulting damage to her genital nerve endings. Boys born with penises that are deemed "too short" (shorter than one inch) may be subjected to surgical and hormonal sex reassignment. These horrific procedures take place in modern hospitals every day, with genital surgery performed on an estimated two thousand American infants a year, often resulting in irreparable harm to sexual responsiveness and/or fertility.

The treatment intersexed people have received at the hands of the medical establishment reflects our profound cultural unease with ambiguity of any kind, particularly gender ambiguity. For decades, doctors operated under the assumption that intersexed individuals couldn't possibly grow up to be healthy adults unless they received immediate sex assignment; many withheld accurate medical information from intersexed children and their parents with the justification that the truth would be too psychologically traumatic. Since the fifties, the prevailing treatment model has been to "normalize" intersexed people with mutilating surgery and then to deceive them about their own medical histories.

Recent years have seen the rise of activism by and for intersexuals. The Intersex Society of North America (ISNA) was founded in 1993 as a peer support, education, and advocacy organization dedicated to ending "shame, secrecy, and unwanted genital surgeries for people born with atypical sex anatomies." ISNA's goal is to reform the treatment of intersexed children, specifically to establish a model in which doctors defer all nonessential surgeries until the individual is old enough to give informed consent. A growing number of pediatric endocrinologists and other medical professionals are embracing reform, but until ISNA's model is universally accepted, it will be up to the parents of intersexed children to defend their children's rights to self-determination. We encourage all readers, especially prospective parents, to visit ISNA's website at www.isna.org for up-to-date information and resources.

The hardest thing for me was telling partners that I had MRKH. People would try to penetrate me with their fingers and I wouldn't tell them not to even though it caused me a lot of pain. I was embarrassed, I was afraid people would think I was a freak, etc. Now I choose partners that I know will not judge me.

that constructing a vagina is less difficult. In penile-inversion surgery, the penis is turned inside out, so that the skin of the former penis shaft becomes the walls of the new vagina, and part of the corpus spongiosum is used to create a clitoris.

Some FTMs opt for upper-body surgery—a double mastectomy—but not lower-body surgery. Some choose to retain their vagina and reproductive organs, while others choose their surgical removal. Those seeking genital reconstruction can choose between phalloplasty—in which a penis is surgically constructed from skin grafts—and metoidioplasty—which involves releasing the testosterone-enlarged clitoris from its hood and creating a scrotum out of the labia majora. The resulting penis is smaller than one "built" through phalloplasty and can't necessarily be used for penetration, but it has full sensitivity, unlike a penis created through skin grafts. In phalloplasty, the clitoris is left at the base of the newly constructed penis, above the scrotum, to allow for sexual sensation.

A thorough discussion of the varieties of preoperative and surgical approaches available to transsexuals is beyond the scope of this book. At this time, sex-reassignment surgery is far from perfect. Postop transsexuals may suffer genital nerve damage, have limited ability to reach orgasm, or have reduced sex drives. Of course, there are a rich variety of sensations available from erogenous zones other than the penis and vagina.

Some transsexuals identify exclusively as their post-transition sex and embrace traditional gender roles. Others identify as *transgendered*, a general term for anyone who challenges binary definitions of sex and gender. The transgendered movement includes transsexuals, cross-dressers, intersexed people (see sidebar), and all those who feel the categories *male* and *female* are inadequate to describe their experience of gender identity.

Despite increasing awareness of transgender issues, our society remains repressively phobic of any blurring of gender lines, and transgendered people face bias, hostility, and even violence simply for being who they are. A grassroots civil rights movement has taken shape, aided by the networking possibilities of the Web. Check out our resource listings for referrals to transgender organizations—ending discrimination based on gender identity will liberate every one of us.

Orgasm

There are many reasons to enjoy sex: It's a celebration of the human body; it's relaxing; it's entertaining; it promotes intimacy; you can do it alone, with a friend, or in a crowd. And you can have orgasms as a result. Orgasms are a simple pleasure, which we'd all benefit from taking less seriously. Orgasm generates more anxiety than any other single topic in our line of work. Men worry that they're coming "too quickly"; women worry that they're taking "too long" to come; and everyone worries that they're not having good enough, strong enough, or simply enough orgasms. We live in a competitive society, and we need encouragement before we can appreciate our own unique responses, without looking over our shoulders to see if somebody else out there is having an even better—or more "normal"—time. If you had never heard another person describe an orgasm, never read a bodice-ripping novel, or never seen a romantic movie, how would you describe your own experience of orgasm?

Some are just a quick hard rush that shoots through my body like a bolt of lightning. Others feel like a slow burn, they build up over time, they tease me, floating up and down my body—spreading out like concentric circles, and then there will be a burst of release.

Orgasms at different times involve different parts of my body—back, buttocks, different parts of my legs down to the calves, feet, shoulders, neck. I must be moving my legs in order to come.

Orgasm feels like water shooting up through the top of a fountain, tickling all the way, then shooting out of the top in electric vibrations through my body.

Orgasm is often for me this very still point; there's lots of movement as I'm getting increasingly excited, but when I come everything is tight and intense and still.

Orgasm feels good. Sometimes it's very concentrated, and sometimes it's totally diffuse throughout my body. Sometimes, if I'm very stressed out, it just feels like a release. When I'm relaxed, I feel like I'm floating in a place where there is no time or space. .

Orgasm for me feels like a release of a spring of love emotions toward my wife. It is mysteriously wonderful, and words are just insufficient to describe it.

Expectations

Orgasm, in the most pragmatic sense of the word, is an involuntary muscular contraction that signifies the release of sexual tension. Yet, as the plum in the pudding of sex, this simple physiological reflex inspires a wide range of emotional, psychological, and even spiritual responses:

I leave everything. I'm conscious only of ecstatic sensation, a universal sensation, warmth and vibrance coursing through me. Freedom from everything mundane rips through me, and I float on the breath of god—so to speak.

I experience orgasm as a minideath, approaching blackout. Psychologically, I have an approach/avoidance conflict. The closer I get, the more afraid I am. My partner has to reassure me.

My orgasms aren't completely reliable, and I often feel like I need more. Maybe I'm afraid of them. Afraid of the intensity or of being so far away from myself.

Before you read any further in this book, you might want to take the time to consider your own internalized expectations of orgasm. Do you share either of the following viewpoints?

Orgasm is always the ultimate point of any sexual experience. Sex without orgasm is like a cheeseburger without the cheese…missing something.

I enjoy having orgasms, but they're not my goal of sexual activity.

We propose that you consider treating orgasm as a possible, even probable, outcome of any sexual experience, but that you try to avoid focusing on it as a goal. When you focus on the end result of any sexual experience, you run the risk of rushing past or even denying yourself some of the more subtle pleasures to be enjoyed along the way. If you're reluctant to embark on a sexual experience unless satisfaction is guaranteed, you're cheating yourself out of the joys of the unexpected. New toys and techniques may not set you on a tried-and-true path to orgasm, but they will open up entirely new horizons of sensation. We hope that you'll approach the techniques described in this book with pleasure, rather than orgasm, as your goal.

Orgasm leaves me feeling energized, refreshed, and beautiful. Sometimes it's a very quick experience, and other times the build-up is so great that it becomes almost like an orgasm itself.

I like reveling in the last minute or two before surrender to orgasm. Often I will tense up all over my body, rise up, and let my partner know how good I feel.

Although orgasm is amazingly pleasurable to me it's the thirty seconds or so before it that are my favorite. My mind disappears and I feel my entire existence has been shifted into my clitoris…like it's a mountain and I'm floating towards its peak, floating around in that blissful place. The actual orgasm itself is frenetic and convulsive and violent for me. There is nothing peaceful about it.

Your expectations of orgasm may manifest as anxiety about what type of physiological response truly "counts" as orgasm. This is more of an issue for women than men, as women are more likely than men to have never experienced an orgasm or to feel a discrepancy between their own physiological experiences and a hazy, romantic ideal of orgasm as an earth-shaking event:

I was around 10 or 12, and would lie in bed and rub myself until I shook. I read my mom's Cosmo magazines and—because I didn't understand what was happening—kept thinking that if I only could get past these spasms, I'd find out what an orgasm was.

I mostly am not quite sure if I've had an orgasm. My current partner once told me, "Well, you're certainly having some kind of climactic experience!" and described several things I didn't remember doing, so it seems like there's some sort of perception error.

However, orgasm envy is not limited to women:

I don't think I've ever had an orgasm the way my wife has. I have come very strongly, but not to the extent that I think I should.

If you are someone who's never experienced an orgasm, many of the toys and techniques described in this book may be of use to you in exploring your sexual responses. Vibrators, which provide sustained, consistent stimulation, are particularly helpful for those women who have not yet been able to move beyond arousal to orgasm. If you're someone who's not sure if she has experienced orgasm, take note of the range of sensations described throughout this book. Do any of the experiences you read about echo your own?

Solo or Partnered

It's quite possible you'll find that your experience of orgasm shifts, depending on whether you're alone or with a partner. You may find more freedom in solitude:

I enjoy coming by myself best because I can float uninterrupted from intensely screeching pleasure into blissful relaxation without worrying about pleasuring my partner.

Orgasm is pretty hard to come by for me. It's easily attainable when I'm alone, but a lot harder with a partner. When I'm alone I can go as fast or slow as I want—I guess I don't feel as much pressure to come right away. I can spend as much time on myself as I want.

Or you may find the presence of a companion gives you more satisfaction:

Orgasm with a partner rocks my whole body, and then there's a wonderful release. By myself, it builds to a height of pleasure and then release, not as intense as with a partner.

In the best of sexual relationships, you'll each feel secure in your unique responses, and you can honestly share each other's pleasure, however it's taken:

I find that since I have been with my husband these past five years I can slow down and truly enjoy orgasm. We like to share each other's orgasm, watching the other person come. Coming together is not a necessity, and it's also okay that I do not choose to come during intercourse. Because of this I feel more free about my orgasm. I use a vibrator, dildo and vibrator, my hands, his hand or mouth—and sometimes I do come during intercourse.

Multiple Orgasm

This term is used to describe the experience of having more than one orgasm in quick succession. We do hope you won't translate the fact that some folks experience multiple orgasms into a performance hoop to jump through in bed. However, if you're intrigued by the idea of expanding the parameters of your sexual responses, read on. Whether or not you experience more than one orgasm in a single session, you can certainly have a good time practicing!

MEN: Multiple orgasms are more common in women than in men, as men tend to experience what's known as a "refractory period" after ejaculation, during which they're temporarily unable to achieve another erection. This refractory period can last anywhere from a few minutes to a few hours. There are, however, men who have reported experiences of consecutive ejaculatory orgasms with only brief refractory periods between each ejaculation. You may have experienced this yourself in adolescence—it occurs fairly infrequently in men over 30. More commonly, men who achieve multiple orgasms have trained themselves to orgasm without ejaculating, thereby sidestepping the "draining" effects of ejaculation and the need for a refractory period.

As noted above, ejaculation and orgasm are two distinct physiological phenomena, and it's possible to train yourself to experience the latter separately from the former. You might undertake this training in the spirit of Taoist sexual practitioners, with the goal of preserving the "vital energy" of your semen. Or you might just want to experiment with new sensations.

How do you train yourself to orgasm without ejaculating? The key is to consciously play with your level of arousal, to learn that responses you may have experienced as "inevitable" do fall under your control. Stimulate yourself until you reach the point where you feel an impending orgasm, then stop for up to twenty seconds and wait for the urge to ebb. It's helpful to hold still, breathe slowly and deeply, and relax your pelvic muscles. Then start up again. Continue to tease yourself, backing off from the verge of orgasm several times.

My technique is partial orgasms. This is when I jack off for a while, and then when it's getting so good that I have to come, I let go of the pressure from my hand, and just let my cum drip out. This gives me about 90 percent of the pleasure of a complete orgasm, but since there isn't a full release of energy, I can continue this cycle of jacking off endlessly.

I sometimes come without orgasm, and often orgasm without coming. The longer intercourse lasts for me before ejaculation, the greater the chance of orgasm without ejaculation.

Experts on male multiple orgasm fall into two slightly different camps when it comes to coming. Both emphasize the importance of cultivating PC muscle tone and awareness. One school of thought advises men to contract the PC muscle at moments of high arousal as a way of "putting on the brakes" to prevent ejaculation—this squeezing should be followed by holding still, breathing deeply, and relaxing all the muscles of the pelvis and butt to back off from orgasm. In this school, men are taught to gradually build arousal until reaching the brink of orgasm, at which point, if they squeeze the PC muscle long and hard, they can launch themselves into orgasm without ejaculation.

The second school of thought holds that contracting the PC muscle will cause, rather than delay, ejaculation, and that the trick to orgasm without ejaculation is to keep the PC muscle completely relaxed. Whichever technique you employ, the bottom line is that voluntary control of the PC muscle can be a great sexual enhancer, so start doing your Kegel exercises today.

Ready for a few final tips? Taoist sexual teachers advocate pressing an acupuncture point located in your perineum when you feel yourself close to ejaculating. This is supposed to halt the passage of prostatic and seminal fluids to the urethra, and to allow you to experience orgasm without any expulsion of fluids. If you're having intercourse with a partner, you may also find it useful to adopt a position that reduces muscular tension in your body (such as partner on top)—so that you can focus on and control your pelvic muscles more easily. Whichever of these tips you adopt, if you take the time to build your level of arousal, you'll doubtlessly be rewarded with at least one powerful orgasm—and maybe many more.

When I was about to climax, my girlfriend took her middle finger and placed the tip of it on my anus, with the rest of her finger resting behind my scrotum, pressed hard against the skin, while she cupped my balls in her hand. I don't know what she did but it took me forever to cum!

I remember jumping out of bed and screaming, "What the hell did you do to me, and can we do it again!!!"

Orgasm without ejaculation is tough to achieve for me, but well worth the extra effort. I have nearly the same feelings as orgasm with ejaculation, but all the sensitivity remains, and I remain horny. This makes sex last longer.

WOMEN: Some researchers have suggested that women are more likely to experience multiple orgasm than men because of differences in genital blood flow. Blood is propelled out of an erect penis during the spasms of orgasm via a concentrated network of veins. There is no such single concentrated vein pathway from a woman's erect clitoris and labia, so blood flows in and out of her erectile tissues more readily, facilitating repeated orgasms. Although every woman theoretically has the physiological capacity to experience multiple orgasms, not every woman will particularly want to have or will enjoy having more than one orgasm at a time:

Usually I feel satisfied and very relaxed after my one orgasm.

I'm lucky if I can manage two orgasms in twenty-four hours, let alone in a row. Never had multiple orgasms happen. After I've come once, it's just too sensitive, and I'm not interested enough.

I experience multiple orgasms. They eventually decrease in intensity for me, and rubbing myself raw isn't really that pleasurable. Quality is more important than quantity.

Of course, if your curiosity is piqued, there's no reason not to explore the possibility of having more than one orgasm in a sex session. The three basic rules of multiple orgasm are: back off, breathe, and move. After your first orgasm, your clitoris may be too sensitive to take any more direct stimulation. Continue stimulating yourself indirectly—switch to a lighter touch. If you're using a vibrator, you might want to move the vibrator to another part of your genitals, or to the back of your hand, while you continue to touch yourself with your hand. Take deep, panting breaths, and rock your pelvis in time with your breathing. Let the energy build back up in your genitals. Within a few minutes, excruciating overstimulation may well give way to excruciating pleasure and you'll find yourself sailing off into another orgasm. Some people find that their second or third orgasms feel more powerful than the first, and some find that their orgasms become progressively less intense:

Multiple orgasms are fantastic, but sometimes I feel my body doesn't know when to quit!

During masturbation, I generally enjoy four to five orgasms—though they diminish in intensity after that. Several times, more out of curiosity than anything else, I have gone out for marathon sessions—between one to two hours long—and continued to orgasm (stopped counting at fifteen to twenty). Hands and fingers finally worn out, but clit still obliging.

When I do have a second orgasm, it is more intense than the first, though a lot harder to achieve. In these cases, my partner brings me off the first time, and I bring myself off the second time (usually manually). When I am alone and masturbating, I normally stop after just one orgasm.

Some people who practice breath work and meditative techniques report experiences of orgasm that last for five or more minutes. One explanation is that these individuals are riding an extended, intense plateau of arousal and subjectively interpreting this experience as extended orgasm. Then again, maybe they're simply having five-minute orgasms. There's no scientific study on the topic as yet, and really no need to demand an explanation. Orgasm is a blissfully subjective response.

I have to work at orgasms, but once they arrive I keep coming, i.e., my clit keeps throbbing, especially with firm pressure.

I used to have something more like multiple orgasms, which occurred after the second or third when they would all blend together into a continuous extremely high state that was almost torturous (but great).

Spontaneous Orgasm

This term refers to the phenomenon of reaching orgasm without touch. A fair number of women report that they can reach orgasm purely through mental stimulation, breathing techniques, and contracting the PC muscle. Wet dreams are better documented in men than women, but both sexes can attest to having orgasms in their sleep. Women and men with no genital sensation because of spinal cord injuries have also been documented experiencing orgasms while sleeping. People with nerve damage can often learn to have orgasmic sensations in other parts of the body. The long and short of it is, there's plenty of proof to the adage that the brain is the biggest sex organ.

Interesting note about orgasms: I can have them hands-free. If I lie or sit pretty still and focus on a fantasy (especially if I've smoked a joint first), I can have intense, mind-blowing orgasms without any kind of physical stimulation. Lucky me!

I was born a paraplegic, so I cannot feel below my waist. This has limited my ability to orgasm through the sense of touch. However, I am very intuned to my thoughts. My vagina does lubricate and I do orgasm when I can concentrate.

The Big O

We realize it may seem a bit contradictory to follow our assertion that orgasms are but one of many reasons to have sex with several pages full of orgasm tales. We do believe that orgasms aren't the be-all and end-all of sexual experience, and we know that many people have great, pleasurable sex without orgasms. But orgasm strikes us as a fascinating and revealing topic because in many ways people's feelings about orgasm serve as microcosms of their feelings about sex in general. If you were asked the question, "How are you feeling about your orgasms?" your response would doubtless include, not only the sensations and the emotions you experience during sex, but also your feelings about your body, your genitals, your relationships, and your desires. Try answering this question, and see what you learn about yourself.

Since learning to masturbate, my response cycle has evolved so that I will come and then shortly after (less than one minute) my crotch will be begging me to do it again. These days I will come once or twice, but for a while nothing less than twice would do! It was an amazing feeling to have the need be beyond my control or creation, in a way. I have had trouble coming with partners and being able to sexually respond well, so there is something special about this.

Orgasm is my elusive best friend. I've been sexually active since about 13, and I only started having orgasms a few months ago, at the tender age of 23. That's when I started to use my vibrator. I really enjoy my orgasms, demure and non-earth shattering though they may be. That warm, warm feeling is just terrific. I try not to think about having one while I'm masturbating, because I think it lessens their intensity. When I'm not masturbating, I do think about them. I remember how my temperature goes up, how I lose sense of time, how these waves pulse through my insides and hips up through my stomach. I like the noises I make.

Sex and Your Doctor

In an ideal world, members of the medical community would be valuable resources for your questions about sexual anatomy and response. Despite the fact that we count on doctors for accurate physiological information, at least as many people have been intimidated, alarmed, or actually misinformed about sex in their doctor's office as have received useful, reassuring advice. It's understandably challenging both for laypeople to bring up sexual matters to medical professionals, and for medical professionals to address these matters. Consider the following limitations and our suggested coping mechanisms:

Lack of Training

Medical schools offer no standardized program of training in human sexuality, and state licensing requirements are hardly strenuous (for instance, in the state of California, medical students are only required to have a total of twelve hours of human sexuality training). There's a growing movement to provide better sex training for doctors, but effects could take decades to trickle down.

Grassroots organizations can provide up-to-date, accurate information for laypeople on a host of medical issues. Sex-information hotlines (see our resource listings for referrals) offer far more extensive human sexuality training to their volunteers than medical schools do to students. If you have access to the Web, you can find a wide range of information online.

Specialization

Doctors tend to have very specific areas of expertise and knowledge. If you're experiencing a specific sexual problem, discuss it with the appropriate specialist. Take your erectile concerns to a urologist. Discuss your vaginismus with an OB/GYN. If your concerns aren't exclusively physiological, you may find that a sex therapist is best equipped to help you.

Most doctors operate from a disease-based model, and are more likely to be able to diagnose medical conditions than to discuss behavioral guidelines. If you're seeking advice on sexual practices, you may find that a family practitioner has a more holistic, better-informed approach than a specialist. Nurse practitioners and social workers can also be valuable resources. The staff at women's clinics are frequently well-informed about sexual matters, thanks largely to pioneering work within the feminist health movement.

Embarrassment

Doctors are raised in the same sex-negative society as the rest of us and aren't necessarily any better equipped to discuss sex than the average person. Don't expect your doctor to be the one to raise the topic of sex. You'll need to be proactive in requesting information. Come to your appointment with a clear idea of what specific questions you'd like answered—it can be helpful to write these down beforehand just to identify what it is you want to know. Even if doctors can't answer your questions right then and there (remember, they may not know the answers), they should either schedule a follow-up appointment or refer you to another professional who can help you.

You may have qualms about approaching the doctor with whom you have or hope to have a long and trusting relationship with a question that might embarrass one or both of you. For example, "You've told me I shouldn't have vaginal intercourse until six weeks after childbirth, but what about anal intercourse?" or "After my heart attack, is it more dangerous to masturbate or to have sex with my wife?"

Well, the choice is up to you. You can ask the question and assume that your doctor will either have a good answer or will have to research the answer, in which case you'll have made a valuable contribution to sexual consciousness-raising in the medical community. If your embarrassment might prevent you from clearly communicating what it is you want to know, you can take advantage of anonymous resource options, such as sex information hotlines and the Web.

Power Dynamic

There's an inherent power dynamic in the doctor–patient relationship. Not only is the doctor an authority figure, but whatever he or she puts into your medical records will be easily accessible to other doctors and insurance companies.

Here again, you can either go public with your concerns for the sake of increasing the general pool of medical knowledge, or you can opt for anonymity (for example, many free clinics offer anonymous HIV testing). In medical emergencies, you need to get to a doctor regardless of what will or won't show up in your patient files. Be aware that there's nothing new under the sun, and that emergency staff won't blink twice at situations that might strike a layperson as unusual.

The bottom line is that doctors are people, too, and you're going to find some who are excellent, sensitive communicators about sexual matters and others who aren't. You deserve access to accurate sex information, and if you can't get this from a doctor, please don't assume you've exhausted all of your resources.

If Not You, Who?

Regardless of the response you may get, we do encourage you to bring up sexual questions and concerns to your doctors; to identify, support, and refer others to the sex-positive doctors you find; and to talk with friends and family about the sexual repercussions of medical and physiological events throughout your life. Bringing sexual topics out into the open is a crucial step toward normalizing sex, which leads in turn to a freer exchange of accurate information. Changing the status quo demands everyone's proactive participation, and you can make an invaluable contribution to raising the sexual IQ of everyone in your community simply by speaking up.

CHAPTER

Sex Over a Lifetime

Everyone is a sexual being. Six-month-old babies and 92-year-old grandmas are all sexual beings, so don't ever think that you are the only one who has these feelings or that any of them are wrong, deviant, or bad.

Each individual's unique sexuality is shaped by developmental milestones and significant life events. Sexual impulses are with us from cradle to grave, and sexual self-discovery is not a single journey, in which we map out our personal terrain once and for all. Rather, our bodies, relationships, desires, and patterns of sexual response are ever-evolving. Change is both chaotic and enlivening—if you approach the inevitable changes in your sexual experience with a spirit of curiosity and adventure, your whole life can be enriched.

Childhood and Adolescence

Anyone who remembers masturbating or playing doctor as a child knows that children are sexual beings. Unfortunately, many adults mistakenly view children as sexless, so when a child demonstrates delight in his or her body or feelings, adults respond with anxiety or suspicion. This stems in part from puritan notions that innocence is a sexless state, but also from a tendency to project adult sexual feelings onto children. While children don't necessarily masturbate or look at naked people with the same intentions as adults, they do touch themselves because it is pleasurable, and they do look because they're curious. Too often these typical manifestations of child sexuality make adults uncomfortable at best and fearful at worst.

Yet it doesn't have to be this way. Children's sexuality should be given free reign to develop naturally, nurtured with information, encouragement, and guidance from adults—not denial, shame, or censorship. How else will today's children become tomorrow's sexually responsible adults? We don't hesitate to encourage our children to cultivate healthy self-esteem, positive body image, and respect for others, and these same values can provide the foundation for a life full of sexual pleasure.

Many excellent book and websites are available to help both parents and educators understand and prepare for children's developmental milestones, along with suggestions for how to impart age-appropriate sex information. We have written extensively about raising sexually healthy children in our own book *The Mother's Guide to Sex*, and we encourage you to seek out as many resources as you can and to maintain an open dialogue with your children throughout their lives.

In this chapter we focus on the sexuality of teens and young adults—rather than prepubescent children—because:

- Statistics show that plenty of young people have sex. We believe in the sexual autonomy of today's youth and want to offer them tools and resources for informed decision-making.

- The current emphasis on abstinence-only sex education not only is unrealistic but negatively affects teen sexual health.

- We hope parents, teachers, and anyone in the position to advise a teen about sexuality and decision-making will find the following information useful.

If you are a parent, we encourage you to take an active role in your child's sexuality education. As we discuss below, the sex education that children receive at school or from peers will hardly prepare them for the difficult decisions they will face once their hormones kick in.

If you are a teen, welcome! One of the reasons we wrote this book is that we wish something like it had existed when we became sexually active in our teens. We applaud your quest for accurate sex information, and we hope you'll find answers to your questions about anatomy, self-image, technique, safer sex, and communication in these pages. However, there are many other aspects of your sexual coming of age that we can't address here, so we encourage you to check out some of the materials that have been written specifically for youth. Books like *Deal With It* (for preteen and teen girls) and *Changing Bodies, Changing Lives* (for teen girls and boys) discuss physical and emotional changes, deciding if you're ready for sex, relationships, dealing with peers and parents, and contraception (among other subjects). The Web is also a terrific source of information, and we highly recommend sites like Sex Etc. and Coalition for Positive Sexuality as sources of straightforward information from other teens. Check our resource listings for recommended books, videos, organizations, and websites.

Teens Have Sex

According to the Centers for Disease Control's latest statistics, 39 percent of teens in the United States have engaged in sexual intercourse by the ninth grade, growing to 65 percent by the twelfth grade. This should come as little surprise to the hundreds of our survey respondents who shared memories of their adolescent sexual experiences.

Clearly, teens have been and will continue to be sexually active, yet most receive little information and no real preparation about sex. Soon after the first edition of this book was published, we learned that it was being used in several college-level human sexuality classes. We were thrilled to think that young adults would be learning that sex was something they deserved to enjoy, and that it could encompass pleasure, experimentation, and safety, rather than danger and disease. Yet it seemed sad to us that the sex-positive message these young adults were receiving was arriving a little late. By college age, most of us have struggled through awkward, demoralizing, or just disappointing sexual relationships, and are already trying to repair whatever damage has been done. Even those who emerge from their adolescent sexual forays with positive memories probably would have benefited from a little more confidence and a lot less fear. It's ridiculous that teens are given very little information about sexual pleasure and technique, yet when they reach early adulthood they're expected to intuitively know how to please themselves and a partner. Imagine if we held this same belief about learning to drive a car!

We respect a teenager's fundamental right to make his or her own sexual decisions, and this right can't be signed away to parents or politicians. Adults are responsible for providing youth with the information and support they need to make responsible sexual choices. Sure, not all teens are emotionally "ready" for sex, but neither are plenty of adults. There is no magical age at which sexual maturity sets in; a great many teens possess the ability to negotiate safe and consensual sex, and will do so whether they have adult "permission" or not. If you're a parent, we're not suggesting that you simply give your teen a fistful of condoms, a slap on the back, and a quick list of how-to instructions. We *are* saying that if you communicate your perspective and values and provide both information and tools, these will be infinitely more valuable to youth who choose to engage in sexual relations than a "just say no" lecture.

I have only grown more vigilant about practicing safer sex for myself and providing teens with the means to protect themselves. I don't want my kids to be having sex until they are adults, preferably in a committed relationship. However, I would rather have my kids practicing safer sex than contracting HPV, HIV, or another sexually transmitted disease! I would rather they do something against my wishes with some form of protection than die!

What Teens Learn about Sex Today

In the United States, teens get their sex information principally from friends, parents, the media, and school. In general (and please note there are always exceptions!), information from friends is inaccurate and judgmental, advice from parents is sporadic and accompanied by lots of blushing, and images offered up by the media are unrealistic and one-dimensional. In school—where you'd expect sexuality to be treated with the respect and comprehensive attention paid to other subjects—all discussion of sex has been reduced to a one-note message: Don't do it.

Today's abstinence-based education teaches kids that sex (usually defined as intercourse) outside of marriage is both dangerous and wrong. To prove the point, lectures focus on the perils of sex—that it can lead to teen pregnancy, STDs, and death (in the case of AIDS). Condoms, when discussed at all, are maligned for being less than 100 percent effective against disease transmission and pregnancy.

In Texas we had sex ed in health class and it was entirely about abstinence. We studied STDs and failure rates of contraceptives. Never was it suggested that one could use one or more contraceptive methods to have sex without getting pregnant or contracting some incurable disease.

Often referred to as fear-based curriculum, abstinence-based education seeks to scare the sexual desire right out of youth. The biggest problem with this model is that kids are still having sex. Only now they've been denied the resources, tools, and motivation to engage in responsible sex, which actually leaves them more at risk than if they'd just been told the facts about anatomy, contraception, and safer sex. "Abstinence plus" programs, which *do* raise the topics of sexual responsibility and safe sex, still focus on the negative outcomes of sex (while stressing abstinence as the most desirable option).

Proponents of abstinence-only education assert that increased information about sex will lead to increased sexual activity. However, statistics have shown no causal link between abstinence programs and reduced rates of teen sex. Teens are having the same amount of sex as ever, they're just doing it with even less guidance. Youth deserve to be taught, not only about safer sex and contraception, but also about alternatives to intercourse (masturbation, oral sex, role play) so that they're aware of options, should they want to postpone intercourse. By focusing on intercourse as the be-all-and-end-all of sex, abstinence educators suppress knowledge of the vast range of satisfying sexual activities that can be enjoyed over a lifetime of changing circumstances.

Teens themselves find abstinence programs totally unrealistic and unhelpful. Few of our survey respondents found anything positive to say about them:

Sex education in school came a bit late for me as anything that they taught us was stuff we already knew. That is hardly surprising, since we were 15 when they offered sex ed in my school!

You have more chance of learning about sex from a parrot than you do from sex ed classes. It makes me sick that parents actually support them, while at the same time all these universities are conducting research to find out why so many girls get pregnant— maybe 'cause no one ever bothered to explain condoms to them.

Amazingly enough, the Catholic high school I attended did teach sex ed, which is where I learned most about technical and mechanical matters. The only problem was that the instructors (a nun and a priest) taught us that doing any of these things before marriage was wrong.

The irony of this state of affairs is that according to a national survey by the Kaiser Foundation, most parents would prefer that the schools provide more comprehensive sexuality education, an approach that teaches kids about sexual responsibility, health, and relationships in a positive manner. However the Religious Right's money, political prowess, and scare tactics have all but killed these programs, with the result that today only 5 percent of American schools provide comprehensive sex ed.

1. Teens have the right to appreciate their own and each other's bodies.

2. Teens have the right to know how things work.

3. Teens have the right to know that sex is about pleasure.

4. Teens have the right to know that sex is more than intercourse.

5. Teens have the right to realistic expectations.

6. Teens have the right to make responsible choices.

7. Teens have the right to sexual equality.

8. Teens have the right to sexual diversity.

9. Teens have the right to consent.

10. Teens have the right to resources.

Teens' Sexual Bill of Rights

Given the dearth of sex information we receive as teens, it's a wonder that we pursue sex at all—let alone enjoy it. It's a true testament to the power of our unquenchable desires that we persist, even in the face of disappointment, disillusionment, or disaster. Yet, once we reach adulthood, plenty of us recall our early sexual experiences with nostalgia and protectiveness toward our younger selves. We wouldn't have wanted not to have these experiences, but perhaps we would have wanted them to play out differently. And that could have been the case if we'd been better prepared and informed. Our survey respondents wrote so passionately and prolifically about their first sexual experiences that we're quoting them here to illustrate how teens would surely benefit from a more open, honest, and thorough approach to their sex education. Consider this a Teen's Sexual Bill of Rights.

1. Teens have the right to appreciate their own and each other's bodies. Both boys and girls deserve access to information about sexual anatomy, along with accurate visual representations. Unfortunately, books for adolescents are usually illustrated with vague line drawings, giving the impression that human genitals resemble those of a cartoon character. In the absence of accurate depictions, many teens develop the misconception that their own genitals are somehow abnormal or deformed (a misconception that can last well into adulthood).

Sex ed class was a joke. The only thing I learned was that my female "parts" looked like a teddy bear.

I don't like my cunt very much, which makes me reluctant to let people see it or touch it. My labia minora hang down a lot, and they're a weird color. I don't arouse easily and I don't produce much lube. I'm very self-conscious about it.

Some kids manage to dig up photos in adult magazines, which hardly depict female genitalia in the most realistic light. Our ideal anatomy lesson would also cover smells and secretions, so that both boys and girls could learn that genitals aren't meant to smell like roses:

I felt extreme approach-avoidance conflict before, during, and after my first experiences with female partners. I had to get to know women's bodies, especially their vulvas, and overcome my fear and ignorance about smell and appearance.

As a teenager, my male friends did not hold such great attitudes about women. They used to criticize how their girlfriends' vaginas smelled. Of course, the boys were just covering up their own insecurities, but it made me self-conscious about my body.

One lover told me I tasted like "swamp water" and he hated it. That upset me and it's been hard to shake, even though I've had other lovers who like my taste.

2. Teens have the right to know how things work. Our sexual anatomy lesson would teach the importance of the clitoris as a source of pleasure for women. Lacking this vital piece of information, couples of all ages down through the years have simply pumped away, assuming that female orgasm should be an inevitable byproduct of penis/vagina intercourse, which it rarely is. Both men and women should know how to locate and stimulate the clitoris, so that women aren't routinely left dissatisfied by sex.

I was 15 when I first had sex. I had been going out with my boyfriend at the time for about a year and we figured it was time. We had been going pretty far with the fondling and oral, but it was time to do it! Alas, it is another tale of a boy thinking that penile penetration does it for a girl. There was some foreplay, but not enough. He came, I didn't.

If masturbation were encouraged as a way to discover (and fine-tune) sexual response, disappointing sexual outcomes like premature ejaculation and elusive orgasms could be avoided.

At 16 I got laid and to be honest I was always coming off too quickly.

I had sex at 15 with my boyfriend. I was the initiator. It was mostly memorable for the bug bites—we were outside. It went from pleasurable but clumsy to consistently enjoyable. I didn't often orgasm during sex at first, but eventually learned more about my physical responses and how they differed in partner sex from masturbation.

Similarly, many couples new to sex know nothing about sexual arousal and lubrication, which can make all the difference between pleasure and pain. Teens should know why and when a girl gets wet, why precome is not an acceptable lubricant, how to use lube with a condom, and how to remedy a dry encounter with a commercial lube.

I was 16. I didn't know what sex was; I thought kissing and hugging was sex. I didn't realize that you need your brain to have sex. I though that if I saw a penis, I would automatically become wet and the thing would slide right in. Wrong! It was very painful, I was not wet, I didn't know what to think. I began reading about having sex and then I discovered how to become aroused.

At 13 I had sex, which was not in any way pleasant! Partner did not know about the wonders of lube. Just ram, ram, ram.

It was the first time I'd ever seen an erect penis, much less touched one. I wound up giving him a friction burn from a hand job because I didn't know how to do it.

In his bedroom under a huge poster of Kurt Cobain, we fumbled around and figured out the condom thing. We both kept our underwear on. He just stuck it through the flap in his boxers, and moved my panties aside. I remember it feeling like I was sitting on a broom handle. It hurt, my eyes watered. We didn't know anything about lube or the importance of foreplay. We had to do it three or four times that weekend before we figured out how to make it feel good.

3. Teens have the right to know that sex is about pleasure. The bulk of what children and teens are taught about sex revolves around unwanted touch, danger, and disease. When youth leave home, after years of indoctrination in sexual shame, guilt, and fear, they're supposed to suddenly figure out how to have good sex and healthy relationships. Let's take a more balanced approach, teaching teens about sexual responsibility while also explaining that sexual desire and passion are natural and healthy.

As a young girl and teenager, I was shamed about my sexual desires. I was "bad" for wanting to kiss a boy. I was worse than bad for wanting to do anything else. Later as I got older, the whole subject of sex and love was ignored. It just didn't exist as far as my mother was concerned and was not an acceptable topic of conversation. So...I got very confused. Wanted sex and love and found it very stimulating...but had no tools for handling the situations I found myself in or the feelings that came up about it. It's taken years to get it all sorted out.

My mom has always been very open with me about sex. From her I got the woman's perspective (and a healthy dose of "If you're going to do it, enjoy it— but be smart"), and the okay to feel sexual.

I began having sex when I was 22, and I had no idea what to expect. I was raised in a household that didn't talk about sex and I never felt comfortable talking about sex with my friends, so the only thing I had to draw on was how the media portrays sex, which is always this explosive, passionate, pleasurable experience. I still consider losing my virginity to be the most disappointing experience of my life. I remember it as boring at best, painful at worst, sweaty, and unpleasant, and after having sex a handful of times I was ready to swear off sex completely.

4. *Teens have the right to know that sex is more than intercourse.* Because intercourse gets touted as the "ultimate sex act," it takes on an importance all out of proportion to its pleasure potential. Many have described the resulting "is that all?" moment during their first experience of intercourse.

> *I lost my virginity at 20, and found the actual act pretty disappointing. Before that, I'd always enjoyed being sexual with a partner because at some point we'd do something that would make me climax. It seems like once penetration entered the mix, the other stuff got left by the wayside, and I didn't get as much pleasure out of it.*

> *I was 15. I was full of raging hormones but most boys were pretty disappointing once it got down to the actual fucking. I think the touching, dry humping, hickeys, and making out were more fun.*

Sex is generally more exciting and satisfying when it involves a variety of full-body activities. If only we all could view intercourse as one option among many, teens and adults could enjoy a healthier, happier range of sexual experiences.

> *I was just 18 and so was she. We were both in our final school year. The early experiences involved oral sex, mutual masturbation, and heavy petting, but no intercourse because we were both terrified of the risk of pregnancy and would have to have relied upon condoms (also, attitudes were very different in 1962). However, we were sexually quite uninhibited and we managed to work in a lot of variety and have a pretty good sex life.*

> *I was 15 years old, and the experiences were mostly wonderful. I "only" had oral sex because I was afraid of getting pregnant.*

> *I first had sex at 14, with an older boy. When I lost my virginity, I thought, "Thank God I finally got that over with! Now I can have some real fun!" In the next few weeks we tried everything I could think of that sounded appealing at the time. I was completely insatiable and wanted to do it with everyone everywhere in every way.*

When sex is defined exclusively as intercourse, many youth are left believing that other sexual activities "don't count" as sex, and are somehow less risky than intercourse. Because they're not getting thorough safe-sex instruction, they aren't learning that unprotected oral and anal sex can transmit a variety of STDs. Currently, one out of four sexually active teens contracts an STD. Let's give our kids the gift of sexual health by teaching them all the facts.

> *I lost my virginity at age 17, with a boy, at a summer college-level program for high-school juniors. We had been given a safe-sex lecture earlier in the week— I bless those organizers every day. Thanks to them I know about the morning-after pill and much, much more. Also thanks to them my roommate had some free condoms in her drawer.*

5. *Teens have the right to realistic expectations.* The media (advertisements, popular magazines, movies, music videos) usually depicts sex as glamorous, effortlessly hot, mutually satisfying, risk-free, enjoyed largely by beautiful people—and perfect when you're in love. It's disconcerting at best, and painfully disillusioning at worst, to discover that sex can be messy, awkward, embarrassing, logistically challenging, painful, one-sided, worrisome, and not always perfect—even with the one you love.

> *My sexual experiences were characterized by the insane thinking that if I felt strongly enough about someone then they would come to feel the same way and all would be good. Rarely…nope…never happened that way. So I spent time chasing a dream and missing out on reality.*

> *My first sexual experience was when I was 18. I hated it. It was horrible…hurried and in the back of a friend's car during a church swimming social. I wondered that religious empires had crumbled and political careers toppled for sex.*

> *I had my first sexual experience when I was about 22 years old. I was very nervous and almost did NOT go through with it. I convinced myself to pretend that I was Ron Jeremy and just go for it! Even after that, I didn't really understand all the "hype" about sex since I didn't orgasm from intercourse for the first few months that my girlfriend and I were having sex.*

6. *Teens have the right to make responsible choices.* What you don't know *can* hurt you, and teens who are not given full access to the tools and information to make their own decisions about sexual health are being abandoned to a game of roulette by the very adults hoping to "protect" them. If teens are told they simply shouldn't be sexual, they're more vulnerable to being swept up in the moment without making adequate preparations for safer sex or contraception. Like all too many adults, teens left to their own devices are willing to take a chance, assuming "it won't happen to me."

> *I wasn't expecting to "get lucky," and needless to say, I wasn't prepared. The young lady and I worried for a week (until her period). But the strain broke up the relationship.*

> *I was 16. Backseat of my boyfriend's parents' station wagon. It was spontaneous, and we had no condoms, but were really wrapped up in the moment. So...we used a baggie that had held his sandwich that day at school. It was great! It only got better (as did our protection)!*

7. *Teens have the right to sexual equality.* The double standard regarding boys' and girls' sexuality doesn't seem to be breaking down: Promiscuous boys are admired by their peers, promiscuous girls are seen as slutty; boys should play the field and gain experience, while girls should save themselves till marriage. Girls are rarely encouraged to negotiate sex on their own terms. This lack of agency, combined with the message that good girls only have sex with someone they truly love, leaves girls vulnerable to being manipulated or pressured into sex.

> *I think my first sexual experience with a partner happened when I was about 13, with a boy who essentially wheedled me into it. I resisted every step of the way, with him whining about how his balls hurt and it was my fault, and he needed to screw me to relieve himself. There was no foreplay involved—I don't remember even knowing about foreplay until I was in college.*

> *My first time was at 17 with my boyfriend at the time. He was my first everything. I didn't want to do it, but he kept bugging me, so I said okay. We did it in his friend's spare room. I was less than thrilled and very disappointed. We never really were sexually*

compatible. He wanted it all of the time, while I did too, but not with him.

Let's foster sexual self-esteem in girls from an early age so that they are able to stand up for themselves. Let's teach both boys and girls respect for themselves and their partners. Let's encourage alternatives to intercourse, so that horny kids can go home and masturbate!

> *I think in the beginning I was too wrapped up in whether or not my partner was having a good time, then I finally thought, "Screw that!" I started making sure I had a good time!*

8. *Teens have the right to sexual diversity.* Many of our survey respondents described their first same-sex encounters as enlightening and affirming.

> *When I was first having sex at age 20, it was surprising and confusing. It only got really great after I came out and realized there was nothing wrong with me. It was the sex of the partner I was with that made all the difference.*

> *I started having sex with a partner at the age of 22. She was also the first woman I was with (I've never had sex with a man). It was interesting because I had had several "romantic friendships" with women that didn't include sexual activity, so the first time I was with a woman who wanted to be sexual I didn't even ask many questions...I practically threw myself at her.*

Teaching tolerance for sexual diversity is not usually included in most sex ed curriculums, and as a result queer youth often find that peers make their lives hell.

> *Teenagers are very sexual, but still unimaginative and not at all accepting of different sexualities. I'm continually surprised by how much something as well covered in the media as GLBTQ [gay, lesbian, bisexual, transgender, and questioning] is handled so immaturely by my peers.*

High schools are notoriously unforgiving places to be "different," which plays a role in the high incidence of depression and suicide among gay teens. With next to no support from politicians, religious leaders, parents, and teachers, teens are left to seek community on their own. Fortunately, today many are finding support and validation on the Web.

At 10 I kissed my female best friend passionately in front of both my parents. They flipped out! That has always stayed with me. The gay male community has given me allies and helped me develop self-confidence.

9. *Teens have the right to consent.* Every individual deserves freedom from sexual abuse and coercion. If we raise our children with self-respect, encourage critical thinking, and provide accurate sex information, they'll be less vulnerable to sexual exploitation by adults or peers. Youth who are sexually empowered are better equipped to say no to nonconsensual sex.

When I was 15 I lost my virginity. I had only kissed for the first time weeks before, and I didn't want to have sex. It was in a park during the day. My boyfriend put a lot of pressure on me, and I was very naive and shy at the time. The next time we did it, I was crying and I asked him not to do it, but he just asked me if I wanted him to come or not.

Sadly, many children are sexually abused and many teens sexually assaulted despite their ability to say no. See the section on Surviving Sexual Abuse and Assault below for a discussion of steps to take toward reclaiming a healthy sexuality.

10. *Teens have the right to resources.* Even adults with the best intentions may never get the opportunity to answer teens' sex questions. After all, parents can be the last people teens want to turn to. One teen expressed this sentiment: "I wanted to hear about sex; I just couldn't figure out how to ask the questions." Make resources available to the youth in your life, whether providing them with books, bookmarking websites, or encouraging them to talk with trusted aunts, uncles, or friends.

Sometime after my "starched sheets" began to appear, I found some sex "how to" books left lying around. I thought I had found secret treasure, of course, but I came to realize they had been planted.

Books that assured me there were other lesbians on the planet literally saved my life. Some brave soul had put a copy of Lesbian Woman *in the school library. At the*

time I knew there was a word for it, but I didn't know there were books!

I read a lot of fiction as a kid, some of it quite explicit, and I found that informative too. Novels and fiction also made it quite clear that sex was meant to be fun and enjoyable. Perhaps the factor that most made "sex is fun" clear to me was the fact that I knew as a kid/teenager that my parents were still having sex.

Positive Experiences

Let's face it: First sexual experiences, like first anything, are bound to be awkward, no matter how well prepared you are. Cut yourself some slack, learn as you go, and don't judge yourself too harshly. As these survey respondents make clear, those discovery-filled, ecstatic first sexual encounters may one day come to hold a very special place in your heart.

The first time I saw a hard-on, I wanted to get down on my knees and worship! It was so powerful and beautiful. I was 16, my partner was 27. Intercourse was like coming home. It was grand!

I was 15—sex was awkward and misdirected, but totally empowering. Those experiences gave me more confidence in the power of my female body and educated me in what I want and need to feel good.

I was 20 years old when I first had a partner. Oral sex was my first experience. It wasn't scary at all but exciting. He didn't "attack me" as some young men tend to do in their enthusiasm. The first time I didn't swallow. The next time, I did. I loved it. This was in the early eighties when we were barely aware of AIDS.

I lost my virginity at 13 to another 13-year-old. It was really, really fun and felt really good. Not mind-blowing, but good.

I was 14, he was 15. We'd played around some, gone down on each other a couple of times, and were very much in love and committed to each other. We had some time alone, and decided we were pretty sure we were ready, so he pulled out his good-luck coin and we agreed that heads he got head and tails he got tail. It came up tails. We were both braced for the first penetration to be painful; I will never, ever, ever forget the look on his face or the feeling in my body when we realized simultaneously that (probably as a result of my experimenting over the last couple of years) there was nothing in the way, and it wasn't hurting at all, and it was glorious. It was exactly what a first time should feel like.

I first had sex aged 17, with my first boyfriend. We'd only been together ten days but I've always been quite uninhibited as far as my body was concerned, and my virginity had never been charged with meaning. It was a very good experience even though there was no "love" involved, I took pleasure and it didn't hurt. Even though I didn't stay with the boy long, I think it was the perfect time for me. I wish there wasn't so much meaning given to the loss of one's virginity, especially with girls, because it just encourages guilt and regrets. I'm glad I was raised in a guilt-free environment when it comes to sex because that's what made my first time so enjoyable.

I was already 19 when I started having sex. The very first time I did it was in a nightclub, in the kitchen, on the wooden cutting board. I had been with the guy for nearly six months and I ached for him from the time we met. We did it for 3 hours straight and I remember thinking that I wanted to feel that pleasure all the time from then on. I remember the feeling of his tongue gliding across my nether regions and shuddering with amazement at how great it felt. I think about it to this day, and he and I are still very good friends.

Where I grew up, early sexual experiences were common. I was 13 and it was in the wash room in the projects with a sweet girl named Ruby. The experiences were clumsy and quick and there was always the chance of discovery. There was no guilt because I guess that was the culture. I didn't really learn to make love until I was in my 40s; before that it was all about sex and myself.

I chose to give my virginity to the first man I truly loved when I was 14 (he was 21). I procured birth control pills and used them. We made love as a goodbye—he was leaving the country to avoid military service. Instead of leaving right away, though, he stayed on so we could try it a few more times and get it right.

My first time was at 16 and was a one-night-stand with a guy I met in a night club—he was very handsome and it just happened. I went back to his place and had a lot of fun. I think I learned a lot of positions in that one night! I was careful and used a condom that unfortunately split, and I had to go to the doctor for emergency contraception, but it turned out okay.

My first sexual experiences were exciting. I was daring and loved to be outdoors at night. I was 18 and still lived at home so we would go drive out in the country and find a secluded spot. There is something so liberating about being naked under the stars.

I started having sex at 14, with a 17-year-old girlfriend, and it was a wonderful experience. We were together a little over two years, and explored all sorts of things— fucking, mutual masturbation, anal sex, oral sex, bondage, pornography, and sex toys. I always keep this in mind when people get in hysterics about teenagers having sex, because I know it was a great experience for me that taught me a lot.

Coming Out

Coming out is the process of openly acknowledging aspects of our sexual natures that we'd been either unaware of or unwilling to accept before. It can be one of the most thrilling, empowering events of our sexual lives—and at the same time one of the most frightening. While the term "coming out" is commonly associated with acknowledging a specific sexual orientation, many of us go through a coming-out process simply in identifying ourselves as sexual beings with our own unique sexual desires.

I feel I've always had a strong libido, but in junior high and high school I suppressed most of my desires and curiosities because I was Mormon. As a Mormon I was taught that sex should be saved for when I'm married and even experimenting was not allowed. Once I got married at 19, I still felt fearful of sex in some ways, though my husband was very loving and patient. When I was 25 I had a close friend show some sexual interest toward me and that was the catalyst to my sexual awakening. It caused me to realize I am a sexual being who enjoys sex and it fueled my desire to discover all I could about sex.

I got on the Internet and read many books and websites and learned all I could.

For some people, coming out is a one-time experience of naming a particular sexual identity.

As I've aged, my sex drive has increased. This may be due to the fact that I didn't come out as gay until I was in my early forties. After I finally admitted to myself who and what I am, I found I could finally enjoy sex.

Others come out in a variety of ways as their sexuality evolves over time. In a culture that expects people to settle on one gender identity and one sexual identity, it takes courage to refuse categorization.

Coming out at 17 was quite painless, no big deal at all. When I met my first girlfriend it was so much better than anything I'd had before that I assumed I must be a lesbian. It was two years before I admitted to myself that I was still attracted to men. The process of realizing I was bi was very hard. My girlfriend was not happy; she felt that she couldn't be enough for me if I wanted men too, and I felt guilty for admitting that I was bi after all.

Whether you are coming out as straight, gay, lesbian, bisexual, transgendered, polyamorous, monogamous, vanilla, interested in S/M, or in any other way, we want to praise you! Coming out is a bold and liberating experience with almost unlimited potential to enhance your life. After all, when you feel ashamed or secretive about a part of yourself as deeply personal as your sexual responses and desires, it can lead to shame and self-doubt in every other part of your life. When you accept, name, and celebrate your authentic sexual self, it can have a profoundly transformative effect on your whole life.

When I started seeing women, jump back world! I got saucy, stopped apologizing for anything, thought I was the best lover in the world—spent some time as a femmy stone butch and loved making women come five, six, seven times in a row...then I grew confident enough to also surrender, to be taken, to laugh and cry. By the time I was 25 I felt pretty confident sexually, and it feels like it just keeps getting better and better.

I was very turned off and frightened by the idea when my online lover first broached the topic of S/M. Since

then, I have come to see it as a most magical way of connecting to another human being, trusting absolutely, focusing on giving and receiving in different ways from the conventional. We talk about each scene for many days afterward, exploring the feelings and insights that we got from it.

Family-Building
Sex and Conception

Whether you build a family "the old-fashioned way," or with the help of reproductive technologies, or through adoption, your sex life will be affected. Trying to create a family is a physiological and emotional process that inevitably has consequences for your sexual sense of self.

If you conceive unintentionally, you may be pleasantly surprised and filled with unexpected pride in your body, or you may feel overwhelmed and betrayed by your body. Up to 20 percent of clinically confirmed pregnancies end in miscarriage, which can result in a devastating sense of loss, guilt, or shame. You should know that sexual activity does not "cause" miscarriage, as most miscarriages occur as a result of chromosomal abnormalities in the embryo or fetus.

My lover and I had a miscarriage a few years ago. I did not know I was pregnant until we miscarried. We had been using birth control. The first time I saw him (long-distance relationship) after the miscarriage, I felt that having sex was wrong. I was utterly floored by the idea that something had lived and died inside of me in the previous six weeks. I felt that sex would be disrespectful to our lost child. My body had become (to me) something that created and killed another soul. Basically, I felt immensely guilty for having had a miscarriage and I was punishing myself for it. After lengthy discussions and crying, I was able to accept that my body was not "bad" for having lost a child, and my sex life went back to normal.

If you're in a heterosexual partnership and trying to conceive, you may struggle with the sense that timed intercourse is oppressively countererotic. If you're conceiving via reproductive technologies, you have to accept that conception involves, not sex, but a whole host of medical personnel. If you're among the estimated 10 percent of men and women in their reproductive years who are dealing with infertility, you face challenging issues of disappointment, failure, anger, guilt, blame, and sorrow that necessarily overlap into the sexual realm. And if you adopt, you have to be prepared to invite total strangers into your home to assess your fitness as a parent. While a discussion of all the ways in which family-building impacts your sexuality is beyond the scope of this book, you'll find it covered it greater depth in our book *The Mother's Guide to Sex*.

Sex and Pregnancy

Pregnancy is a time of enormous physical change and more than its fair share of discomfort. Your entire body is in a state of expansion: Your heart pumps more blood; your lungs take in more air; the ligaments in your pelvic girdle soften and stretch; your uterus increases in volume a thousand times; and your breasts swell with developing milk glands. The first trimester can be accompanied by nausea and fatigue, while subsequent months can bring leg cramps, backaches, water retention, heartburn, hemorrhoids, and more. Plenty of women find that their interest in sex nose-dives during pregnancy.

I thought both morning sickness and my low sex drive could be conquered by mind over matter. Well, guess what? You can't fool Mother Nature!

During my pregnancy, I didn't even want a man to look at me, much less touch me in any sexual way.

Others find that their sexual desire ascends to new heights. Levels of estrogen, which enhance feelings of well-being, libido, and general sensitivity, rise during pregnancy. Freedom from birth control, a greater sense of connection with a partner, and pride in your new-found body's creative potential can all be highly arousing:

My daughter changed everything for me. During my pregnancy, I was insatiable when it came to sex. Maybe it was the hormones, maybe it was the knowledge that I couldn't get "more" pregnant. Whatever caused it, my poor husband thought I was going to kill him. My skin was more sensitive, orgasm was so much easier, and so much better for me. I think another part was that I didn't have a reason to be self-conscious about

my body. The weight I gained was for our child, not because I sat around eating bonbons all day.

Being pregnant was a wonderful experience sexually for me and my husband…we really started building the trust then, I think; and I found the hormones during the middle to late months made me feel aroused quite often. My husband loved my shape, the breasts, the belly.

My breasts went from a size 36B to a 38EE. We joked about my porn-star boobs, but boy were they fun to play with. Suddenly they were everywhere—I could drag them all over my lover's body. I didn't have to bend over so far to get them in his mouth and he loved fucking them with his cock.

During both pregnancies I became very horny—I think it had a lot to do with not worrying about getting pregnant. Plus my breasts were bigger and more sexually sensitive. It didn't hurt that my partner found me irresistible and was always caressing me.

As an added bonus, the physiological and hormonal changes of pregnancy effect an erotic transformation of your genitals. By the second trimester, increased blood flow engorges the erectile tissues of your vulva, while increased levels of estrogen pump up your vaginal secretions. If you're willing to experiment with the new methods of stimulation that your temporarily "new" genitals might require, you may enjoy new realms of sexual sensation. Many pregnant women report that the increased blood flow to their genitals results in greater arousal and stronger orgasm. Others become aware for the first time of uterine contractions during orgasm—these grow stronger throughout pregnancy as your uterus grows more sensitive to oxytocin, a hormone released during orgasm, which also later initiates the contractions of labor.

When I was pregnant, I came during penetration, which was the only time that ever occurred in my life and it hasn't happened since. (That was FUN!!!) Sex was much better after I had a child, and now at 35, it's even more enjoyable even though my body is less "objectively" beautiful from pregnancy and aging.

During pregnancy, my orgasms were sublime— especially in the last two or three months. I can't describe the feeling of a pregnant orgasm. The entire uterus is involved; peaceful waves of pleasure radiate from just under the breastbone down.

Of course, pregnancy also presents challenges. Anxiety about the life changes you're facing may short-circuit desire. If you're partnered, you may face desire discrepancies. Your best bet is to cultivate compassion and to recognize that both you and your partner have the right to your individual feelings. If you can approach your different desire levels with a spirit of flexibility, you're more likely to come up with ways to get your needs met and sustain intimacy.

I turned 30 and was pregnant with my third child. After the first trimester, I couldn't think about anything but sex. Unfortunately, my partner was on a different wavelength, so I went through a lot of batteries.

One of the benefits to being pregnant was being forced to discover new ways to have sex. We tried out an inflatable pillow, which we still use, to keep pressure off my back. When I wasn't in the mood for intercourse, we'd strike provocative poses and masturbate for each other. And often just having my partner stroke my body while we kissed was a powerful form of erotic intimacy.

Keep in mind that each pregnancy will be different:

During my first pregnancy, I was so hormone driven I would wait at the front door most days to pounce on my husband. During the second one, I had no interest. I thanked him for the sperm donation and then met with him after the delivery!

Whatever your level of desire during pregnancy, you should know that sexual activity poses no threat to a normal healthy pregnancy. The fetus lies cushioned by amniotic fluid and well-protected by the uterus, and won't be harmed by penetration or orgasm. An exception would be if you're at risk for premature labor, in which case you'll be advised to avoid vaginal intercourse and orgasm during the last trimester of your pregnancy, as there's a slight chance the uterine contractions of orgasm could induce labor. Similarly, if you have a history of miscarriage or a medical condition such as placenta previa, you'll be advised to avoid both penetration and orgasm.

Sex Postpartum

Childbirth is a physically grueling process, and your body deserves time to heal. The only sex advice most parents receive after childbirth is to abstain from "sex" for six weeks. Sex in this case means vaginal penetration, and the caution refers to the fact that until your uterus has completely healed, penetration could result in infection. Obviously, there are plenty of ways of being sexual that don't involve vaginal intercourse, and we would encourage you to follow your desires wherever they lead you—surveys show that up to 60 percent of couples ignore the six-week waiting period in favor of enjoying some form of sexual intimacy.

On the other hand, it's common for new mothers to feel low sexual desire for some time after birth. You are dealing with a dramatic decline in estrogen and progesterone levels and a surge in prolactin, the hormone of milk production, which is a natural tranquilizer. Prolactin will continue to suppress your estrogen levels while you breastfeed, reducing vaginal lubrication and genital sensitivity. Many women also report that it is harder to become aroused or to reach orgasm for up to a few months following birth. If you've had a cesarean birth or complications with your vaginal delivery, you need time to recover from surgery. Nerve damage from an episiotomy or obstetric intervention could make genital stimulation painful for as long as a year. And of course, you're also dealing with the challenge of regaining ownership of your body and navigating huge changes to your lifestyle, all of which may serve to make sexual activity less than compelling.

Parenthood adds the fatigue and distraction factors into the mix. I find I still have desire at nearly, but not quite, my usual level, but sometimes have a harder time getting to orgasm. My mind skips around to parenting issues and has to be brought back to matters at hand. Also, I am breastfeeding, which I understand tends to decrease lubrication; I have noticed that to be true in my case.

Prioritize your postpartum healing by taking regular sitz baths, doing Kegels to regain strength in your pelvic muscles, enjoying whatever relaxing exercise makes your body feel good, and masturbating. Masturbation can be an ideal, low-pressure way to reacquaint yourself with your genital anatomy and sexual responses. Do not engage in partner sex until you've identified any genital trouble spots—for instance, scar tissue from a tear or an episiotomy, or bruised areas in your vagina—to ensure that you can communicate to your partner what you discover about your changed body.

When you are ready to engage in sexual activity—whether it's genital massage, oral sex, or intercourse—make sure to incorporate plenty of lubrication and relaxation into your encounters. If you want to try vaginal penetration, experiment with positions, such as side-by-side and woman-on-top, that allow you to control the depth and angle of penetration. Don't feel you have to rush back into intercourse; experiment with other ways of expressing sexual and sensual intimacy.

When my child was little, I have to say sex was not one of my favorite pastimes, because of lack of sleep, time, and privacy with spouse. Thank God children grow up. With time, my desire has come back, and I have a little more zest. I have become more selfish and interested in trying more things.

After my daughter was born, my desire went down, mostly due to exhaustion and stress. It really hasn't gone back to the way it was before she was born, even though she sleeps through the night. I am now a full-time housewife and part-time student, and sex has kind of gone to the back burner for now.

Above all, give yourselves a break; parents often find it takes as long as two years to get back to their prebaby sex lives. Respect your feelings, take your time, and do what feels best for you. You may find that the physical strength, emotional resilience, and generosity of spirit required to parent all translate into greater sexual confidence and assertiveness:

For quite a while (over a year) after I had my baby girl, I didn't want anything to do with sex. Now, however, the desire is coming back, and I'm finding that I am much more demanding in getting what I want! And much more vocal about things!

You'll probably find friends to be your best source of support and encouragement during this time. Unfortunately, doctors aren't trained to be forthcoming with information about sexual matters, and your OB/GYN is unlikely to offer much guidance about the possibilities for sexual activities or the vagaries of sexual desire. We encourage you to compare notes with other new mothers, as grassroots information-sharing will probably yield a more reassuring range of responses than checking in with your HMO.

I talk about sex with strangers for a living, but when it came time to ask questions about sex of my nurse practitioner—who had been very motherly during my prenatal visits—I procrastinated and conveniently "forgot." My partner would come along and prod me to ask the questions we both wanted answered.

I don't know where I'd be without my mothers' group. Five of us got together when we had our first kids and we're still fast friends seven years later. We share all kinds of information and can talk about things we're too embarrassed to bring up even with our partners.

Sex and Parenting

Parenthood presents numerous logistical obstacles to your sex life, as well as the emotional obstacle of reconciling your identity as a parent with your identity as a sexual adult—mothers, in particular, are hardly encouraged to identify as sexy babes. But if you're willing to summon up a little initiative and creativity, you can reinvent your sex life in richly rewarding ways. Here are some tips.

PLAN FOR SEX. You may look back fondly on the days when you could drop everything and get nasty whenever the spirit moved you, but the reality is that once you become a parent, it's unlikely you'll have sex unless you plan for it. What you lose in spontaneity, though, you can gain in erotic anticipation. Try scheduling a regular date time during the week when your baby's with a sitter or your child's at a play date. If you're partnered, use this time to relax and reconnect with each other—whether or not you engage in an erotic encounter during every weekly date, you'll be building intimacy that reaffirms your sexual connection. As always, communication is vital. Share your concerns, your desires, your needs, your preferences, and your expectations with your partner.

And be prepared to take advantage of opportune moments. If your child takes a regular nap, or watches cartoons every Saturday morning, use that time to share adult pleasures. If your baby's schedule is unpredictable, grab your partner the minute the baby falls asleep—you may rediscover some spontaneity after all.

Being a parent has made us realize that quality of love-making is very important. We sometimes only have little windows of opportunity and we need to make the most of them. It was a challenge when our kids were younger because they needed more of our attention, but now that they are older we can lock our door and they will leave us alone.

Now that we're parents, time is an issue. So we take care of business when the baby goes to sleep or when we find ourselves alone. It's usually not as romantic or long as it used to be, but it's still just as nice!

ASK FOR HELP. Call on family, friends, and neighbors to baby-sit so that you can spend time with a partner. If you feel overwhelmed by the scarcity of time, privacy, and energy, know that you're not alone. Connect with other parents to pool resources or to get advice, suggestions, and a friendly ear.

TAKE CARE OF NUMBER ONE. Your sex drive will stay on permanent hiatus if you're completely run down. Try to get plenty of sleep, eat regular meals, and remember to exercise (this doesn't have to mean a grueling aerobics regimen; try yoga or stretching, taking regular walks, or simply dancing around the house to your favorite music). The more energy you have, the more likely you are to want a good roll in the hay. And speaking of exercises, both men and women can benefit from keeping up with their Kegels; not only does a strong PC muscle improve your experience of sex, but simply doing the exercises can raise genital awareness and arousal. Masturbation is a great way to stay in touch (literally) with your sexual self.

I have two young children and don't often have the pleasure of sex with my husband, so masturbation has become nearly a daily activity. It's a chance to appreciate my hard-working body, and it gives a real lift to my day.

Find ways to relax and build a bridge between your busy day as a parent and your private time as an adult. Take a warm bath, request a massage, or have a glass of wine.

BE CREATIVE. If you're too exhausted to get hot and heavy but want to keep your sexual batteries charged, try a quickie masturbation session. If one of you is in the mood but the other is not, rent an adult video and watch it in bed together. If you're feeling short on inspiration, play an erotic board game, read erotica aloud, or experiment with sex toys.

Since becoming parents, we have had to become creative!!! We've learned how to get a quick thrill while keeping our clothes on. Sometimes we make out in the car while our son's asleep in the back seat. It has added a level of excitement and romance.

We both enjoy oral sex and touching, and often we spend our time in bed engaging in activities that don't lead to intercourse. Parenting sometimes leaves us too tired for energetic sex, but we are very affectionate and often our quiet closeness at bedtime leads to fondling and tender lovemaking.

GET AWAY. Sometimes just getting away from it all does wonders for the libido. Go to a romantic inn, take a camping trip, offer to house-sit for someone— just do something to get out of your own environment. If you can, bring a friend along as a sitter, or leave your child with relatives for a couple of days.

After becoming a dad, sex happened a lot less often and was less fun (because we were stressed and tired)— perhaps that's why we only had one child! Seriously, things did get back to normal but only because we had lots of help from our parents and from friends in looking after our baby daughter so that we could go away for weekends and longer holidays. We have managed to maintain sexual desire in a long-term relationship, which lots of people seem to find very difficult. Going away together a lot has been a major help with that, I think.

CULTIVATE PERSPECTIVE. Bear in mind that the logistical challenges of today will be gone tomorrow. Childhood passes quickly, so it's wise to cultivate the long view.

Being the mother of two teenage sons, I can say that I've had my ups and downs sexually. My teens and twenties were great, lots of sex. I was pregnant and raising children in my thirties, so there was a definite lack of libido, augmented by sheer exhaustion. My forties saw a resurgence of my desire for sex and as the boys get older, my husband and I have more free time to pursue nookie. We are just now coming into "our time!"

TEACH BY EXAMPLE. If you're worried that prioritizing your sex life is somehow selfish or inappropriate, keep in mind that your kids deserve to see you modeling the kind of pleasure-filled life you want *them* to grow up and have. While it's natural that sex may recede in importance, particularly if you have young children, don't allow societal messages about the virtues of self-sacrifice (usually directed at mothers, not fathers) to bully you into feeling you're no longer entitled to sexual pleasure. Your identity as a sexual being is nonnegotiable.

When I was 28 years old I had a baby and for four years I did not have sex. I was completely celibate because I thought of myself as "a mother" and that I had to focus on my child. I recently began experimenting with sex and have discovered a whole new side of my sexuality. I'm older now, more comfortable with my body, and willing to try new things. I really love this stage in my life. I do feel like sex is the priority in my life right now. It's seems like that is all I think about. I'm being very selfish, which is generally okay except sometimes I feel conflicted because I have a young child, but so far I have been able to balance my newfound sexuality and motherhood.

Midlife Changes

Menopause marks the end of a woman's reproductive years, and occurs on average in her early fifties (though some women reach menopause as early as age 44 and others as late as age 56). Perimenopause describes the period of several years leading up to the complete cessation of menstruation, a period marked by the symptoms we associate with menopause: mood swings, hot flashes, insomnia, headaches, and so on.

At menopause your ovaries no longer produce progesterone or estradiol (estrone, a weaker type of estrogen, continues to be produced in fatty tissue). The decline in estrogen levels results in the reduction of vaginal lubrication, genital blood flow, and elasticity of genital tissues, as well as a thinning of the vaginal walls (often given the somewhat alarmist name "vaginal atrophy"). However, menopause by no

means marks the end of a woman's sexual years. Although some postmenopausal women experience diminished desire, decreased genital sensation, or less intense orgasms, most report no loss of libido, and many enjoy sex more than ever.

Now that I am menopausal my drive has increased, and my orgasms are wonderful.

Orgasm has become far more intense and deep-seated. I used to be able to jump up and run around after sex but my orgasms are so intense now that we have had to put in double glazing to keep the noise down, and my legs don't work properly for ten minutes after.

I never experienced masturbation or orgasm until I was separated at 36. My counselor asked me about masturbation, gave me a book, I tried it and wow! My sexuality is blossoming now that I am past menopause. I want to explore my sexuality in a new, curious, open way.

If the sexual side effects of menopause are causing distress, or if symptoms such as hot flashes or insomnia are worrying you, you may consider hormone replacement therapy (HRT). It would be pointless even to try to summarize the pros and cons of HRT here, as new data on its risks and benefits are published nearly every month. You and your medical professional can make the best decision based on the specifics of your own health history. If you do opt for HRT, you needn't consider it a permanent commitment; only about 20 percent of women who start HRT stick with it for more than five years.

Perimenopause and menopause are transitional times, accompanied by numerous physiological and hormonal adjustments. Just as some women find pregnancy sexually depressing while others find it sexually inspiring, you can expect that your experience of menopause will be unique and that it won't last forever. Menopause isn't *the* capital-C Change that will shut the door on your vibrant sexy youth; rather, it's one of many changes in your life that can lead you to new discoveries about your sexual self.

I'm on the road to menopause, and for a time about two years ago I experienced the complete disappearance of libido that some women report. Oddly, I didn't experience it as loss or frustration, just as if someone had turned a switch to "off." In a sense, it reminded

*me of how I felt as a child, before I started realizing that
some pleasurable feelings carried a label reading "sexual."
During the libido-free time, I didn't even miss being
sexual, other than in an intellectual, "I wonder if it
will come back?" sort of way. I'm pleased, though,
to report that it did, in spades.*

Certainly, HRT is not the only way to address the sexual side effects of menopause. Love your vulva and it will love you back. If you keep having orgasms, you'll maintain a nourishing flow of blood to genital tissues. You can help maintain vaginal flexibility and tone with Kegel exercises, vulva massage, and masturbation with dildos. Of course, you may decide that you'd prefer to pass up vaginal penetration entirely—plenty of women of all ages have happy sex lives without it.

If vaginal dryness makes sex less fun, use water-based lubricants. Some postmenopausal women find it helpful to apply a daily lubricant (such as Replens) to nourish the vulva. Others use topical estrogen creams or rings, which are in lower dosage than estrogen patches or pills.

Testosterone levels decline at midlife for both men *and* women. In fact, a man's testosterone levels begin a gradual decrease after young adulthood, falling to about a third to a half of their original high by the time he's 80. Testosterone levels in women decline after menopause, but not significantly. If you have noticed declining libido, you may be intrigued by the notion of testosterone replacement. We would never recommend the casual use of testosterone patches, gels, or injections. Serious side effects from testosterone include increased cholesterol levels, sleep disorders, and liver damage, while less serious side effects include acne and increased facial hair. But we have heard reports from people who have benefited from supplements of testosterone and other androgens such as DHEA. Just proceed with caution and with medical supervision.

*I'm on estrogen/testosterone hormone replacement
since I hit menopause; the testosterone makes me
really, really horny!*

Although men don't reach the end of their reproductive life in middle age, they face most of the same midlife sexual changes that women undergo. With increasing age, most men find that they require direct physical stimulation to attain an erection and that mental arousal or visual stimulation will no longer suffice. Many men report that erections take longer to attain and, due to reduced elasticity of erectile tissue, are less firm. It may take longer to reach orgasm, and the refractory period between ejaculations usually lengthens. The good news is that losing the sexual response pattern typical of his teenage years can be hugely beneficial to an older man's experience of partner sex:

*The nice part about getting older is being able to last
a long time and choose when I want to climax, i.e.,
to time my orgasm to coincide with my wife's. The
downside is that my ability to perform is diminished if
I'm tired or not sufficiently aroused; if this is the case,
sometimes I cannot reach orgasm. Also, when I do
have an orgasm, I don't shoot nearly as far as I used to.*

*A few years ago I noticed that I did not get erect as easily
as before. My urologist told me that I could use that for
my good and my partner's good. Many women only see
the penis when it's erect; they tend to think it's always
that way. Now my partner has the opportunity to get
my penis erect, which can be very arousing for her.*

*I'm glad I don't suffer from premature ejaculation any-
more. And up until age 40 I used to walk around with
an erection most of the time; now that's not an issue.*

Senior Sex

*I don't hear enough about sex over 60. We still like to
do it, you know!*

Our youth-obsessed culture treats sex as the exclusive birthright of the young, beautiful, and fit. The reality is that not only do older men and women deserve to have a sex life, chances are they're having an altogether better one than they did in their well-toned youth.

Age brings the self-awareness necessary to a flourishing eroticism. Many women don't gain the sense of entitlement required to name and act on their own desires until later in life. Assertiveness can open the doors to newfound passion:

*I call myself a "sleeping beauty"; I didn't discover
what an orgasm was until I was 52. Before that, I
had sex with my inept wham-bam-thank-you-ma'am*

ex-husband for 30 years. I did what I thought I was supposed to do but always woke up very grouchy the next morning. It wasn't until I started playing around on the computer that I learned what an orgasm was. My online sexual partner was into S&M. He taught me how my nipples had a lot to do with my pleasure. So, I learned how to use a vibrator and to use rubber bands on my nipples. Wow!! A very powerful sensation occurred when I pulled a rubber band off my nipple. I never met my online partner but I give him the credit for waking me up. It took a very long time to really enjoy sex with a human being until I met my current, 62-year-old partner. Now I have the best sex I ever had. Who says old farts are dead!

Men often report that aging frees them from the tyranny of intercourse, and simultaneously allows them to explore a full-bodied, more imaginative sexuality:

As I have gotten older, I find that I do not have to get off each time in order to enjoy sex. When I was younger the physical pressure to get off was extreme but as an older person there is not the physical pressure. I'm not the "gun and run" type anymore.

One definite advantage of getting older is that it now takes me longer to come. Intercourse lasts much longer, and I can enjoy fellatio much, much longer. I have also become a more considerate lover, engaging in much more foreplay than in my younger years.

As I get older, I need more touching, more kissing, more direct affirmation that I'm wanted. Intercourse is no longer a goal in and of itself.

As you age, your repertoire of physical responses will expand. You can explore sensual massage and a range of techniques that aren't strictly goal-oriented. Masturbation provides an excellent tool to explore how your body and its responses are changing. You may switch to having sex in the morning if you're less energetic at night, or to having sex in the afternoon if your joints are stiffer in the morning. After retirement, you may delight in having your days free for long, leisurely sexual escapades, alone or with a partner. We ourselves cherish the dream of retiring from our labors and moving to a community house by the seashore, where we'll sit on the porch in our rocking chairs, surrounded by friends, with vibrators and lubricants close at hand.

When I was younger, physical conquest was the objective. Today, it is more an intellectual melding.... Today I find that "going to bed" starts much earlier in the day, involves more sweet connections beforehand, and is a warmer joining later. Although much less intense now, sex today is much more satisfying.

Disability

The sexuality of people living with disabilities is all but rendered invisible in our society, but you'd better believe that men and women with disabilities are sexually active. And they're exploring varieties of erotic response that all too many able-bodied folks miss out on.

Sexual expression among people with disabilities takes many different forms, just as physical limitations take many different forms—varying not only from one disability to another, but also from one individual to another. If you have spinal cord injury, you may or may not experience genital sensation, erection, or orgasm, but you don't lack for erotic sensation. Nipples, necks, and ears can be highly responsive erogenous zones.

Since the accident, my orgasms are different than they used to be, though it is hard to describe or qualify them to someone else. There are places on my body that are much more highly sensitized (like the inside of my thighs, my neck, my tits)—I think to compensate for where I have less feeling (like on my butt). Fortunately I can still feel my clit and pussy.

It's possible to focus so intently on touch in one part of the body that it feels exquisitely as though the entire body is being touched. Orgasm is as much an experience of the mind as the body. While the stereotype is that people living with disabilities default to oral sex (which, needless to say, can be a huge source of sexual satisfaction for those with and without disabilities alike), mobility issues don't necessarily preclude intercourse—or becoming a biological parent.

If you have a disability, spontaneity is not always an option, particularly if intercourse is involved. You and a partner may need to make preparations for a sexual encounter, whether making sure bladder and bowels are empty or ensuring that you have ample time and privacy. But the rewards are obvious. Simply navigating the logistics of daily life can be so physically stressful for people with disabilities that the chance to relax into an erotic exchange can be particularly precious.

My sexual experiences changed when I became disabled (paraplegic) at the age of 25 as the result of a spinal cord injury. I really needed to do a lot of sexual exploration after that. I have an incomplete injury and still have genital sensation. I still am easily aroused and experience desire pretty much the same, but the objects of my desire are different: I now have to feel comfortable with, not just attracted to, the one I desire.

People with physical disabilities benefit from an articulate activist movement, but those with developmental disabilities tend to lack community empowerment. Well-intentioned parents and caretakers usually deny the sexuality of individuals with developmental disabilities. At the same time, men and women with developmental disabilities are particularly vulnerable to sexual abuse, and advocates estimate that anywhere from 30 to 90 percent of those in group homes or residential facilities are sexually abused, usually by staff. People with developmental disabilities have the right to adult sexual and romantic relationships. Advocates for sexual rights have began to create training and education tools, such as classes on sexual anatomy, masturbation, communication, and abuse prevention.

For a far more comprehensive discussion of this topic, we heartily recommend *The Ultimate Guide to Sex and Disability* by Cory Silverberg and Miriam Kauffman. See our resource listings for other publications and websites related to sex and disability.

Medical Issues

Anything that affects your physical health and ability is going to affect your experience of sex, yet illness need not slam the door on your sex life; in fact, if you listen to your body, it may *open* the door to a whole new range of pleasures. If the debilitating pain of arthritis makes sex seem unappealing, take the time to warm up your joints with a warm bath, a massage, or gentle stretching, and experiment with different positions to find those that are more comfortable.

A heart condition may make you leery of sexual activity—but the good news is that if you can handle normal physical exertion, such as climbing stairs, it's perfectly safe to have sex. Studies have found that the risk of having a heart attack during sex are comparable to the risk from getting out of bed in the morning (so stay in bed and have sex!)

High blood pressure (and the accompanying medications) and adult-onset diabetes can produce erection problems—we address some recommended coping mechanisms in the Sexual Anatomy 101 chapter. Women with diabetes can experience loss of vaginal lubrication and sensation, which can be ameliorated with lubricants, vulva massage, and playing with vibrators.

If you have a chronic illness, you're familiar with the challenges presented by limited energy. Open communication with a partner becomes more crucial than ever.

I'm HIV-positive, and during a low T-cells week, I fell asleep in the middle of hot sex with my partner—ouch. Have recovered with help of medication. Now I can have sex in the evening again. For awhile had to be in the morning only. My partner was very understanding. But it's been hard to lose the "sex is always there to do" feeling and know this life won't go on forever.

I tend to go through spurts. I am a sex fiend one day, and I couldn't want sex less the next. This is due to my problems with my thyroid gland and depression. It's a horrible feeling, knowing that you don't want the person you love more than anything to touch you—wishing that you could make love to him, but your body just isn't willing. I still love sex and I love my partner, but sometimes my body chemistry gets in my way.

People who face a sudden dramatic illness, such as cancer, have to confront the sense that their bodies have betrayed them, along with an often grueling treatment regime. Obviously, pain of this variety is libido-depressing, and sex may take a back burner to getting well. Yet many people who recover from cancer develop a perspective on life's priorities that can truly enhance their sex lives.

My sexual self-esteem actually got raised by a near brush with death due to cancer. I began wondering, How long am I going to disrespect myself? Until the day I die?

Abdominal surgery, such as a hysterectomy, may affect a woman's sexual responses. Hysterectomy is the surgical removal of the uterus, and sometimes the ovaries and fallopian tubes as well. Removing the ovaries is becoming less routine, as it puts a woman into what's called "surgical menopause," which is often accompanied by worse symptoms than natural menopause.

Some women report that hysterectomy has negative effects on arousal and orgasm. After all, the uterus is intimately involved in sexual response; it produces a hormone (prostacyclin) that is believed to play a role in orgasm, it's connected to the same pelvic nerve pathway as the vagina, and it contracts rhythmically during orgasm. Removing the cervix during hysterectomy can be particularly distressing to women who enjoy penetration and pressure against the cervix.

I had a hysterectomy about five years ago, for cervical cancer. About a year and a half after that, I had intercourse for the first time since the surgery. The man penetrated me and I found I felt pretty much nothing, and my arousal plateaued and dwindled. At first I didn't know what was going on, then I made the connection with my surgery and started to cry. I freaked him out. I was terribly upset. I didn't know if I'd ever be the same. I still don't, actually, because though it seems as if overall sensation has improved, I still have yet to have an orgasm during intercourse, which I was able to do before the surgery. I lack data, though, since I haven't had much sex since then. I am certain my libido has been affected. Certainly I can still get turned on, but not as easily. I used to be able to turn myself on quite readily, whenever I wanted to. Now if there's no outside stimulation, I often find I can't turn myself on. I can go as long as a month without much sexual feeling. I am convinced it is due to the loss of my womb. I miss her.

Be proactive in discussing your current sexual response pattern with your surgeon so that you can request appropriate options, such as a supracervical hysterectomy, in which the cervix is retained. As long as your vaginal nerves and muscles are left intact, hysterectomy may even have a positive effect on your sex life. Many women who have hysterectomy due to uterine fibroids find the release from pain erotically inspiring.

I had a hysterectomy seven years ago and sex has never been better. No more pain from the fibroids, no periods to plan around, no pregnancy worries. It was completely liberating for me.

Since undergoing a full hysterectomy when I was 42, my sexual peak is at its highest. I could have sex at least three times a day, I am always way above average for wetness, and my partner said that he has never ever tasted anything so sweet as when he has oral sex with me.

Whatever medical issues you are facing, you may well discover that tapping into your erotic energy has the potential to be profoundly healing. We're not just talking about the considerable physiological benefits of sexual arousal and orgasm, which boost the immune system, release endorphins, relieve tension and stress, serve as a mild cardiovascular workout, and promote general well-being. We're talking about the emotional and psychic benefits of acknowledging yourself as a sexual being. Whether you're fantasizing about the cute U.P.S. delivery person, enjoying the sensation of sun on your skin, cupping your partner's genitals in your hands while you fall asleep, or pursuing a roof-raising orgasm, you're accessing an important source of human creativity and connection. That's some powerful medicine.

Depression

Chronic depression affects close to twenty million adults in America, while situational depression affects millions more. Depression is a disease characterized by despair, feelings of worthlessness, inability to experience pleasure, disrupted sleep and appetite, poor concentration, and more. Loss of libido frequently accompanies these symptoms, though that's not the case for everyone. Some studies show that depressed people are more likely to engage in unsafe sex. Maybe you know what it's like to seek unsafe sexual situations out of a desire to harm yourself, or a yearning to break through a cloud of despair with strong sensation, or simply because you don't care anymore. Making the effort to seek out safe and satisfying sex presumes a level of self-esteem and self-assertion that a depressed person can't necessarily muster.

Fortunately, recent years have seen enormous strides in the treatment of depression. The class of drugs known as SSRIs (selective serotonin reuptake inhibitors), which were introduced in the late eighties, has proven to be highly successfully in treating depression. Unfortunately, certain sexual side effects affect many (though not all) people who take SSRIs: Both men and women report reduced libido, genital sensation, and lubrication, along with difficulty in reaching orgasm. If orgasm is achieved, it can be muted or less intense.

When I was taking Prozac it completely killed my sex drive. I would attempt to masturbate for extended periods of time but I could never climax. It turned me into a raging psychopath. It would seem like a roller coaster ride where I was stuck at the top of the hill and couldn't come down. I wound up sobbing, and nothing I tried was very helpful.

One of the things that I've had to deal with for many years is the way that orgasm is often muted, buried, or nearly impossible on my medications. It doesn't seem to make any difference to my experiences of desire or arousal—I still have those in spades. I find that I walk around much of the time these days in a state of high arousal. It's just that getting to the point of orgasm is difficult on antidepressants, no matter what I'm doing or with whom.

Be aware that not everybody experiences these particular side effects. If you do, and your depression is situational, you may take SSRIs on a short-term basis to help you through a difficult time.

I took Paxil for ten months for a depression I suffered around the age of 32—was desperate at the time, so I suppose I'm glad it's out there— but I almost forgot about sex during that time. As a point of pride I masturbated with a vibrator to make sure I could still get off. (Sigh) Glad that's over.

When I was taking antidepressants for a year, my libido DIED. It was great to not be depressed but when my libido went away, that made me a tad depressed anyway (paradox, eh?). I eventually stopped the medication and got back to a manageable state of lethargy, but with the ability to once again achieve sexual pleasure and masturbate.

For many people living with chronic depression, going off treatment is simply not an option, and for them the benefits of taking SSRIs far outweigh the sexual side effects. And of course, the absence of depression can be libido-enhancing in and of itself.

My antidepressants lower my sexual desire a little, but I feel so much better when on them, so the effect is offset.

Furthermore, many people find that any sexual side effects abate with time as their bodies adjust to the medication.

My sexual desire decreased when I first went on Prozac, but since I've been on it for some time, I have been feeling more sexual.

If you are taking antidepressants, we encourage you to be proactive about your sexual satisfaction. Discuss with your doctor your experience of sexual desire and arousal. He or she may advise you to experiment with lowering your dosage or switching drugs. For many people, Wellbutrin, an antidepressant that's chemically unrelated to SSRIs (it's also marketed under the name Zyban as an aid in quitting smoking), not only has no negative sexual side effects but has the advantage of boosting libido. Your doctor may also recommend switching among the various SSRIs (such as Prozac, Paxil, Zoloft, Luvox, and Celexa), as your individual body chemistry will interact in different ways with different drugs.

Surviving Sexual Abuse and Assault

Estimates vary, but there's no question that a significant minority of boys, and an even higher minority of girls (anywhere from one in three to one in eight), experience child sexual abuse. And one report from the National Center for Victims of Crime estimates that one in three women will be sexually assaulted in her lifetime. Obviously, women are at particular risk for sexual abuse and assault. Ours is still not a culture in which women are allowed to walk as freely or take up as much space as men. Even those women who never experience sexual assault encounter an atmosphere of casual disrespect in public settings that can challenge their sexual self-esteem.

Exposure to the world undercut my pleasure in being a sexual person. It's not that I suffered any kind of attack or anything, but I suffered from the lack of respect for women and the attitude that "women are there for men to prey on" that seems to be prevalent on the street.

Reclaiming a healthy sex life can be a lifelong process for survivors of sexual abuse or assault. Most abused children are assaulted by adults close to them: parents, relatives, coaches, or teachers. Assault victims are often assaulted by people they know: friends or lovers. Naturally, adult survivors find it challenging to feel safe and to trust, particularly in an intimate sexual situation.

When I was 15 my boyfriend molested and tried to rape me. Before that, I had been comfortable with sexuality, but wasn't ready to be involved. Afterward I was seriously disturbed by sexual emotion being directed toward me, and didn't even let myself enjoy sex until a few years later. Now I'm having a great time with sex toys and my partner.

Survivors may compensate by always saying no to sex, by suppressing desire, or just by avoiding sexual situations. Or they may compensate by being unable to say no to sex, using sex to bolster their sense of self without making conscious choices based on consent and desire.

I was sexually abused as a child, so, though I had numerous sexual experiences as a teenager and young adult, it wasn't until my thirties, after seven years of celibacy, that I was able to adequately explore my own sexual desires and learn what I need to become truly aroused and experience orgasm. I also found a partner with whom I felt safe enough to experiment and learn new things.

If you're a survivor, you've probably experienced "dissociation," or checking out during sex: One minute you're feeling your partner's hands on your skin, the next you're feeling detached from your body or making a mental shopping list—anything to avoid being present in the moment. To heal, you'll need to learn what Staci Haines, author of *The Survivor's Guide to Sex*, refers to as "embodiment," the ability to get back into your own body and experience a range of emotions and sensations, including sexual pleasure.

Like anyone who has suffered trauma, you can be "triggered," flooded with emotions, sensations, or images related to your abuse that make it difficult to stay in the moment. Certain sexual situations may be particularly strong triggers, catapulting you into the past, as perhaps when a partner strokes the inside of your thigh a certain way, or wakes you in the middle of the night. Sexual healing involves learning to identify and work through your triggers so that they no longer have the power to hijack your sexual encounters.

I was molested as a child and had never been able to discuss it. When I began to work on the many problems and issues that I had as a result of the abuse, I met my current girlfriend. It turned out that she had also been sexually abused. She had been working on her issues for years. She was very open and shared with me. I was able to also open up to her. We are able to share our triggers, needs, desires, and fantasies. My sexual self-image has become positive. It is no longer uncomfortable or scary to have sex. I relish the joy of giving and receiving physical pleasure with her.

For practical help with sexual healing, we recommend *The Survivor's Guide to Sex*, the first book ever written on cultivating an empowered sex life after child sexual abuse. This thoughtful, compassionate guide offers women invaluable advice on cultivating an embodied sexuality by learning how to develop boundaries, navigate triggers, embrace their own desires, and communicate with a partner.

I was very sexually active from my teens into my thirties, but as a survivor of early sexual trauma, I found that I was either an untouchable, or when touched was not really present with what was going on with my body. I find that by getting more in touch with my own body and being more comfortable with who I am, I enjoy sex in my fifties with much more personal awareness than I did as a promiscuous young woman. I still have issues that come up for me, but I can deal with them knowing what it is I am dealing with and get on to the enjoyment part again.

Maturity Has Its Rewards

Are you getting the sense that we delegated the writing of this chapter to our survey respondents? The truth is, we only wish we had room for more quotes!

We were bowled over by the passionate outpouring that resulted when we asked our respondents to describe how their experience of sexual desire had changed throughout their lives. We'll close by letting these articulate women and men explain some of the many advantages to sexual maturity.

You understand the mind–body connection

I've met some great women who have been able to help me fulfill my deepest and darkest fantasies. By doing this, I've found there is really no end to my sexual desire, and I've started to realize just how much of sex is really in the mind. I've also been exposed to Tantra and find my views toward sex and intimacy have changed because of it. I'm much more into establishing a good "connection" instead of trying to be some porn star stud all the time.

I guess that since I first became active I have always enjoyed sex physically. The difference has been in maturing to enjoy the mind-fuck aspects of sex…of getting off in the head as well as the body—that I find makes orgasms and sex better and more completely fulfilling.

When I was younger I used to get wet by just the mere sight of certain lovers. As I've gotten older I notice that I want more mental stimulation from my partner. I want to wine and dine them or have them wine and dine me.

You value intimacy

I see sex as so much more complicated and complex than I used to. It's so much less about hormones and bars and craziness. I used to cavort around, flirting and drawing people into bed with me. It was fun and short-lived. Now, I see myself as a partner in a quest. I really understood this when I was with a man who had problems with premature ejaculation. We worked together fixing the problem. In the end, I felt like I understood sex, his body and my body, so much more. I'm looking for sexual experiences that are less superficial and based more on trust.

This might seem corny but being involved in a long-term relationship with the same woman (twenty-two

years) has made sex even more incredible. We know what turns each other on, we experiment with various sexual toys and products, and things keep getting better and better. I can't imagine how having random sex with someone else could be nearly as good. This other person would have to be an incredible communicator to leave both people satisfied. I think with one-night-stands one person probably gets off more than the other. So getting older and monogamy seem pretty damn good.

You accept yourself and your desires

I think that women finally learn, somewhere in their late thirties or forties, that they can enjoy sex, too, and let go of their girlish fears and inhibitions to enjoy what's between their legs. All in all, my sex life has never been better. It's amazing and gets better all the time because we're constantly expanding our horizons, trying new things.

After our second child, my ex-husband complained often that I was no longer "tight enough" for him, and began to pursue anal sex almost exclusively. He seemed unable to come without it. He also began to lose interest in me altogether (although this may have been a gradual drifting apart that sometimes happens in marriage) and I lost all sense of myself as a sexual being. Now, in my new marriage, my husband is very loving and passionate, very attracted to me, and our sexual relationship is amazing (to me, after having lived for so long without one).

I was a late bloomer in terms of acknowledging and enjoying my sexual feelings. I grew up with a feminist consciousness, and I had (and sometimes still have) a hard time sorting out strong sexual attraction to girls and women from sexist objectification. The result was a lot of shame around my use of pornography for self-arousal. As I grew older and became more self-confident, I realized that I could respect and love a woman and want to have sex with her, without necessarily objectifying her. From that realization (which came through a dream) I was able to develop, ever slowly, into integrating my sexual and emotional feelings about women.

You know how to assert yourself

As I get older, sex is much more enjoyable. It seems to me that experience is everything! I'm not nearly as shy about things as I was in my twenties, and I'm not afraid to take control or tell my partner exactly what I want and like! Sex in my forties is so much better for me that I hope it just keeps getting better.

As I've gotten older, I experience orgasm more often. I think a big part of it is because I'm not as nervous or overwhelmed by sex as I was when I was first learning. I'm more relaxed, and just let it happen. And sex is a great stress-reliever, if I can look past the initial "I'm too busy" to get there.

CHAPTER 5

Communication

The key to any successful sexual relationship is communication. We know you've heard it before, but if some of the activities described in this book tempt you to expand your sexual repertoire, we hope you'll take the time to make sure your communication skills are in good shape. After all, you can acquire all the toys, lotions, and manuals in the world, but they're useless in a relationship unless you can talk about what you want to do with them. You can study your anatomy, learn 101 different positions, and read about new techniques, but if you're unable to describe where it feels good and why, you're headed for disappointment and frustration.

And since communication is a two-way street, your years of sexual experience or open-mindedness won't do you any good if you aren't attuned to your partner's needs. Discovering her or his needs, anxieties, and desires, as well as learning to share your own, will open doors to greater understanding, experimentation, and healing, ultimately leading to overall greater sexual intimacy.

Unfortunately, there are a million and one things that get in the way of effective communication. In this chapter we'll examine some of these barriers and suggest ways to move beyond them.

Common Challenges

Our primary goal as sex-toy saleswomen is to get people to articulate their sexual needs. Without this information, we are unable to help a customer find something that will satisfy her or his particular need. However, this crucial first step is also the most difficult one, simply because so many of us are too embarrassed to talk about sex, with either lovers or total strangers.

Our discomfort with sex is ironic. Although we live in a society where we are bombarded daily by sexual images and references to sex, speaking intimately with someone about our own sexuality is extremely challenging. At Good Vibrations, we routinely discuss strangers' sexual needs with them without ever raising an eyebrow, yet when it came to interviewing our friends about their sex lives for this book, we balked and procrastinated, imagining our mutual embarrassment.

We are all motivated by an intense curiosity about sex, but thwarted by our inability to discuss it. We seek information, elucidation, titillation—note the commercial success of the daily talk shows, sex manuals, advice columns, and the *Sports Illustrated* swimsuit edition—but our curiosity is far more restrained when it comes to discovering a partner's needs or sharing our own.

You don't have to look very hard to uncover reasons for this behavior. From the attitudes and morals instilled in us at a young age to the conflicting messages about sex that society imposes on us as adults, it's no wonder we're a tad repressed. Here are just a few examples of communication inhibitors:

Social Conditioning

Think about your intimate relationships. Is it true that one of you usually wants to talk about sex and "the relationship" more than the other? There's an automatic imbalance when you begin a relationship, simply because you've each developed your own approach to communication. Many things influence individual communication patterns: gender differences, family dynamics, traumatic experiences—and figuring out which ones are relevant to you can be a starting point if you want to change something.

Inadequate Sex Education

No one teaches us about sex when we're kids because we're not supposed to have it, yet when we reach adulthood (at some arbitrary age), we're expected to magically know how to expertly please ourselves and our partners. After a certain age, our curiosity and inquisitiveness become a liability—a sure sign that we're inexperienced, poor lovers, or virgins (take your pick)—so we quit asking and start faking.

What we *do* learn about sex as kids comes sporadically from parents, school, friends, and the media. Depending on the accuracy or depth of the information, we may end up more confused, misinformed, or intimidated by our discoveries. Formal sex education in school usually deals with prevention of disease and pregnancy—downbeat lectures emphasizing danger and disaster. How do we learn sexual self-esteem and respect, let alone how to talk about sex, when we're taught to fear the consequences of our own libidos?

Beliefs, Attitudes, Stereotypes

Each one of us was raised with a unique set of moral beliefs about sex, usually informed by myriad cultural stereotypes or religious doctrines, or both. How we incorporate these into our adult sex lives is directly related to how, what, and even whether we communicate. Guided by whatever we have come to view individually as "acceptable sexual behavior," we're bound to run into a few problems exploring or experimenting with someone who holds even slightly different views. Consider these few examples:

- Perhaps you don't want to tell your partner you masturbate because you think it's wrong and you're trying to quit—remember when the priest told you masturbation would lead to blindness?
- Maybe you're really intrigued by anal sex, but you've always heard that anal sex is a gay practice and you don't want anyone, including yourself, to think you might be homosexual, so you never explore this activity.
- You might be a gay man who feels that your erotic dreams about women are inconsistent with your practices, so you keep them a secret from your lover.

We deny ourselves and our lovers access to different facets of our sexual personalities when we practice this kind of self-censorship. Getting at the root of some of these attitudes can help you overcome the inhibiting ones or clarify those that are very important to you.

Fear

Fear of rejection or of the embarrassment that comes from revealing our ignorance or beliefs is an enormous deterrent to communication. Our fragile egos often prevent us from making a simple inquiry or confession, one that might lead to greater sexual self-awareness.

It's not uncommon at Good Vibrations for a clerk to approach every individual in the store and offer to answer questions, yet be turned down by each one. But should she start explaining the differences in vibrators or dildos to just one customer in the store, those very same people will gather around to eavesdrop on the rest of the instruction. Remember your schoolteachers telling you that "there's no such thing as a dumb question"? You still didn't ask because you thought everyone else probably already knew, and you weren't about to make a fool of yourself. The fear seems even greater when it comes to questions about sex.

Many customers confide in us because they're afraid to tell their partners what they want, certain they'll sound kinky or stupid or demanding. We act as a sounding board, reassuring them that their curiosity is natural and encouraging them to talk to their partners.

People also worry about deflating their partners' egos by suggesting a change. Perfectly harmless suggestions can be misinterpreted as dissatisfaction with previous performance:

When I was married, my husband hated it when I masturbated—he couldn't understand why I needed to do that when he was around.

This woman probably deprived herself (or masturbated on the sly) instead of attempting to disabuse her husband of the notion that her solitary enjoyment reflected poorly on their sex life. She could have explained why she enjoyed it, perhaps even suggesting they try it together.

Goal-Oriented Sex

Many of us have specific requirements for a satisfying sexual encounter. For some it might be a minimum of two orgasms each, for others it might be hour-long foreplay or a new position. How rigidly we adhere to these requirements can increase our own and our partner's performance anxiety.

The more proscriptive and goal-oriented we make our sexual activity, the more we set ourselves up for anxiety and frustration. Talking with a partner about our expectations can help relieve the pressure, while allowing us to push back the boundaries we've set up around our sex lives:

I like to negotiate beforehand, clearly stating each person's limits. My husband and I talk about what we feel we want to do on any given night. It doesn't deter spontaneity, just keeps us in synch.

Language Considerations

The differences in our relative comfort or discomfort around sexual terminology can affect the way we communicate. While one person might say, "I'm dying for you to plunge two wet fingers in my juicy cunt and pump," another might say, "Please put two fingers in my vagina" and hope for the best, while yet another

may hate having to spell out what she wants, perhaps spreading her legs and raising her hips to encourage the activity. Finding a common, comfortable vocabulary to share, including clear nonverbal signals, can minimize this confusion and add an erotic edge to your sex play.

If you need a little assistance developing a sexual vocabulary, you have several options. Make a list of words you like or find particularly hot (flip through a sexual slang dictionary if you need help with terms). While you're alone, practice saying them aloud and using them in sentences—after a while they won't sound so foreign coming out of your mouth and you can start reciting them more dramatically. When you masturbate, try imagining the words you'd like to say to heighten arousal. You and your partner can create separate lists of preferred words or phrases and then compare them to see what turn-of-phrase works for each of you. You can also build a shared language by reading a variety of erotic stories out loud and discussing which turn you on most—some folks favor Victorian euphemisms, others prefer urban slang, while some employ flowery prose. Similarly, watching X-rated or educational sex videos can show you how others use sexual vocabulary. For more on talking dirty, refer to the Fantasies chapter or pick up a copy of *Talk Sexy to the One You Love* or *Exhibitionism for the Shy*.

Prerequisites to Good Communication
Know What You Like

Something often overlooked in discussions of sexual communication is the importance of articulating our needs to ourselves. While this may sound a little obvious, it's actually a crucial first step in the communication process. We don't expect people to go supermarket shopping without first having some idea of what they want—and if they can't find something, they must be able to describe it to someone who can assist them.

The same goes for our sexual needs. It's going to be pretty hard to tell a partner what we want if we aren't sure ourselves.

It has been difficult for me to let him know what I like. Sometimes I don't even know, myself.

Ask yourself a few questions about what you want to change: Is your partner touching you in a way that is unpleasant? Is it the motion or the spot? Would you prefer being touched somewhere else or in a different way? If you aren't sure, you could do a little homework—are you confused about anatomy, sexual response, certain fantasies? Try reading, chatting with a friend, calling a sex-information line, talking to a therapist, or visiting a sex toy store.

The very best way to pinpoint what you like is to concentrate while masturbating. Pay attention to what does or does not feel good so that you can show your partner.

Know What You Need

Your commitment to pursuing what you like in a sexual relationship is just as important. We all have specific sexual needs, so it does no one any good to assume that there is a standard way to have sex. The chance that your lover will know instinctively what you like is slim, so expect that you're going to have to get vocal at some point. You might want to practice alone first, saying out loud, with specifics, what you want. Imagine different scenarios and practice how you would introduce your concerns. If you've got highly specific physical or emotional needs that your partner may not be aware of, don't assume that he or she will figure them out—be up front and honest, and you'll both be more comfortable negotiating sex.

> When I was pregnant for the first time, my sexual desire dropped off drastically, but my need to be held, caressed, and spoken to lovingly increased dramatically. My partner was incredibly understanding—I got to dictate the terms of our sex life and there was never, ever any pressure from him. In the end, we discovered a new way of being sexual.

This self-assertion is especially vital when orchestrating new sexual relationships, particularly when it comes to issues like safer sex and contraception:

> I'll admit that when I have a new partner I have to negotiate safer sex because most of the women I've slept with aren't used to latex.

If you have familiarized yourself with safer sex practices and have decided ahead of time what activities will or will not be included in your sexual encounters, you are much more likely to get what you want.

Improving Communication

You know what you want—and now you know how to initiate a discussion about sex—but how to tell your partners? It sounds so much easier than it is. There's always some reason, in the heat of passion, that you decide to keep it to yourself: You don't want to hurt your partners' feelings; you don't want to seem greedy; you're afraid your partners won't want to do what you want; you don't want to shock someone you just met; you don't want to shock someone you've been lovers with for fifteen years. The excuses are endless! But the alternatives to being honest are grim—frustration, boredom, resentment, irritation, and so on.

Some people find it easier to communicate their sexual desires to strangers because their desires aren't enmeshed with the emotional intimacy experienced with a long-term partner. Others may not feel comfortable sharing the same information until they've known someone for a while. Whatever your experience, we hope you'll benefit from the following suggestions.

In the Bedroom

If you're fond of the relatively direct, but often misunderstood, nonverbal method, make sure your partner understands what you're trying to convey. Your lover is rubbing your clit and you moan. Is it a moan of pleasure or irritation? Your lover continues, and you moan louder. Are you signaling encouragement or annoyance? Obviously, moans are not universally understood. Lend a hand to this confusing situation—literally. If your lover is not pleasing you the right way, take your hand and guide your lover's. If this still doesn't do the trick, show your lover just how you like it by masturbating while she or he watches, and then have her or him try it again.

> During sex I often masturbate and let my partner "help." This works well and is very satisfying and intimate without the performance anxiety I get when trying to come for somebody else.

Remember that communication also means letting your partner know when the stimulation is oh-so-perfect. Try cheerleading—a simple, one-word exclamation goes a long way. Use your body to convey appreciation in a clear way—arching your back, breathing hard, grabbing hair!

The alternative verbal route is more direct, though often more difficult for people. We're afraid to add to our lover's already intense performance anxiety or to appear too demanding. But remember, your partner wants to please you, so your suggestions will most likely be met with enthusiasm. And expressing your needs doesn't have to be done in a critical way. Compliment your lover on her or his performance of the activity you like, and then ask for more. "Your mouth on my penis feels great, and I'd really love it if you sucked on it a little harder." If it's an activity that just doesn't feel good at all, gently guide your lover's hand or head somewhere else and say what does feel nice:

I hate to say anything that could sound critical or unappreciative to a woman who is trying so hard to give me pleasure, but it is important to just say "softer," "slower," "harder," or "let's do something else for a while." I've learned that simple words like these are real easy and effective ways of communicating; they can be used either as a request or as a question. I learned this from a woman who liked to know she was doing it right.

If your partner is not very responsive to your ministrations, ask for feedback or signs of encouragement. Give your lover options, moving from one body part to another, varying pressure or movement, asking what feels good, great, or bad.

It is hard to communicate exactly what I want sometimes, because when I'm aroused, I usually don't want to talk. And it's hard to constantly say, "harder, softer, left, no, right, up, down a little." It's just hard to be specific enough. I am very sensitive, so there is a fine line between something feeling wonderful and it feeling painful. I have many, many times wished there could be a machine hooked up to me, and it would register whether my pleasure level was up or down, so, without talking, my lover could see what was working or what wasn't!

Aural Inhibitions

I would like to use my voice more—to allow moans, sighs, and cries to come out naturally rather than suppress them because I'm embarrassed.

You may share this person's concern. Are you afraid your roommates or neighbors might hear you? Just turn up the volume on your sound system. Are you afraid your partner will think you're odd if you make noise? If your lover emits pleasurable sounds, chances are he or she will be turned on by yours. To practice, try giving free reign to your vocal chords while masturbating. Have your partner watch, if you like, and then describe to you afterward how it felt to watch you. Or during your next lovemaking session, follow up your partner's moans with your own sighs of passion. This can be good practice for you, and the "duet" effect can increase excitement for both of you. If your partner is also the silent type, you may discover you're both suppressing sound for fear of what the other will think—try addressing the subject in a nonsexual setting. You can both engage in the exercises just described. You might also watch a porn video (or a sexy mainstream movie) together. Watch the love scenes with the sound on and then hit the mute button—once you discover how much those sighs of pleasure enhance your viewing, you may be inspired to incorporate them into your personal X-rated moments!

Outside the Bedroom

Of course, there's far more to sexual communication than just lying in bed and moaning loudly when something feels good or flinching when something annoys you.

Discussing change and introducing new sexual activity can be difficult for couples, yet the rewards are obvious: variety, experimentation, growth, self-discovery—all of which can contribute to a more satisfying relationship. This book is all about exploring new kinds of sexual activity, but it is essential for you to think carefully about the hows and whys behind your desire to change. Here are a few things to consider:

MOTIVATION: Why are you contemplating a change in your sexual repertoire? Are you dissatisfied with something? Why do you feel the need to upset your routine? Are you trying to save your relationship? Does your lover feel the same way? Are you trying to change something about your partner? How will your partner react to this suggestion? Are you hot for this activity because everyone else on the block is doing it?

It's very important to consider the effect your suggestion might have on your partner's sexual self-image or how you might be adding to his or her performance anxiety. Are you buying your girlfriend a G-spot vibrator because you want her to learn how to have orgasms during intercourse? How does she feel about this? Does it diminish the value or importance of the clitoral orgasms she has? Encourage her to tell you what she thinks about the activity. What do each of you expect to get out of it? Clarifying what you're really after, and why, should help you figure out the best way to approach your partner.

I tried using a vibrator with a longtime girlfriend. However, she was very shy about it and couldn't really get into it. It was very awkward introducing it. I think it began by us talking about masturbating and I asked her if she ever used a vibrator. She said no, so I brought one out. We fooled around with it for a while, but it didn't seem natural.

It sounds like these two were off to a good start, but their embarrassment got the better of them. Perhaps they could have acknowledged their mutual discomfort and talked about what was causing them to feel shy. Perhaps the girlfriend felt intimidated or pressured by the focus on her arousal. It also sounds like the vibrator was a surprise, which might have taken her aback. If they'd been able to clarify their expectations with regard to the vibrator, they might not have approached the experiment so halfheartedly.

INTRODUCING THE SUBJECT: Unless you're absolutely certain that your lover adores the element of surprise, it's best to bring the subject up when you're not in a sexual setting. Just because you think something sounds fun doesn't necessarily mean your partner will.

Take the example of a woman buying a dildo to use on her girlfriend. She's been penetrating her lover for years with her fingers, and she figures her girlfriend will love the feeling of a dildo. Plus, she thinks, if she buys a dildo harness to go with it, her fingers will be freed up to explore other areas of her girlfriend's body. However, when she dons her new garb that special night, her girlfriend recoils in horror, saying she doesn't want to be fucked by a man.

Had they talked about it first, our intrepid shopper might have explained to her lover that it didn't even occur to her to impersonate a man; she just wanted to free up her hands, and at the same time please her lover the way she likes. They could have discussed the dildo/penis association and what to do about it, possibly avoiding the whole misunderstanding and ending up with a great new sex toy.

When you *do* bring up your ideas in conversation, try not to be confrontational or demanding. You might introduce the subject by making an observation: "I noticed that you really like having me hold your wrists down during sex. Do you think you might want to be tied up?" Or take the playful approach: "I had this terrific fantasy about the outdoors, some trees, some rope, you…me." If you're trying to change a pattern, you might just inquire how it got to be a pattern: "I dreamed about doing it in the stairway, which made me wonder why we always have sex in the same place." Listen carefully to your partner's reactions; try to get to the bottom of any reservations or feelings your suggestion may have elicited.

Of course there are times when surprising your partner can pave the way for an explosive sexual encounter. If you've discussed the desired activity before and ascertained that it's something your partner is interested in, by all means take the initiative and plan the event. Just make sure that your partner likes surprises and that you're planning something he or she might actually enjoy experiencing, not something that's best kept a fantasy.

You don't always have the opportunity or the desire to discuss your sex concerns with a partner. If you only recently met someone and aren't planning on seeing her or him again after an afternoon or evening of sex, you obviously won't know that much about the person. While it's still in your best interests to be as direct and specific about your desires as possible, you obviously can't follow our advice to find out how your partner feels about sex toys before whipping one out from under your bed. There's certainly nothing to stop you from suggesting the toy or technique to your partner, but obviously if he or she is not receptive, you're more likely to enjoy the encounter if you're willing to compromise. You could ask what the reservation is, which might be something you could alleviate quickly with a thorough explanation or reassurance. For example, someone's eyes might bulge when he or she sees the Magic Wand vibrator, but assurance that it's not meant for penetration might elicit a sigh of relief.

BE SPECIFIC: It can never hurt, and it's usually infinitely more helpful, to be specific about what you want from your partner. Avoid saying, "I want you to pay more attention to me," if what you really want is for your partner's lips to linger lovingly on your breasts.

She has a hard time describing exactly how she needs something to be done to her to reach orgasm. I keep telling her that I flunked ESP 101 in school and that if she doesn't help me, then she isn't going to get the most out of the situation. Communication: It works!

If you find yourself dissatisfied with a routine— perhaps you would like your partner to initiate sex more—offer some suggestions. "I'd devour you on the spot if you ever propositioned me in a public place." Or create a nonverbal vocabulary that you can both use— a signal or a modification in your dress, for example.

FOLLOW UP: If you try something new, by all means talk about your experience afterward. If you both had a great time, tell your partner in detail what you found so exhilarating. It may have been more fun for one of you, and this will give you an opportunity to acknowledge that and fine-tune your sex play so that one of you doesn't feel left out or shortchanged. This couple could have benefited from such a discussion:

When I first got the Wahl two-speed, I got the guy I was dating to consent to include it in our lovemaking once. It was, for me, EXCELLENT: I mounted him from the top and used the vibe on my clit, and it was one of the most pleasurable experiences I remember. He, however, never wanted to use it again—threatened? I don't know.

Tips from the Trenches

Our readers were just as forthcoming with positive suggestions for initiating conversations about sex with partners. We're sure you'll find that many of these tips will help you get the dialogue flowing in your own beds.

FIND THE RIGHT TIME AND PLACE: *We're usually in the living room after our daughter is in bed asleep, and sometimes a show on TV will bring up the subject or one of us will just start in. It's important that neither person judge another's fantasy or idea, and not being in the bedroom is an excellent idea.*

TEST THE WATERS: *I start out talking about the movies or a TV show I'm interested in (like Queer as Folk) and see what kind of response I get. I shy away from judgmental people and this is a safe way to weed them out before it's too late.*

REALLY LISTEN: *I find that letting the person I am talking to "off the hook" is most successful. What I mean is, sometimes we get too caught up in words and spend less time on meaning. Political Correctness is our generation's greatest sin. I have had people call me "crip" or "gimp" and I know that it wasn't an insult, while other have said to me "I admire you so much" and I could feel the dig of their prejudice. Sexual discussion for me is the same way. Just spit it out (don't swallow) and we'll sort out the meaning together as we go along. If people aren't afraid of saying the wrong thing, or being insulting, crude, or perverted, it is easier to communicate.*

LOOSEN UP, RELAX: *I like to talk about sex when my husband is massaging my feet when things have quieted down for the evening. Do not try to talk about issues during, right before, or right after sex.*

BE CONSTRUCTIVE: *A question I always ask is, "Anything you want me to do more of or different in the encore?" This focuses on the positive and not the negative. This way a person tells me what they want me to do rather than what they did not enjoy.*

KEEP IT FUN: *In the "question game" we take turns asking each other questions. The rules are—don't ask anything you don't want an honest answer to, don't lie, you get three "passes" where you don't have to answer, and it doesn't count as a question if you ask the same one you just answered.*

AVOID ABSOLUTES: *Don't use the words "You Never" and "You Always"!*

TAKE BABY STEPS: *I started emailing him some erotic stories that weren't too intense, but had some of my fantasy elements, and then increased the erotic nature of them and approached trying it out with him, if he was comfortable. He was very comfortable...just never wanted to make me uncomfortable!*

COMPROMISE: *For so long, "compromise" has meant giving up my own thoughts and desires to avoid conflict. When I would raise an issue, I would have to ignore my desires, try to justify the fact that I had desires at all, or simply give up on trying to talk about them in the name of peace in my home. Now I have more autonomy and self-esteem and stand up for myself in the bargaining process.*

WRITE IT DOWN: *Once we wrote down a list of all the somewhat outré things we wanted to try and then traded lists, so we wouldn't have to deal with the embarrassment of saying them aloud. Imagine our joy when we discovered some of the same things on both lists!*

NEGOTIATE: *When my current partner and I discuss sex, we usually do it in a your turn/my turn kind of way. Whenever I ask for something different or say I want to quit doing a particular act, I always make sure I phrase it in a way that encourages him to propose something new he wants to do or decline something he doesn't want to do anymore.*

PROBLEM SOLVE (AND REAP THE REWARDS): *When we talked about sex during her period we determined she can have her oral sex (clitoral) while wearing a tampon, and after she finishes her climax, she does not mind pulling it out and letting me finish mine. Had we not discussed this, we would have just stayed away during those 5–7 days…and to tell you the truth sex during periods has become very satisfying for us both.*

TAKE A DEEP BREATH…AND JUST SAY IT: *Just coming out and saying it is the best way. The more I try to be tactful and considerate, the longer it takes to get to the subject, and the more nervous the other person gets. Never say, "Honey, we have to talk," and then pause. That sends people's blood pressure through the roof, regardless of what follows. Better to just say, "You know, I'm feeling rather insistent that you don't sleep with the football team without using condoms," or "I'm concerned about the fact that we haven't had good sex in two months." Bluntness works. And if I scare off a partner that way, better that they leave me after I've been honest with them than stick around so we can mislead each other.*

SHOW AND TELL: *I usually start small by discussing what he likes, where he's sensitive. I ask him to stroke himself so I can see what he likes. If he's comfortable with this, he'll open up about what he likes.*

MAKE IT ABOUT DISCOVERY: *We learned a great deal about one another's sexual past and preferences before we even touched each other. It made it much more easy and fun once we started kissing. I told him I knew he wasn't a mind reader, I let him know that my vibrator was a tool and not a replacement for a real person, and I was just honest about my feelings.*

TAKE ACTION STEPS: *We have to make a plan to actually start trying the things we do talk about. Sometimes it seems that waiting for the perfect moment means it never happens. And waiting for it to just "happen naturally" can mean it doesn't, either!*

SEE THE BIG PICTURE: *Putting the emphasis on more physical intimacy without sex in our relationship has made us both feel safer to discuss things we haven't been able to discuss before.*

Common Concerns

We asked our survey respondents what subjects they found the most difficult to discuss with partners. Their answers ran the gamut—from insecurities about physical characteristics, to contraception, to exploring fetishes. Many of the responses fell into some general categories, which we've listed below. Perhaps recognizing that many people struggle with similar issues will give you more confidence broaching these subjects in your own life.

STDs and Safer Sex

With one out of five people diagnosed with a sexually transmitted disease, it's not surprising that many people mentioned this as a troublesome issue. Not only can STDs impact one's self-esteem, but they also put the burden of education on the person with the disease. They are so commonplace that it's in everyone's best interest to be more aware, which ideally would make us all more sensitive to a partner's disclosure. Some excellent websites and resources on STDs offer various scenarios for discussing the subject (see our resource listings). You might also refer to our Safer Sex chapter.

It's tough to talk about my genital herpes—difficult with my current partner, but I brought it up very early in the relationship to get it out of the way.

A partner unknowingly gave me an STD, and I unknowingly gave it to another partner. The series of conversations that I had with the two of them were more unpleasant than root canal surgery. Compared to that, the inevitable "Just because I can't be monogamous doesn't mean I don't love you" conversation was EASY!

Speaking of Sex

Many communication barriers would cease to exist if we were more comfortable talking about sex. One way to increase our comfort level is to practice discussing sex with a partner when we're in a nonsexual setting. This removes sex from the impassioned, volatile setting of the bedroom.

Imagine sitting for an hour each day with your partner and just talking about sex—sharing your thoughts, feelings, what pleases you, what scares you, with no judgments, no defensiveness, no ulterior motives. Gradually you'd be able to understand one another's desires and demands. Eventually sex wouldn't be nearly so mystifying.

Most of us, however, are unable to discuss sex so routinely and good-naturedly. Most likely, sex doesn't come up spontaneously in your everyday conversations, so you may need to practice just getting the subject on the table. Here are a few ways you could introduce the topic:

FANTASY AND IMAGINATION: "I had the most incredible erotic dream about you, me, and some aliens." Your dreams can spark discussions of fantasies, taboo behaviors, or secret desires. You might discover that your penchant for pornographic science fiction is shared by your partner.

FACT FINDING: Conduct sexual histories of your partners. Pretend you're from the Kinsey Institute, and you want to know what your respondents think about masturbation: When did they start? How did they feel? Were they ever discovered? How often do they masturbate? Don't judge, just listen. Make up your own questions, or use Kinsey's.

NEWS COMMENTARY: "I read the most interesting editorial today about condom distribution in public schools." A news item can lead into discussions of safer sex, sex education, your sex history, etc. Or, "Today on *Oprah*, she interviewed female pornographers." A TV talk show might create an opportunity to exchange views on women's sexuality, erotica, and porn.

READ A SEX BOOK: You could agree to read a self-help book or visit an informational website together and discuss the issues this raises. Or try some erotic fiction, sharing your reactions to the passages. This will expose you to the language of sex and help you find a comfortable sexual vocabulary.

CORRESPONDENCE: Several of our customers cited letter writing and email as an informative and erotic way for partners to share their thoughts with each other:

I am always eager to talk to my partner about sex. I like writing him suggestive letters and enjoy letters he gives me.

Leaving judgment and dogma behind will make it both easier and safer for you and your partner to talk honestly about sex. Once you find yourself tossing around sex terms, expressing yourself and your needs may come more naturally. And in addition to being good practice, the background information you gather will be helpful when you or your partner wants to try something different.

Considering I'm back in the arena of looking for a partner/sexual partner, I realize there are many subjects I'm not so comfortable bringing up. I think diseases and condoms and number of previous partners isn't that easy for me to discuss, but it's a necessity.

Trying a New Sexual Activity

How boring life would be if we didn't try new things! The same holds true for sex, yet we find it incredibly difficult to chart this territory with lovers. We're afraid of being considered kinky or perverted, we're afraid of hurting a partner's feelings, or we're simply so embarrassed by our own desires that we never initiate the conversation. But how will we know if we never try?

I would like to try some things to pleasure him (like anal penetration on him with a dildo), but I know that he has a "mental block" toward anal sex. I really fear that even bringing it up (only to find that the idea is revolting to him) will damage our sexual relationship.

I still struggle with asking a partner if I can be on the receiving end of oral sex. It's been browbeaten into me that men don't like doing it, even though my husband does.

I'm still terrified of coming out as kinky. I got into BDSM and kink in my last relationship and now I have absolutely no idea how to bring it up with new crushes or potential dates.

So many men find anal stimulation difficult to discuss. They think it's only for gay men, which is silly. Every man has the same nerves and prostate that can be aroused, but some can't admit it.

Sexual Performance or Compatibility

Critiquing a lover's performance, no matter how gently or constructively we may try to do it, is never easy. We keep quiet for many reasons—we harbor our own insecurities about performance, we don't want to alienate our partners, or we're reluctant to seem demanding or aggressive. Yet the alternatives are equally unpleasant: sexual frustration, resentment, and poor self-esteem.

It is very difficult to raise the issue of me not being sexually satisfied. I have a high sex drive and my boyfriend's got a very low one. It brings up a lot of conflict, so I don't like to bring it up.

It is really hard to tell someone when I don't like something they are doing, because it so easily can feel like an attack on a very sensitive place in them.

I have trouble expressing my need for longer stimulation during traditional intercourse. I feel like I am attacking his ability to last.

I found it really hard to tell a man he was selfish in bed. This was compounded by the fact that I enjoy a submissive role, because people tend to think that means I don't want to orgasm or be attended to at all! It is difficult to explain it is a role and underneath it I'm still me.

Illness or Disability

People with illnesses or disabilities have to routinely explain their specific limitations or needs to partners. On top of this, they often find themselves tackling common assumptions or stereotypes about sex and disability. Dealing with your own or a partner's issues of self-esteem can make it even more difficult to initiate sexual conversations.

Explaining to a partner that I'm not in the mood, due to medications, illness, physical pain, or exhaustion, has often been difficult. It seems that most people want an excuse—they need a reason beyond "I really just don't feel up to it today." I guess this probably has a lot to do with their own self-image, and the idea that if I don't always want them, there must be something wrong with them. Of course, this isn't true, but I can see how some folks would take it that way, particularly partners who don't have a strong sense of their own self-worth.

My lack of libido is due to the antidepressant medication I take. Even the most sensitive guys seem to look upon it as a challenge. I'd rather have someone look for other ways to pleasure me than become obsessed with showing their prowess.

The most difficult subject for me to raise with a partner is vulvodynia. I'm very lucky to have recovered almost fully, but there are still painful times, particularly around my period. This is very difficult for me to discuss because it has so impacted my sexual self-image. I don't want my current lover to view me as "damaged."

Fantasies

They're called "fantasies" for a reason—they belong in the realm of the fantastic. Like dreams, they needn't be safe, politically correct, or coherent. Because our fantasies can fall so far afield of what we'd consider doing in our "normal" lives, many couples are reticent to share them with each other, out of fear they'll be judged. There's nothing that says you need to divulge your fantasies, and, for many couples, keeping them private is the key to their erotic charge. Yet many others find that sharing their fantasies introduces new erotic terrain to explore mentally, or in some cases physically. See the Fantasies chapter for more on this subject.

It's hard to talk about fantasies or new things I want to try. I'm usually afraid either that I'll be thought of as weird or sick, or that he will turn me down.

My partner has had a hard time feeling safe to divulge her more "out there" fantasies with me because I have had none to share in return, I guess because I just don't really fantasize.

What about the physical aspects of fantasy? It's one thing to fantasize about trying anal sex or introducing a third person to our sex play, it's totally different when the finger actually touches or the person is in front of you.

Sexual History

While it isn't necessary to divulge your entire sexual history to partners, when there's information that's vital to the success of your current encounter, it's certainly a good idea.

How much I divulge about my past sexual abuse depends on how deeply I get involved with a partner. There are certain physical triggers that occur during sex that I let my close partners know about so that they can avoid them.

I think things would have gone a lot better in my last relationship if I hadn't been too embarrassed to communicate my lack of experience, both sexual and romantic. It created a block, and we really didn't talk about sex at all.

I was pleasantly surprised to find most people have had profound respect for my flashback triggers and so on.

Troubleshooting Problem Areas
Negotiating Differences, Compromising

If you suggest something to your partner and meet with total resistance, you have a few options. If you're with someone you aren't planning on seeing again, you're better off not pushing. If you're new to the relationship and would like it to continue, you could wait until you're a bit more familiar with each other before exploring your suggestions. In either case, if the activity you're proposing is necessary to your satisfaction, and your partner is unobliging, you probably ought to find another place to hang your hat.

If you're interested in trying something but your partner isn't, try talking together—examine the reasons behind your curiosity and your partner's resistance. Talking about it might break down some attitudes, stereotypes, fears, or anxieties. You might also find a way to compromise. You can evaluate how important it is for you to pursue this particular sexual activity. Is it worth jeopardizing the relationship?

A textbook example is the man who wants his wife to perform fellatio on him, but she's not interested. Once he explains how much pleasure it would give him—perhaps offering to reciprocate something she desires—they can explore the reasons she's hesitant, and perhaps reach a compromise. Does she think it's a dirty practice? Maybe he can shower first, or use a condom. If she doesn't like him coming in her mouth, he can tell her when he's about to come, and she can finish with her hand. Or he can wear a flavored condom on his penis. If she doesn't like the feeling of having her mouth filled with penis, perhaps she can take just the tip of the penis in her mouth, and stimulate the length of his penis with her hand.

Your partner might be resisting your suggestion merely because the activity is unfamiliar. Try reading a self-help book or some erotic literature together. Give it time; sometimes all one needs is a little time and space to get used to a new idea.

Desire Discrepancies

One of the most common sexual concerns expressed by couples today is something sex therapists refer to as desire disorder or desire discrepancy. In short, your sex life feels out of synch because one of you wants sex more or less frequently than the other does.

Here's a simple example: When asked how often they'd each like to have sex, Bill claims he's comfortable with once a month, but Ted would prefer twice a week. Ted is always initiating; Bill starts feeling pressured. Bill may also feel like the one with the problem; he may eventually lose any desire to have sex. Both just get more frustrated.

If this situation sounds familiar, it's in your best interest to start talking. Here are some things you and your partner can discuss:

Share your definitions of desire and sex. What does sex mean to you? Is it intercourse, orgasm, genital stimulation? Perhaps one of you has a broader definition of sex—more touching or emphasis on the sensual side of sex, role-playing, or experimentation. Use this as a basis for negotiating sex play.

Maybe one of you defines sexual desire as the urge to have intercourse, while the other associates desire with any sort of erotic feeling. The latter might actually be experiencing greater sexual desire than either of you think; she or he just needs practice channeling it into partner sex. It might even come as a relief to realize that one of you hasn't lost desire—it's just being experienced differently.

What are your expectations? Where do they come from? Is there some statistical average you and your partner are aspiring to? Are you trying to keep up with the mythical Joneses or the leads in the latest romantic movie? It will help to examine your expectations about frequency of sexual desire, and whether you as an individual are comfortable with that.

Unfortunately, it's not uncommon for the person with less sexual desire to feel like the one with the problem. It's good to remind ourselves that there is no standard for sexual frequency. It's about as absurd to expect two people to have the same desire for sex as it is to expect them to have the same craving for chocolate or exercise or reading material. But since sex for so many of us is integral to our primary relationships, it makes sense that we'd have to work on negotiating our differences. (Just as we would balance other lifestyle dilemmas, like how to raise kids, religious differences, contrasting cultural tastes, etc.)

When desire discrepancies trouble a relationship, it's crucial that both partners work toward an acceptable middle ground.

Talk to your partner about what affects your desire. Exploring the various elements—both positive and negative—that affect sexual desire can help both of you understand and work with these issues. Stress at home or work, a history of sexual trauma, pressure from a partner—these are a few of the many things that can inhibit us. If you are the partner who wants sex more frequently, you might ask yourself whether you use sex to satisfy other needs (for example, gaining attention, seeking acceptance, relieving job stress).

It's just as important to discover, share, and explore those things that enhance our sexual desire. Visual imagery, a certain smell, or a particular fantasy may activate your desire. By identifying these stimuli, you can learn how to access, cultivate, and channel them into partner sex.

Use this shared information to reach a compromise. Fueled by the information you gather through these discussions, you and your partner can begin to explore your options toward mutually satisfying sexual encounters.

Let's use our original example. Perhaps after discussing their views on sex and desire, Ted learns that Bill is annoyed by their goal-oriented, orgasms-required lovemaking routine. Bill would rather do without the performance anxiety or sexual acrobatics. Ted might agree to trade in or expand their routine to one more inclusive of sensual touching or verbal gymnastics.

Bill may also have felt that since he was never going to want sex as much as Ted, there was no point in trying at all. Perhaps he stops initiating because he knows Ted will do it eventually, or he's afraid that if he shows interest he and Ted will be having sex all the time. The two could agree to exchange roles for a period of time, so that only Bill will initiate. This may take some of the pressure off Bill and give Ted something to anticipate.

Maybe Ted confesses that he sees each sexual encounter with Bill as a confirmation of Bill's love for him. They might explore this further and devise substitute ways for Bill to express his love for Ted, thereby reducing the sexual demands on Bill.

The two can work toward being more accepting of their desire discrepancies, adapting their sexual activity to accommodate them. For example, Ted could masturbate while lying in Bill's arms, or Ted could massage Bill with no sexual expectations.

Obviously, depending on the specific circumstances, there are numerous ways to work on desire discrepancy. The only requirement is your willingness to discuss it with your partner. You may be able to work out quite a few things yourself. Should you require further counseling, there are some excellent self-help books available, or you may find it helpful to work with a sex therapist.

Keeping the Flame Alive

If you've ever been in a sexual relationship that's lasted longer than a year or two, or are in one now, you're probably well aware that one of the biggest challenges facing any couple once they walk off into the sunset together is attempting to sustain a hot and happy sex life. In the first flush of a relationship, effortless passion is just a kiss away as the two of you revel in the excitement of getting to know each other, uncovering secrets, and sharing confidences. That you aren't yet secure in your relationship adds an element of dramatic tension that heightens arousal, and can lead you to seize every erotic opportunity with abandon, for fear that it might be your last with this partner. If you settle into a long-term relationship, you may find that once the first wave of erotic exploration subsides, you and the person who's now your domestic partner are having sex less and less often.

Studies have shown that the frequency of sex drops over time for couples of all sexual orientations, a phenomenon sometimes ominously labeled "bed death." One popular theory holds that couples who "merge" together, sharing every aspect of their lives in a cozy cocoon, aren't getting the distance required for sexual sparks to fly. While it's true that settling into a predictable shared routine can dampen your libido, some therapists are beginning to point out that "bed death" is hardly the result of two people's knowing each other too well. In fact, hot sex with a long-term partner requires both intimacy and self-disclosure, and many couples would rather maintain a boring, but non-threatening, status quo than expose their true sexual selves. "Merged" couples may be intertwined in the practical, emotional details of each other's daily lives, but they often stop well short of sharing their sexual hopes, dreams, and aspirations.

In the early days of a relationship, you may trust your partner less, but you also have less to lose if he or she lets you down. Many of us find it easier to take sexual risks—to assume the active role of seducer, to explore brand-new sexual activities, and to share fantasies—during the heady time when everything's slightly off-kilter and you feel powerfully attractive. As the dust settles, we become not only habituated to each other, but also habituated to making certain assumptions about each other: "Oh, I'm sure he doesn't really like going down on me" or "She wouldn't want to watch porn with me—it would offend her political sensibilities."

For every assumption we make about the other, there's an accompanying fear: "Maybe it really turns him off to get close to my genitals, and he just doesn't want to tell me" or "Maybe she'll think that real lesbians shouldn't even *like* watching porn." Paradoxically, being open about sexual desires and fears doesn't necessarily get easier the longer you're in a relationship—in truth, it can be harder to expose yourself, because you risk offending, disgusting, or disappointing the person you care about most. It's natural to have the unconscious fear: *What if the scales fall from my lover's eyes and she or he discovers what a pervert I really am and stops loving me?* All the sexual shame that melted away in the heat of your first combustion comes creeping back in to silence you. And in the hustle-bustle of domestic living, it's easy to think: I'm sure we'd be having sex if only her in-laws weren't coming to dinner, or the dog didn't need walking, or he hadn't had such a long day at the office.

Of course, being in a long-term relationship doesn't mean you have to settle for infrequent, routine sex. But if you want to get yourselves out of a rut, you will need to take some risks. Your first step will be to communicate: Address your fears, regrets, sorrows, and longings head on, and share them with your partner. Keeping the spark alive takes a certain amount of initiative. We sometimes fall into the trap of assuming that if our partner hasn't requested a certain activity by now, it must mean he or she is not interested in it. But if you're both thinking this, imagine what fun you could be missing out on!

Consider some of the suggestions in this chapter on improving both your self-awareness and your awareness of your partner's preferences. Look for books that flesh out these ideas in greater detail and include tips for people in long-term relationships. *Hot Monogamy*, primarily geared toward heterosexual couples, offers exercises designed to help you and your partner identify your individual emotional and sexual needs and effectively communicate what you want. Jack Morin's *The Erotic Mind* (see sidebar for more about Jack) provides unexpected insights into the sources of sexual passion and offers a road map of ways to inject dynamic excitement into an intimate relationship. His book is valuable reading for individuals of all sexual orientations, whether partnered or not. It addresses the complex nature of sexual arousal and guides the reader toward a better understanding of what it is that turns him or her on, and why. With this information under your belt, you'll be well-equipped to keep the home fires stoked and burning.

Initiating Sex

It can be challenging to communicate your desire to be sexual with another person, whether a complete stranger, a new acquaintance, an old friend, or a long-time partner.. You're risking possible rejection while trying to satisfy your own sex drive. Whether you're successful depends, of course, on whether the person is interested in you or sex, but you can improve your prospects by tuning in to your partner's preferred approach. If you are with a new lover, you can either ask what approach pleases or go with your instincts. In longer relationships, you'll eventually become familiar with each other's preferences.

It's not unusual in most couples for one person to initiate sex more often than the other. If this is a dynamic that works well for you, great. If it's a source of frustration, you may be experiencing the desire discrepancy discussed above and now have an idea of what areas need work. If you've simply fallen into a rut, talk about it and see if you can't find a way to break the routine. Perhaps one partner just needs encouragement that he or she won't be rejected, or the partner who normally initiates just needs to practice taking turns. Maybe you'll recognize that you like sex initiated in different ways, and sharing your requirements will give you each a better understanding of what will please the other.

You're not always going to get the response you hope for when you initiate sex. If someone turns down a sexual proposition, rather than perceiving it as a blow to your self-esteem, why not congratulate yourself for having had the courage to pursue your desire? Celebrate your sexual feelings in a different way—masturbate. If your lover simply isn't "in the mood," and there's not much chance that will change, respect that and find an alternative way to be sexual. You can't expect to be sexually in synch with a partner all the time.

We thought you'd enjoy seeing the many unique ways people enjoy having sex initiated. For some it can vary with their moods; for others, the requirements are quite specific. We asked survey respondents to describe their favorite ways to have sex initiated, and their answers varied immensely. Maybe you'll come up with a few new ideas the next time you've got sex on your mind!

Many people are fond of the nonverbal method:

If I'm really driven, I like to communicate physically— just reaching over or coming up from behind and grabbing. Not talking is much sexier.

A lustful look and touching. Lots of words are unnecessary. I like a certain look that says, "I wanna fuck you."

I like my partner to initiate by slowly undressing me or turning baths for two into a lovemaking session.

Others prefer the verbal approach:

I like to express that I want this or that in a way that's friendly, loving and HOT.

With a new partner, it needs to be verbalized.

I initiated my most recent encounter by saying, "Can I touch you? Can I kiss you?"

Double entendre is big with me; wit and a quick mind are a turn-on.

Some enjoy planning ahead so that the anticipation can enhance the sex:

I like to talk about it long before we actually get down to it. It's wonderful to spend an afternoon or evening together, knowing that it's going to happen.

I love to whisper and tease my partner along, often for hours, over dinner.

I like some very intentional setting–up, like "I want to make love tonight, why don't you put on perfume only and I'll be over later."

Others relish the element of surprise:

I like them to be spontaneous. If I'm sitting in a chair reading, I want the book taken from me and my glasses removed and my mouth covered with wet lips.

I like to be caught off guard, for my partner to start massaging, fondling, stripping, or teasing me while on the phone.

I like my lover to come up from behind, grab my breasts, and bite my neck while I'm doing something boring like the dishes.

And some respond better to force:

I like to be grabbed in a darkly lit club and dragged outside for a good time!

Since I'm a pretty aggressive female, sometimes I like my partner to be forceful with me so I can be passive for once!

Others are partial to a slower or gentler approach:

I like to start with a kiss, then get into heavier and heavier groping to the point where I feel like I'm going to die; then I like for my partner to undress me slowly. I like to be teased into a frenzy.

Others have their own methods of initiating:

More often than not, when I initiate it's either by kissing or stroking or sometimes by just fellating my partner as a way of saying Hi.

In the past I would initiate sexual encounters by reading someone's palm and telling them some great sex was in their future!

Usually I grab him by the balls and growl!

One Last Example

As a way to illustrate some classic communication pitfalls, here's a description of a not-uncommon transaction at Good Vibrations:

A woman shyly enters the store and looks around surreptitiously. She heads over to the vibrator section, where she gazes in bewilderment at the many sizes and shapes. A clerk approaches her:

"Is there anything I can help you with?"

"Oh no, no. I'm just looking," she says, clutching her purse, visibly embarrassed.

"Do you have any questions about the vibrators?" the clerk persists.

"No. I'll let you know if I do. Thanks."

The clerk retreats. After some time and consideration, the woman selects a large, very realistic-looking penis-shaped battery vibrator, makes her purchase as quickly and discreetly as possible, and makes a hurried exit.

The next day the woman returns. She whispers to the clerk that she'd like to return her vibrator,

perhaps saying something like "It didn't work out" or "My husband didn't like it." She's disappointed; at this point she'll either elaborate on the problem, and perhaps the clerk can help her choose a more appropriate toy, or, being too embarrassed or defeated, she'll give up on sex toys for good.

HERE'S WHAT PROBABLY HAPPENED

At some point this woman (let's call her Ellen) decided she wanted to try a vibrator. Maybe while talking to a friend about her difficulty having orgasms, Ellen learned of the wonders of vibrators. Maybe Ellen read about vibrators in a book or a magazine and decided it was worth a try. So, she pays a visit to Good Vibrations.

It's the first time Ellen's ever been in a sex shop and, like most newcomers, she's embarrassed. Once she finds the vibrator section, she is overwhelmed by the variety of sizes and shapes. Understandably, her brain is firing questions: "What does that do?" "Where does this go?" "Do women really like that?" She probably begins questioning what she plans to do with her vibrator once she buys it.

When the clerk approaches to offer help, Ellen's shyness and embarrassment render her speechless, so she doesn't ask her questions. Maybe she's not sure what she should ask. Eventually she purchases a vibrator that looks vaguely familiar to her—the penis-shaped battery toy.

That night during lovemaking, she pulls the toy out from under her bed to surprise her husband. He's shocked, confused, threatened, defensive. He questions his performance. "Don't I satisfy you?" He questions her need for him. "Won't that fake penis eventually replace my real one in your affections?" She might try to explain, to express her needs, but most likely the toy goes back under the bed, and both of them give up.

WHAT WENT WRONG?

How could this have been avoided? When Ellen decided she wanted a vibrator, she could have asked herself, "What specifically do I want it for? To stimulate my clitoris or to use as a vibrating dildo?" Ellen could have talked with her friend about how she uses her vibrator. Maybe she could have even borrowed her friend's vibrator. Then Ellen could have talked to her husband, perhaps saying, "I have a friend who uses a vibrator, and she says her orgasms are really different.

I'd love to try one; would you like to help me experiment?" This might have opened up a discussion on what her orgasms were like at the time, and whether the vibrator would complement their sex play or be used solely by her. If either of them felt uncomfortable about toys, they could have talked about that. Discussing their issues in a nonsexual, nonthreatening setting might have provided Ellen the opportunity to reassure her husband about his performance and her affection for him.

But instead, Ellen set out for Good Vibrations with the vague notion that she wanted a vibrator for something. When she walked in the door and was instantly overwhelmed by the variety, she began to wonder what she really *was* going to do with the thing. She felt foolish, ignorant, and just plain embarrassed. She became increasingly uncomfortable, but since she came with a mission, she purchased the phallic model that looked most like a vibrator to her.

Had Ellen talked about her sexual needs with her friend or her partner, she might have been able to articulate what might satisfy those needs. Perhaps she could have conveyed her questions to the clerk, who could then steer her in the right direction. She might have seized the moment to ask the clerk for feedback or information on any of the issues that came up during her conversation with her husband.

Since Ellen never let her husband know that she was at all interested in vibrators, he was shocked by the abrupt change in their routine and figured she was trying to tell him something about his performance. His defensiveness, combined with her confusion over the sex toy, ultimately killed any enthusiasm Ellen had for trying something new. If they had discussed it first, or if at any point along the way Ellen had figured out what she wanted out of that vibrator, she might have been able to explain it to someone: herself, her friend, her husband, or the store clerk, any or all of whom might have offered some useful information and some much-needed encouragement.

Benefits

The benefits of good communication are infinite. New relationships can prosper from early sharing of likes and dislikes, not to mention discussions on safer sex and contraception. People in longer relationships can troubleshoot problem areas if they're able to discuss sex comfortably. And people at all stages of a relationship can benefit from the chance to experiment with new kinds of sexual activity. Talking about sex enables us to break old patterns, eliminate arcane attitudes, and explore the many sides of our sexual selves.

"The messy reality is that it's harder to have good sex with someone you love," explains Jack Morin. Huh? But what about the idea that finding one's true love will automatically lead to a lifetime full of satisfying, combustible sex? Jack, a psychotherapist, simply refers to this as our "hearts and flowers" mentality. In truth, relationships, sex, and eroticism are infinitely more complicated.

In his groundbreaking book, *The Erotic Mind*, Jack explores the many paradoxes intrinsic in eroticism, offering readers much-needed perspective and validation for the complexities of their erotic natures. After years of counseling clients in his therapy practice, Jack realized something was amiss with Masters and Johnson's–style sex therapy, which was based on the premise that removing all the obstacles within a relationship would lead to great sex. Jack noticed that this "neat and clean" approach to relationships ignored the reality that, in many cases, obstacles such as guilt or anxiety could actually function as aphrodisiacs. "Anything that turns us off can potentially turn us on, and vice versa," explains Jack. In other words, eliminating all problematic elements from one's erotic life can rob it of its zest.

For example, many people associate sex with guilt as a result of growing up in a sex-negative culture. One might think eradicating guilt would benefit our sex lives, but in fact the guilt that accompanies rule-breaking is a powerful aphrodisiac— think about the intensity of sexual experiences that involve the fear of getting caught (children exploring masturbation, adults enjoying sex in a public place). Learning to embrace or incorporate some of these turn-ons in a healthy way can help couples keep the spark alive.

Couples in long-term relationships are often perplexed by the fact that sexual desire can dissipate rather than escalate as they become closer and more compatible. According to Jack, some individuals begin to lose their sense of "otherness," fore-going controversy for the sake of keeping the relationship on an even keel. "One of the best things you can do for your sex life is to not downplay differences, to not shy away from disagreements and arguments," says Jack. "It reminds you that you're not with a reflection of yourself, there's another person there. It's that otherness that is so fundamental to attraction."

Identifying these seeming contradictions and coming to terms with them is incredibly difficult for people, according to Jack. "It's very disturbing to people, because if we could, none of would design sex this way. We would make it so that when we developed more intimate relationships with higher cooperation and mutual respect, sex would get better!"

In addition to exploring the origins of some of our more powerful turn-ons, Jack also offers advice for couples on honing their communication skills. Learning how to tell your partner what you want sexually is one of the most challenging and rewarding skills couples can develop. Many people find it difficult either because they harbor a romantic notion that their partner will intuitively know how to please them or, more commonly, because they're afraid of hurting a partner's feelings. "Part of this comes from a natural protectiveness that we feel toward our partners. We don't want to hurt them or put them down, so we keep our mouths shut, to the detriment of the sexual relationship." As a way of getting couples to share the information, Jack encourages his clients to describe one or more ideal scenarios of a sexual encounter.

Curious about what Jack's currently up to? Visit his website, www.malebeautyproject.com.

PROFILES *in* PLEASURE:

Jack Morin

"The messy reality is that it's harder to have good sex with someone you love."

CHAPTER

Masturbation

You would be hard-pressed to find anyone more enthusiastic about masturbation than we are. Why sing the praises of an activity most people can't even admit doing?

We think masturbation should be the national pastime: It feels good; it's healthy; it's natural; it's free; it's legal; it's your birthright; it's easy to do; it's convenient; it's voluntary; you can do it alone; you can do it with someone; it's educational; it's a unique form of self-expression; it's relaxing; it's invigorating; it builds self-confidence and self-esteem; it's creative; it's ageless, colorless, genderless—the list could go on for pages.

These days, masturbation is often referred to as "solo sex" or "self-loving." While we appreciate the existence of a larger sexual vocabulary, and we will use these words for variety's sake, we're standing up for the word *masturbate!* Enough of those clinicians or authors who find the word dry, technical, or tainted by a sordid past. We're liberating it from its oppressive history and embracing it in word as well as practice!

To Know Me Is to Love Me

Here are just a few excellent reasons to masturbate regularly:

It's Natural

Despite a wide range of cultural taboos, there is nothing unnatural about masturbation. You're born with all the equipment. Ultrasound images have shown a fetus masturbating (touching his genitals with fingers) in the womb. Children, those little barometers of all things biological—that is, unlearned—do it with no instruction and often before they're even talking. They touch their genitals because it brings them physical pleasure, just as scratching an itch would:

> *My earliest memory of touching myself is when I was still in a crib, on my stomach, with a blanket rolled between my legs—rocking myself with my hand underneath me on my genitalia through the blanket. My mom said she caught me doing this at six months old!*

At age five I discovered this great way to feel good.
I called it "tickling" myself.

My sister, who is five years my senior, taught me to
masturbate when I was around 5. I had no concept
of sex at the time and used to masturbate to the
alphabet!

Unfortunately, many of us were raised with misinformation, guilt, and pleasure-phobic attitudes about masturbation. As adults, we'd do well to note childhood experience (either by affirming our own children's practice or by conjuring up memories of our own, or both) in our efforts to embrace masturbation. Our survey question that resulted in the most voluminous as well as the most colorful, enlightening, and humorous responses asked people to recount their earliest memories of self-pleasuring.

If you are still not convinced that masturbation is natural, remember that in 1972 the American Medical Association declared masturbation a normal sexual activity.

Masturbation Is the Basis for Good Sex

What better way to learn about your anatomy and sexual responsiveness than by masturbating? We are all unique sexual beings, and masturbation will teach you just what type of stimulation feels good to you. In fact, sex therapists and other health professionals routinely prescribe masturbation to women and men who want to increase their sexual awareness, desire to break through sexual barriers, or may be experiencing some type of sexual dysfunction. Preorgasmic women are encouraged to masturbate regularly, to experiment with various types of stimulation. Masturbation allows women who are unaccustomed to paying attention to their own sexual responses the time to explore their unique sexual rhythms. Men can gain control over the timing of ejaculation with masturbation methods such as the squeeze technique and the stop/start technique. And partner sex gets that much better when your partner delights in your own pleasure.

The first time I masturbated while my husband fucked
me, it was liberating. Letting him watch me do that
and seeing that it turned him on, I came so hard that
I cried afterward, and he was really moved by that.
The lovemaking that followed was just as memorable.

You can improve your own sexual awareness by experimenting with masturbation. Many of the techniques and toys we discuss relate in some way to masturbation. Adding Kegel exercises to your masturbatory ritual will have positive effects on both solo and partner sex. Women pursuing multiple orgasms and men trying to orgasm without ejaculating may enjoy experimenting alone free of performance anxiety. In Betty Dodson's masturbation training video for women, *Celebrating Orgasm*, she sagely notes, "To get really good at sex, we need to practice for a couple of hours at least once a week."

Almost all the toys we discuss can enhance or add a new dimension to solo sex. If you're planning to introduce a toy into partner sex, you might increase your chances of success by playing with it alone first. If you're buying a toy for a partner, you should encourage her or him to play with it alone as well as with you.

By playing with a toy or practicing a new technique alone first, you spare yourself performance anxiety, frustration, or disappointment when your fondest expectations aren't fulfilled. One woman's first masturbation story confirms this:

In my twenties a man friend/lover bought me a
battery-operated vibrator and wanted to teach me
how to masturbate. He went very slowly and was
very patient, but I was embarrassed. Once I
relaxed and practiced on my own, I loved it.

Alone, you're responsible only for your own pleasure, so you're free to go as slowly or as quickly as you like. You're more likely to give yourself the time and permission to practice until something works for you. Once you've discovered the secrets of success, you can approach partner sex with more confidence.

For instance, let's say you're the proud new owner of a Hitachi Magic Wand and would like to use it with your partner, but you're not quite sure how. Play hooky from work to try your toy out alone (how liberating to take a day off to masturbate!). Use it as many ways as your imagination permits, but wait to use it on your clitoris or penis last. Press it against different parts of your body and notice where you get an erotic charge. Maybe on the back of your neck, the inside of your thigh, or your nipples. Vary the speed and pressure, stop and start the vibrator, lie on top of it. When you place the vibrator on your genitals, pay as much attention to what doesn't feel good as to what does.

After you've had a delightful afternoon (or several) with your new toy, you're in a better position to orchestrate a fun toy tango with your partner. You can begin by describing all the ways you like to play with the toy. Let your partner maneuver the vibrator while watching your reactions, or vice versa. Try exploring the unique ways two bodies can enjoy a vibrator. Two women can nestle the vibrator between them. A man can enjoy indirect vibrations if he uses the vibrator to stimulate his partner's clitoris while he is penetrating her. Are you catching on?

Here's another example: Perhaps you've always wanted to dress your penis up in one of those sexy leather cock-and-ball toys, but you're not sure whether you'd be comfortable showing it off to your partner. Plant yourself somewhere comfortable and try it out. Practice putting it on and removing it so that it becomes second nature; if it's adjustable, try out the different options till you discover the right fit. Admire yourself in front of the mirror, don't be afraid to strut your stuff! Use a variety of touches, caresses, and strokes on your penis and testicles, so that you can share these with your partner later. You're discovering the pleasure potential of your new toy and gaining confidence using it, putting you in a much better position to introduce the "new you" to your partner.

Are you ready to call in sick? Well, if that doesn't seem likely, remember that another advantage of masturbation, as one woman reminds us, is that you can do it discreetly almost anywhere:

When I go to lunch at work, I'll go to the nearby park to eat and listen to the radio in my car. Several times now I've started thinking about my "needs" and I've masturbated in the car in the park. There aren't many people there, but the thought of someone "catching" me or "watching me" really excites me. The orgasms from that are a great stress relief in the middle of the day.

Masturbation: Freedom of Sexual Expression

I like to be sexual every day, with either myself or someone else.

When I'm in a relationship I masturbate regularly as a gift to myself.

Every time you masturbate, you're asserting your identity as a sexual person. Masturbation is sex. If you believe you're only being sexual when you're with a partner, you're missing out on an entirely satisfying, fulfilling aspect of your sexual self.

And every time you masturbate, you actively cast off those repressive attitudes about sex instilled in you by parents, teachers, friends, priests, aunts, uncles, counselors, therapists, politicians, and the media. You're not going to go blind; you aren't "wasting your seed"; you're not frigid; you aren't being punished; you won't get a disease. You're celebrating your sexuality *and* practicing safe sex. Give yourself a hand! For many of us, it was a strong sex drive and a sense of humor that helped us survive our formative years:

During my elementary-school years, I was in Catholic school, and comments made by the nuns made me feel I was committing a sin. So I prayed for God to forgive me while I rocked and rubbed!

I went to a Catholic school where the only sex education we ever received came from a nun one afternoon during the eighth grade. She advised us to try and distract ourselves when we were experiencing "impure" thoughts. Her suggestion (which she admitted worked for her) was to picture, in great detail, a juicy hamburger with all the trimmings! For years, every time I saw a hamburger I got turned on, and every time I got turned on I got hungry!

Masturbation Is Healthy

Don't you wonder why we never see newspaper headlines about the health benefits of masturbation? Every other month you hear of a study proving that a daily glass of wine or a brisk walk through the park is good for the heart. Considering how the media loves sex, it's surprising that we haven't seen the headline "Study Shows Daily Masturbation Reduces Stress, Invigorates Heart, and Prolongs Life." It's just another example of the taboo shrouding this simple sexual activity, because all of that is true!

Next to running, masturbation is my favorite way to clear my brain.

People have been obsessing for so long over the mythological health risks of masturbation that they don't stop to think about these health benefits:

- Relieves stress and tension
- Releases endorphins
- Relieves menstrual cramps
- Fights yeast infections by increasing the blood flow into the pelvis
- Exercises and flushes the prostate gland, reducing the risk of prostate infections
- Strengthens pelvic muscles
- Provides a good cardiovascular workout and also burns up calories

We wouldn't be surprised if masturbation was even good for your complexion! What's more, this simple act of taking responsibility for your sexual needs is bound to improve sexual self-esteem and self-confidence:

I love masturbating—it makes me feel more sexual and therefore better about myself.

Another advantage of masturbation is that whether you're young, old, partnered, or single, masturbation allows you to remain sexually active throughout your entire life.

Masturbation Is Popular and Creative Sex

When you masturbate you disprove the myth that heterosexual sex in the missionary position is the most widely practiced sexual activity. Far more people regularly masturbate than engage in sex under that narrow definition.

As you will see later in the chapter, there are hundreds of ways to indulge in this exciting recreation. You can spice up partner sex with masturbation or choreograph a slow self-loving ritual:

I make a double-handed fist and lie on my front on top of my partner with the pressure indirectly on my clit, directly on hers. I move in a familiar rhythmic pattern; the pace picks up and I usually come in less than three minutes. I have nice arm muscles because of it!

I used to be a quick-and-dirty gal, but now I've learned to take my time. I like to come home before my housemate gets off work and grab a few various erotica books and flip to all the really hot parts.

I like to get myself as aroused as possible just using one hand on my clit and then at the last moment toss the book aside and insert my left middle finger into my vagina to feel the pulsing. I love that!

The bottom line is that masturbation can work for you almost anywhere, anytime. Whether you're single or partnered, low on libido or hormones-a-raging, weathering temporary changes to your sex life or dealing with permanent physical limitations, masturbation is a rewarding sexual outlet:

As a pregnant single mom, I got tremendously horny. I had wild dreams about sex with celebrities and former lovers and would wake up and engage in some of the hottest masturbation sessions of my life.

Reasons to Masturbate

As part of Good Vibrations' celebration of National Masturbation Month in May, we invite our customers to submit their top ten reasons to masturbate. We've printed a few of our favorites here.

- You never have to tell yourself, "A little to the left, a little higher, and a whole lot harder."
- It's a really good "pick-me-up" in the middle of the day when decaf is all that's available in the office coffee room.
- Every time you do it you're part of the world's largest simultaneous experiment proving that masturbation does not cause blindness.
- What better way to have fun, keep the birth rate down, and reduce stress...all in just minutes a day.
- It's a great way to sound animated on the phone while the parents are telling you about the latest goings-on in "the old neighborhood."
- Self-serve is always cheaper.
- It's less embarrassing if you call out the wrong name.
- Gets you into the mile-high club without too much hassle.
- You'd go insane if you didn't do it.
- It's always there when you need it.

Historical Perspectives

Why do we need to give you all these fantastic reasons to masturbate when according to the Kinsey Institute's statistics, 94 percent of men and at least 70 percent of women already indulge in this marvelous pastime? Because most won't admit it! Partly this is because we're inherited a lot of negative misconceptions; we'd like to reveal some of the infamous history that has made masturbation a taboo activity down through the ages.

Masturbation in the Bible

In the Western world we often assume that all sexual proscriptions have their basis in the Bible. In fact, the Bible adopts no particular stand on masturbation. However, the story of Onan, which is found in the book of Genesis, is frequently interpreted as an injunction against masturbation. The story relates how Onan's brother died childless. According to the customs of the time, if a married man died childless, it was the duty of the male next-of-kin to attempt to impregnate the dead man's wife, to ensure the continuity of the family name and property rights. Any child born this way would be considered the offspring of the deceased. Onan was not inspired by this idea, "…so whenever he slept with his brother's wife, he spilled his seed on the ground so as not to raise up issue for his brother. What he did was wicked in the Lord's sight, and the Lord took his life" (Genesis 38:9–10). Onan's spilling of seed (semen) has been interpreted as either masturbation or coitus interruptus, and just to be on the safe side, the Christian church has condemned both activities for centuries as sins against God.

The Economics of Ejaculation

The taboo against masturbation has its roots in the time-honored religious rejection of any sexual activity that is nonprocreative. It's bolstered by a widespread tendency to apply an economic metaphor to the "spending" of bodily fluids. The notion that men have a predetermined, fixed allotment of sperm, and that every ejaculation depletes a finite store of this precious fluid, can be found in many cultures. Chinese Taoist sexual practices are based on the notion that female yin energy is inexhaustible, while male yang energy

must be hoarded. Therefore, Taoist sexual techniques involve men controlling ejaculation and channeling semen back up to the brain. Aristotle wrote that semen is a valuable nutrient and that the loss of even a little of this nutrient results in exhaustion and weakness. This philosophy lives on in the modern superstition that male athletes shouldn't weaken themselves by having sex the night before a big game.

The classic tract against masturbation, and one that influenced popular thinking on the subject for over a hundred years, was published by a Swiss doctor, S. A. Tissot, in 1758. His *Onanism: Treatise on the Diseases Produced by Masturbation* argued that the loss of a single ounce of semen was more debilitating than the loss of forty ounces of blood. Following this logic, a man who masturbated consistently gradually depleted his life force, becoming enfeebled, ill, and mentally deranged—ultimately, the madman could masturbate himself to death.

Despite the obvious fact that they do not produce semen, women were not exempt from Tissot's theory of the destructive forces unleashed by masturbation. Tissot argued that masturbating women developed symptoms ranging from hysteria to lengthened clitorises, and were ultimately driven to uterine fury, "which deprives them at once of modesty and reason and puts them on the level of the lewdest brutes, until a despairing death snatches them away from pain and infamy."

Nineteenth-Century "Cures"

Tissot's work was first translated into English in 1832, and during the second half of the nineteenth century Europe and America saw an explosion of treatments designed to curb masturbation in children, men, and women. Doctors designated masturbation as the cause of most ailments that could not otherwise be explained or cured. Masturbation was blamed for mental illness and consumption. In a stunning display of circular logic, masturbation was blamed for the constitutional invalidism of Victorian women (who, had men allowed them to get out of the house and out of their corsets, would doubtless have been in excellent health).

Treatments for preventing masturbation ranged from the pathologically violent to the absurd. Turn-of-the-twentieth-century magazines featured advertisements for penile rings that were spiked on the inside so that any boy who experienced an erection during the course of the night would be woken in pain. Bondage belts, restraints, straitjackets, cauterizing irons, and even clitoridectomy (the surgical excision of the clitoris) were all methods used to dissuade young women from masturbating. These methods lived on into the new century in the more benign form of mittens put on children at bedtime so that they couldn't easily play with themselves during the night.

American health reformers of the nineteenth century tackled masturbation as part of a larger problem of excessive excitation of the senses. Radical reformers felt that physical excitement of any kind—even the seemingly innocent pleasure of spicy food—was a dangerous drain, robbing one of the energy necessary for productive labor. Sylvester Graham assured young men that they would be capable of self-restraint if they followed a course of cold baths, fresh air, and bland, vegetarian food (such as the whole-grain cracker named after him). John Kellogg treated visitors to his Battle Creek Sanitarium with continence-inspiring cereals, and lectured that masturbation was "the vilest, the basest and the most degrading act that a human being can commit." Graham and Kellogg were, however, at the extreme end of a continuum of medical literature. By the beginning of the twentieth century, attitudes were beginning to shift to an acceptance of sexuality as a force that needed only to be properly channeled, rather than totally reined in.

Twentieth-Century Acceptance

Sigmund Freud has had a tremendous influence on sexual attitudes in the modern world. On one hand, Freud normalized the varieties of sexual experience with his theory that every human being goes through homosexual, oral, anal, and narcissistic phases during childhood development. And yet, by decreeing penis-in-vagina sexuality to be the ultimate goal of sexual maturation, he effectively dismissed the enjoyment of all other sexual activities as proof of immaturity and inhibited development. The interpretation of masturbation as an immature activity lives on today, as does the equally unfounded Freudian theory that arousal from clitoral stimulation is somehow less mature than arousal from vaginal stimulation.

It was Alfred Kinsey, the trailblazer of sex researchers, who contributed the most to a destigmatization of masturbation. In interviews with thousands of men and women, Kinsey focused on gathering data on the precise sexual activities his subjects were actually engaging in. He was unique for his time, and ours, in treating all sexual activities with equal respect. Kinsey noted that masturbation was the activity most likely to result in orgasm for women, and spoke out against the Freudian notion of masturbation as an immature activity.

Yet even with the statistics to prove the ubiquity, and therefore presumably the "normalcy," of masturbating, a stigma remains to this day. This isn't surprising—for, despite the fact that there are countless excellent reasons to masturbate, there are just as many widespread fears and anxieties around doing so.

Why Is Masturbation Still a Four-Letter Word?

While it's true that some people still believe the masturbation-leads-to-insanity myths just discussed, most are aware that these claims are untrue, serving only as a reminder that science and "morality" make dangerous bedfellows. What, then, is it that keeps masturbation, even today, cloaked in secrecy and denial?

A Tenacious Taboo

In many ways, the taboo against masturbation is the most long-standing and tenacious of sex taboos. We see this every day in our store. Individuals who are comfortable with the idea of buying sex toys to share with their partners become skittish, embarrassed, or downright irritable when it comes to buying a toy for solo use. The notion that masturbation is an immature activity or a second-rate substitute for partner sex has a powerful hold on the popular imagination. "If I were having enough partner sex, or good-enough partner sex," the myth seems to go, "I wouldn't need to masturbate."

Apparently, the pure self-interest implicit in masturbation makes many people uncomfortable. Countless sex manuals acknowledge the universal practice of masturbation, yet it is often presented as a useful tool in the building of a better sex life, rather than as a pleasurable end in itself. It's certainly true that masturbation provides valuable information about an individual's sexual responses and preferences, and this information can in turn enhance sex with a partner. However, we question the notion that masturbation is, at best, a necessary means to the exalted end of better partner-sex. A lot of people who consider themselves free of sexual hang-ups have simply rewritten the equation "Sex is only good if it involves procreation" to read "Sex is only good if it involves two loving people." This myth gets exploited, not only by authors of sex books (though they can be the worst) but also by novelists, advice columnists, and screenwriters—think of the sex scene in the last movie you saw.

The philosophy motivating our work and this book is that sexual pleasure, whether arrived at alone or in a crowded room, is a perfectly valid end in itself. After all, it's delightful to take a bath alone, eat a good meal alone, go for a bike ride alone, listen to music alone. It's equally delightful to have sex alone. We like to think that there's not a person alive whose life wouldn't be greatly enhanced by masturbation.

Addiction Fears

You know that popular cliché, "You can never have too much of a good thing"? That about sums up our feelings regarding masturbation and addiction. If you do it and you like it, keep doing it, with our blessing and encouragement. It's true that if you masturbate, and you enjoy it, you're probably going to come back for more, which conceivably qualifies you as an "addict." It's the negative connotation behind the word *addiction* when used in the same sentence with *masturbation* that causes our hair to stand on end.

Some people maintain that it's bad or unhealthy to rely on one activity or behavior as the primary source of one's pleasure. But if this were true, couldn't we just as easily be adversely addicted to our hobbies: reading, fishing, traveling, jogging? Can you imagine the mind-boggling array of recovery groups that would spawn? Masturbation is natural, is healthy, and brings us pleasure—so why deny yourself? As long as you are not hurting yourself or anyone else (which is difficult to imagine, with a solitary habit), you can get off till the cows come home, for all we have to say about the matter. We suspect that, behind folks' fear of masturbation, a few other factors are at work, often disguised as addiction anxieties.

Guilty Pleasures

Many of us have a long association of sexual pleasure and guilt. We feel guilt because we're doing something we were told was bad throughout our youth, or we feel selfish or greedy for putting our sexual needs first:

I feel a little guilt, when I masturbate, that I should be having an orgasm with my husband.

I feel guilty about having more than one orgasm.

Guilt was easy for me as a Catholic, so masturbating under the tub spout left me with horrible images of suffering an embolism while playing with the gushing water, and my dear old dad coming in to find his eldest child dead with rigor mortis setting in, my legs frozen in pretzel position around the faucet head, while cold water spewed out over the tub and flooded the bathroom.

Because it's difficult for many of us to enjoy our pleasures guilt-free, we tend to look for something that might be "wrong" with them. For example, if you eat too much chocolate you'll get acne; if you jog too much you'll get overly fond of the endorphin high. In reality, these fears function as unnecessarily negative ways to control or moderate our pleasures. Some people might not "give in" to the temptation to masturbate because they fear that once they try it, they'll quit their jobs and stop seeing friends just so that they can stay home and masturbate all day. In fact, once people "give in," they'll probably start going to work with a better attitude!

Sometimes we just need a reminder or reassurance that what we're doing is okay. For the gentleman who won a contest we held at Good Vibrations asking folks to submit their top ten reasons for masturbating, all it took was a pat on the back to liberate his guilty conscience:

Thank you for picking my list as the "most universal" ten best reasons to masturbate. I think this means that I am now completely able to leave behind any left-over guilt I might have felt about masturbating when I was an adolescent. I am no longer a pervert! I am a normal, masturbating person! Yahoo!

Frequency

People are constantly questioning whether they are masturbating "too much."

Too much for whom or what? There's no magic number measuring "normal" frequency. Some folks masturbate several times a day and feel just fine about it, while others masturbate once a week and are wracked with guilt. If you fall into the latter category, try to determine what questions or attitudes are fueling your concern. You might seek answers or support from a friend, book, or professional. Sometimes hearing or reading about the habits of other people is all the reassurance we need that we're "normal":

I got the good news early on that masturbation was okay! Liberating Masturbation *by Betty Dodson and the original* Our Bodies, Ourselves *were important texts. Rita Mae Brown helped me think more outrageously about the right to jack off!*

I used to wonder if my masturbation methods were sick, but books by Betty Dodson, Shere Hite, and Lonnie Barbach reassured me that many other women had my orgasmic patterns.

Perceived Danger

Masturbation is not dangerous as long as you exercise good judgment and use common sense. When it comes to masturbation, there are lots of "do's" but only one "don't"—don't endanger yourself. We've all heard stories about boys inserting their penises into vacuum-cleaner hoses with gruesome results. And while we're constantly assuring people they can't electrocute themselves with a vibrator, we're assuming they aren't planning to use it in the bathtub.

Some people express concern over their rapid heart rate when they become increasingly sexually excited. One woman even joked about it:

My only anxiety now is having a heart attack and being found with all my delightful toys!

Let us assure you this is extremely unlikely. The *Journal of the American Medical Association* reports that men with heart disease are at a lower risk of having a heart attack after sex (1 percent) than they are upon simply waking up (10 percent), exerting themselves (4 percent), or getting angry (2 percent).

Those movie scenes of men having heart attacks during sex are convenient plot devices so that the young wife can inherit all the money!

Hang-Ups

People incorporate a variety of anxieties about sex into their masturbation practices, either consciously or unconsciously. Folks who find their genitals "dirty" might only masturbate through clothing. Those afraid of "getting caught" might wait until they're alone in the house, or have learned to masturbate without making a sound. One of our most common requests at Good Vibrations is for a quiet vibrator, "one that can't be heard through the walls in my apartment." Still others might turn these limitations into necessary ingredients for their arousal; many people enjoy masturbating in situations where there is a greater possibility of getting caught. There's nothing wrong with any of this; it's just helpful to be aware of these dynamics, in case you come face to face with an anxiety that's limiting your enjoyment.

Masturbation and the Next Generation

Unless we make a concerted effort to reassure kids that touching themselves is okay, we continue to perpetuate the stereotype that it's not. We do our kids a disservice if we remain silent or feign ignorance—for without positive reinforcement and understanding from parents, kids are left to sort through the conflicting messages being broadcast around them. Sitcoms refer to masturbation as a joke, advertisers flaunt it to sell product, and politicians condemn it (one president fired the surgeon general over her promasturbation stance, and another described the activity as "pathetic").

Most parents find masturbation one of the more awkward and difficult topics to address with their kids. According to Meg Hickling, a respected Canadian sex educator and author of the book *More Speaking of Sex*, "Many parents realize that masturbation is normal and healthy, but they don't know what to say to a son who's sitting in front of the TV playing with his penis." Meg points out that scolding or embarrassing kids for their behavior simply sends the message that masturbation is bad, and she encourages parents to stress the difference between things done in private (like going to the bathroom or picking your nose) versus those done in public.

> I can remember getting caught a LOT when I was a child, but no one ever told me it was bad or that I shouldn't be doing it, just that I shouldn't be doing it in the living room or at my grandmother's house.

Kids are never too young—or too old—to read your feelings about masturbation. Young children don't masturbate with sexual intent, they're just doing what feels good. Infants and toddlers may not yet be ready for the privacy discussion, but they will pick up on your attitude about self-pleasure if you swat their exploring hands away during bathtime or after a diaper change. Adolescents and teens grappling with sex education courses about STD and pregnancy prevention would probably welcome an upbeat reminder from you that masturbation offers a safe and pleasurable way to release sexual tension.

> I don't have any anxieties about masturbating. My mom encouraged me to masturbate when I was younger. She said it would help me learn what I liked sexually.

> When I was little (6 or 8), I was sure there was something terribly wrong with me for having what I now know were orgasms. I finally gathered my courage and asked my mother about them, and she was fantastic. My fears died down after that. In reaction to the turmoil I felt then, I have fought inside myself and in the community to foster good feelings and clear consciences about self-pleasuring.

As these women show, discussing masturbation with your child in a direct, permissive manner lays the groundwork for a healthy sexual self-esteem. However, this isn't something that comes naturally for most of us, so it's in your best interest to do a little planning and research to sharpen your communication skills. Fortunately there are some excellent websites and books for parents and kids that can prepare you for questions children are most likely to ask. Our own book *The Mother's Guide to Sex* explains the various stages of children's sexual development and offers age-appropriate advice on talking to kids about sex.

> I was 13 when I read a book about sex that belonged to my parents (I found it and managed to sneak a read). This book was very explicit about the clitoris and about masturbation, so I decided to try it and did so, very successfully, that night after I went to bed. I had my first-ever orgasm after only a couple of minutes and even that first time I remember I had to stuff my face into the pillow to stifle my cries. I thought the whole thing was wonderful, absolute magic—I was completely hooked.

How Do I Love Me? Let Me Count the Ways...

So you've made it this far in a chapter on masturbation, and now you're ready for a little action. Before we describe the most common ways folks masturbate, we'd like to encourage everyone—whether you're a seasoned masturbator or new to the activity—to spend a lazy afternoon exploring your body. The following section is geared toward women who need a little practice masturbating, but we invite you all to participate!

If You're Preorgasmic

"Preorgasmic" is the word used to describe women who have never had an orgasm before. Sex therapists generally prescribe a series of masturbation exercises, which, if performed regularly, succeed in teaching most women how to achieve orgasm. The best and most thorough do-it-yourself book is *For Yourself* by Lonnie Barbach. Betty Dodson's videos *Selfloving* and *Celebrating Orgasm* demonstrate techniques for increasing arousal and achieving orgasm. Most programs suggest that you set aside at least an hour a day for several weeks for a masturbation session. During each session your goal is to free yourself from distractions and to focus your attention solely on your body and how you're making it feel good. Here are some basics:

GET IN THE MOOD: You should be completely alone during your session. It's important to relax as much as you can. Let go of all those distracting worries about work or family. If you've got any guilt feelings about masturbating, try to check them at the door. Let your mind wander to images or thoughts that you find arousing. You may want to replay an exciting past sexual encounter. Perhaps you have a favorite fantasy, or even an image of yourself in some erotic environment. If watching yourself in a mirror turns you on, try that. If music, videos, or reading material help, try those. Remove your clothes if you like, and explore the sensations of sun, soft sheets, or water against your skin. Run your hands along parts of your body, noticing which areas are more sensitive than others. Try a variety of touches: tickling, stroking, pinching, massaging.

GET TO KNOW YOURSELF: When you feel ready, touch your genitals, using the same variety of caresses that you did on the rest of your body. If you aren't familiar with the different parts of your vulva, get out a hand mirror and take a good look at yourself. Identify all the parts of your genital anatomy, and then gently touch the inner and outer lips, the clitoris, the vagina. Begin experimenting with different movements: try one finger or many, the palm of your hand, knuckles, anything to elicit a number of sensations. (If you are a man, alternate lighter and heavier pressure on parts of your penis and your testicles.) Stroke or squeeze, fast or slow; use fingers, knuckles, the palm of your hand, or both hands:

I like to lie on my back and stroke my breasts, squeeze my nipples gently, and stroke my thighs. Sometimes I use lotion. I then massage the lips of my vagina with my first two fingers, insert fingers into my vagina, and then when I feel really excited I put my two first fingers on either side of my clitoris and squeeze, and move them up and down—so the clitoris slides in its hood.

Lying back on my bed, I get excited touching my breasts, my stomach, my vulva, bringing the clit smell up to my nose—I love the wetness and moving my hips in a rocking motion. I can fantasize myself coming, or pick a book with arousing material and allow the words to guide my thoughts and my body.

The important thing is to experiment with these sensations, repeating the ones that feel especially good. Let your mind pursue erotic thoughts as your arousal heightens. Continue in this manner until you feel like stopping or until you orgasm. If you don't orgasm, that's okay—what's important is your discovery of what feels good. You can build on this the next time you masturbate.

KEGELS: Insert your finger into your vagina and explore all around the inside in a clockwise manner. Try

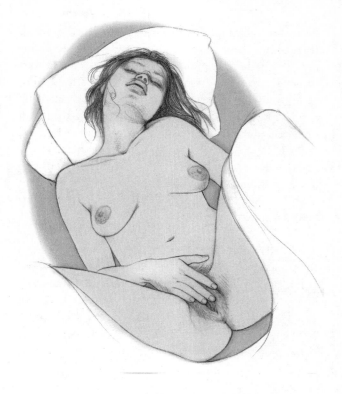

Masturbating with fingers

squeezing your PC muscle (this is the muscle you use to stop a stream of urine) and watching it contract around your finger. Building up this muscle can help you experience greater sensation and stronger orgasms. For more on Kegel exercises, see the Sexual Anatomy 101 chapter.

BREATHE: Many women hold their breath during sexual arousal, but are surprised to discover that deep breathing can result in stronger orgasms. Take regular deep breaths, and exhale through your mouth. As you approach orgasm try to time your exhale with your orgasmic release, and you'll feel the contraction ripple throughout your body. It's fine to hold your breath if this works better for you, but as you get more comfortable with your orgasms, experiment with inhaling and exhaling. You might also find that timing your breaths with some regular pelvic rocking (rather than remaining rigid) helps circulate the sexual energy throughout your body.

BE PATIENT: Try not to get too fixated on the orgasm or else "trying too hard" might kill your arousal. It's not unusual for it to take an hour of stimulation to bring you to the edge, so remaining patient and focused is important. If you find you're easily distracted, try reading some erotica or looking at a video to maintain your state of arousal. Take little breaks if you start to get frustrated. When you resume the stimulation, you'll find your place again. If you find you get really aroused but are having difficulty letting go into an orgasm, reduce the intensity of your stimulation and build back up. You'll find that stopping and starting again will get you nearer the orgasm than applying a steady stimulation, which only desensitizes you after a while. Try to relax other parts of your body and concentrate on your genitals.

TRY TOYS: You can also try adding some toys for a little variety. Vibrators are ideal for women whose hands tire easily or who need more intense stimulation, and many have the added attraction of more than one speed (see the Vibrators chapter). A stream of water from the tub or a shower hose can be a welcome alternative, offering variation in temperature and pressure.

FOLLOW THROUGH: Once you slide into orgasm, don't stop the stimulation unless it's too sensitive to continue. Many women experience a more satisfying orgasm this way, and in some cases it can even lead to a second one.

What's it like? Many women will tell you that you'll know an orgasm when you have one (see the Sexual Anatomy 101 chapter for descriptions).

> The very first time I masturbated, and actually had an orgasm, it was the most wonderful feeling I had ever had. I finally knew what all the hubbub was about, because I was standing in my bathroom, and my knees almost collapsed under me.

This isn't true for everyone, however, and first orgasms don't always come off like bombs bursting in air. A slight bump in your sexual response might leave you wondering "Was that it?" It may or may not be; we can only advise you to pay attention to the signs: engorged genitals, uterine contractions, sensations that shoot through your body. If you think you've had an orgasm, but were disappointed with the results, take a break and try again another time. Whatever your experience, try not to worry, for there are plenty of ways to enhance your experience of arousal. If you can enjoy the ride rather than focusing all your energy on the goal, you're more likely to make progress.

Changing Your Style

Perhaps you have no difficulty orgasming but would like to change your routine. Most of us have one tried-and-true method of masturbating—which is perfectly fine—but you may want to experiment with a little variation at some point. Masturbating with a variety of methods has several advantages.

For one thing, you increase your options for pleasure and learn more about your sexual responses. A vibrator-induced orgasm will feel different than one brought about by your finger, just as a penis positioned under a flow of water will experience different sensations than one thrusting in and out of your hand. This, in turn, will allow you more freedom when it comes to deciding where and how you want to indulge in solo sex. It might be hard to masturbate on the roofdeck of your apartment if you only know how to come in the bathtub.

For another, masturbation can have some pretty nice ramifications for partner sex. As a boy you may have had to masturbate on the sly, so coming quickly was key. While there's nothing wrong with coming quickly as an adult, you might want a little more control over timing so that you're not always beating your partner to the punch. Similarly, if you're able to get off from a variety of methods, it'll probably be easier for your partner to please you in many different ways.

Finally, the more ways you learn to come, the better equipped you'll be to adapt to the ways in which your sex life will change over the years. Women often find that their orgasmic patterns change during pregnancy, postpartum, and after menopause. Age, injury, and various medications can all affect your sexual response, but if you're not completely dependant on one method of achieving orgasm, you'll be able to slip into a new routine with little anxiety or stress. For more on this subject, see the Sex Over a Lifetime chapter.

How to go about altering your pattern? It's important to get in the mood, go slow, vary the stimulation, and practice! Hard as it sounds, you might try depriving yourself of your favorite technique. This will help your desire build, which could make you more receptive to different kinds of stimulation. Who knows, you may one day find yourself capable of masturbating to orgasm without ever touching yourself at all:

> The most memorable time I ever experienced masturbating was when I accomplished my first orgasm without the help of any stimulation. I lay on my bed and mentally stimulated my thoughts and body.

How To

There is no single "right" or "best" way to masturbate. Really, can you imagine someone telling you you're masturbating the wrong way? A lot of people have a favorite method, but this changes from person to person, and your favorite way today might be old hat tomorrow. During one of our continuing education nights at Good Vibrations, eighteen of us went around in a circle and described our favorite way to masturbate. It was astonishing, because though many of us used the same toy, or stimulated the same general area, no one masturbated in exactly the same way. Think about all the things that can vary from person to person, like *position:* sitting, squatting, standing up, lying down on your stomach, back, or side, knees up or down, legs open or closed; or *pressure:* fast or slow, stop and start, or continuous, hard or soft. Toss in a variety of toys or different locales, and you've got endless possibilities for a good time.

Sitting naked, watching gay pornos, right-hand "jacking," left hand on the remote, fast-forwarding to the good parts. I enjoy a basic up-and-down motion—basic but beautiful.

My favorite method is a toss-up between hand or vibrator on my clit, either in a car or in the dark. I also like to masturbate in a pool with the water from the jet hitting my clit.

I strip naked, lie on the bed, then warm myself up by playing with my nipples, rubbing my thighs, and fingering myself till wet. Once excited, I use a dildo to fill me up and, at the same time, use a battery-operated vibrator to play with my clit.

I like manual stimulation (my first two fingers moving in circles over my clitoris) while I'm kneeling. Sometimes I put a finger inside me and use my thumb on my clit. My girlfriend rubs her clit while she's driving and has an orgasm with her pants on!

I enjoy using a vibrator and sometimes a dildo or candlestick at the same time. I also like oral stimulation: eating a banana or Vienna sausages while masturbating. I am very oral, used to smoke while doing it, but have quit for health.

We can't emphasize enough the individual, experimental approach to masturbation. Unfortunately, in all the hoopla over the clitoral-versus-vaginal orgasm and the endless quest for the G-spot, we tend to lose sight of the fact that any way you come is the best way! What follows are brief descriptions of a few different methods, with quotes from people telling it like it is for them!

Women

Studies suggest that at least 70 percent of women masturbate. Many women like to combine a variety of activities as part of their solo sex ritual. Use one hand to stimulate yourself while caressing your body with the other. Alternate or combine clitoral, vaginal, or anal stimulation. Try doing Kegel exercises, taking deep breaths, and rocking your pelvis in time with your breathing to see how this enhances your arousal. Add a little lube for a different sensation but especially if you'll be inserting your toys. Get off on a good fantasy or enjoy some porn as you play with yourself.

Clitoral Stimulation

HAND, FINGERS: This involves stimulation (rubbing, stroking, pinching) of the clitoris with one or more fingers or the palm of your hand. Some find direct contact with the clitoris too intense, and prefer stimulation near or around the clitoris more pleasurable. Others prefer to have a layer of clothing or some other fabric between the hand and clit. Alternate touching your clit with stroking your labia, your vagina, or your anus.

I prefer manual stimulation with the flat of my hand and fingers inside my vagina.

I love fingering my clitoris with my index finger and thumb while reading or watching porn.

I lubricate my vulva with baby oil and rub my clit with two fingers until it gets hard. I often use a dildo in my vagina or a butt plug.

The middle finger of my right hand rubs my clit. I start rubbing just to the right of my clit, then quickly move to the left side where it remains for most of the session.

My left hand is holding the wrist of my right hand. I'm lying on my back, with my legs spread, but sometimes I prefer raising my knees to my head.

Lying on my back with my legs as tightly together as possible. Tickling my clitoris with one finger kind of bent-up very lightly.

WATER: A shower massager with a hose attachment will render any tubless shower a masturbation den. The added attraction of the shower massager is the versatile control that switches the water from a steady stream to a pulsating jet spray. Keep one hand free and adjust the temperature or water pressure for even more variety. Hot-tub jets are fun, too.

I lie in the bathtub on my back and spread my legs beneath the faucet. I turn the water to a small but steady warm stream and let it flow onto my clit. I hold my lips open and move my hips up and down. Absolutely magnificent. It feels a lot like a good licking.

I can't begin to count the times I was lolling in a swimming pool somewhere, ostensibly reading a paperback and sipping a cold drink, while really positioning myself over the heating jets, always keeping a straight face...ah, bliss!

I had a very close relationship with my shower head when I was growing up. I used it every time I took a shower. I remember my mom commenting on my excellent hygiene!

RUBBING AGAINST AN OBJECT: Press against some object to stimulate the clitoris. Many discovered this pleasure by lying on top of a pillow or a piece of furniture, while others found it by pressing against the washing machine during the spin cycle or rubbing against the crotch seam in a pair of jeans!

I was going to sleep one night and the duvet rubbed up against my clitoris when I lay down and I had this urgency to get up and start right away!

I love to balance myself on a corner of the ottoman in our living room. I rub my clit on the corner and periodically lift my hands and my feet off the ground. This gives me an exquisite feeling of flying when I come.

VIBRATORS: These are used primarily for clitoral stimulation, though many women also use these electric or battery-powered toys for vaginal or anal stimulation. They can be combined with different toys and used in any number of positions:

I prefer lying in bed with sexy music, rubbing my body with scented oil, fingering my nipples, and using the Hitachi Magic Wand on my clit.

I enjoy lying on top of my vibrator and whacking myself on the butt.

I most enjoy vaginal penetration with firm, fast strokes, usually using a vibrator. I like to have one hand playing with my nipples.

Clit Pumps

Pumps have traditionally been thought of as men's toys, but lately women have discovered the pleasures of clit pumping. A little cap for the clitoris is attached by a tube to a pump—squeezing the pump creates a vacuum and suction that can temporarily engorge your clit with blood. Some pumps also offer vibration. Use lube to make a good seal, and release the suction every few minutes. You can also use clit pumps on nipples.

G-Spot/Vaginal Stimulation

Inserting a vibrator or dildo into the vagina offers a feeling of fullness and can feel good alone or in conjunction with clitoral stimulation.

Some of my most memorable masturbation experiences involved strange phallic substitutes in the years before I got my first dildo: travel toothbrush holder, toothpaste tube, hammer handle, screwdriver handle, Coke bottle, corn on the cob.

You can also try to locate and stimulate your G-spot (see the Sexual Anatomy 101 chapter) by inserting your fingers into your vagina, though you may find it difficult to get adequate stimulation through manual masturbation alone. Women who enjoy G-spot stimulation often use insertable toys—look for ones made of a firm material, especially those with a curved shape or a bend at the tip.

Anal Stimulation

The anus is extremely sensitive to touch. Many women enjoy stimulation of this area during masturbation or partner sex play. You can experiment with your fingers or anal toys either by themselves or in conjunction with clitoral or vaginal stimulation. Use plenty of lubricant!

I push a lubed-up dildo in and out with one hand, and either rub my clitoris or use a vibrator on my clitoris with the other hand. If using a vibrator, I'll also hold the vibrator against the dildo and up against my anus. Yeow!

Men

An estimated 94 percent of all men masturbate, many by the time they reach puberty. The penis, being a prominent, external organ, practically begs to be handled. You can heighten your pleasure by using a bit of lubricant (or saliva). One popular product is designed specifically for male masturbation. Developed by a concert pianist (what busy hands he must have!), Men's Cream is an oil-based cream that lasts a long time, heightens sensation, and cleans up easily. Men who've tried it rave about it. Look for it in sex stores and catalogs.

You might also like to combine a variety of activities as part of your solo sex play. Use one hand to stimulate yourself while caressing your body with the other. A lot of men like to massage or tug on the testicles while masturbating. Experiment with pinching your nipples or inserting an anal plug while masturbating. Try doing Kegel exercises, taking deep breaths, and rocking your pelvis in time with your breathing to see how this enhances your arousal. Get off on a good fantasy or enjoy some porn as you play with yourself.

Penile Stimulation

STROKING: Place one or both hands around the penis, and stroke up and down along the shaft. Variations include using a few fingers, using just your palms, changing your hand position, limiting your stroking to a certain section of the shaft or glans (particularly the frenulum), stroking in a specific direction, or encircling the head of the penis with

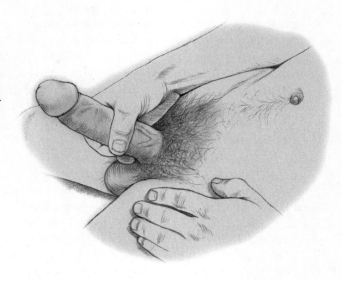

Masturbating with hand

each stroke. Another variation involves pressing your hand against your penis so that it rubs against your stomach as you stroke it. Or you could try wrapping your penis in a piece of clothing or fabric:

I often like to wrap my cock in a soft cloth to stroke it.

I like to be up on my haunches so that I can pull on my balls while stroking my cock gently. Most men like to stroke vigorously, in my experience, but I like it slow.

I lie in a recliner and apply some lotion. I use one hand on the shaft and rub the head, testes, and the area toward my anus with the other hand.

I put my thumb and two fingers of each hand around my dick and move up and down until I reach climax.

I like to cup my balls in my left hand and move up and down the shaft with my right hand whilst fantasizing of someone I love. I vary the speed and go to the verge of orgasm and then usually back off and approach orgasm a few times until I'm really anxious, and then I cross into orgasm.

I prefer rapid stroking with my hand encircling my penis—I usually take some pleasure in delaying orgasm. Occasionally I use lather or oil.

I love to tie off or stretch out my balls and look in the mirror at myself while I lube the head of my dick.

I much prefer to lie on my back and use my right hand to stroke the entire shaft of my penis. I may masturbate as much as an hour before orgasm.

I use a little shampoo or lube around the head and prefer straight wrist-pumping on my cock shaft. I also like a little nipple rubbing and a little fingering of my butthole.

SLAPPING, BEATING: This involves a steady slapping of the penis back and forth between two hands, or against the stomach or another object.

RUBBING AGAINST AN OBJECT: This is similar to the technique of women who like to rub their genitals against pillows or furniture. Try rolling over onto your stomach and rubbing your penis against the mattress, a pillow, clothes, or whatever you find does the trick!

I enjoy reading a dirty book and lying on my stomach pushing my cock against the surface I'm lying on.

I use a pillow underneath my stomach, thrusting between the pillow and sheets.

A pillow, a porn movie, and a couch. I usually fast-forward the porn tape to a section where entry and penetration of a woman is graphically shot. Next, I'll fold the pillow so that it engulfs my penis and, with sufficient pressure, match the porn stars in the movie "stroke for stroke." I'll either come on my stomach or towel off if I choose not to wear a condom.

INSERTING OR THRUSTING: Just as women have appropriated many a household appliance for insertion, so have men found a variety of things and places into which a penis can be inserted—socks, watermelons, warm banana skins, toilet paper rolls, soft eyeglass cases, and plastic blow-up dolls, to name just a few. Just remember to exercise caution and avoid getting stuck! One very popular sex toy for men is known as the Fleshlight. It's a sleeve sculpted from a very lifelike material called cyberskin, which is encased in a hard plastic shell. According to the Fleshlight's fans, this toy comes closest to simulating the feel of a real vagina.

Men with intact foreskins know that they are highly sensitive and may enjoy pulling the foreskin over the glans, so that it serves as a type of sleeve though which the penis can slide. The foreskin reduces friction between the glans and the hand as it thrusts into the hand.

One of the nicest toys for masturbation consists of a very soft latex sleeve, open at both ends, looser than a condom, but tight enough to stay on my erect penis even in the presence of lubricants.

I slick up my hand with water-soluble lubricant, grasp my penis, and try to simulate the feeling of a wet cunt, thrusting and caressing.

I sometimes put tissue around a knot hole in the floor and fuck through the floor.

PENIS PUMPS: Pumps have long been popular with men as masturbation devices. A generic pump consists of a long cylinder that fits over the penis and is attached to a pump. The pump creates a vacuum around the penis and pulls in blood to temporarily enlarge it, a feeling many men find pleasurable. Men who enjoy this type of stimulation play with varying degrees of pressure and suction. You should be sure to follow the recommendations for proper use and avoid using the pump at high pressure for longer than fifteen minutes at a stretch. Use ample amounts of a water-based lubricant inside the cylinder, as well as around the base of the penis, as this helps create a seal. Attachments for nipples and clits are available for some pumps. Penis pumps vary drastically in quality; if you're in the market for one, it pays to shop around for the good ones.

My husband LOVES his pump! He likes it the best for masturbation, but we also get off on admiring his ample member.

VIBRATORS: A variety of vibrators provide penile or anal stimulation. Back-of-the-hand models, vibrating sleeves, spot vibrators, and cylindrical and anal vibrators can all provide intense stimulation:

I like to slide my wife's battery vibrator along the shaft of my penis.

When I use a dildo inside me, I usually stimulate my penis with the other hand or with a powerful vibrator.

WATER: Women aren't the only ones who can spend suspiciously long periods of time in the bathtub! Many men have discovered the joys of placing the penis under a steady stream of water. Jacuzzi jets, pulsating shower-head attachments, or the stream from the tub faucet can all do the trick. Experiment with different areas on the penis. Many men report enjoying water stimulation the most when they are about two-thirds erect and often prefer a direct spray on or below the glans. Some uncircumcised men enjoy directing the stream of water underneath the foreskin.

Masturbating at age 14 involved bathing in a tub and stimulating myself using a hand-held shower head, directing the spray at the glans of my penis to give me curiously pleasurable and powerful sensations. I would lie on my back in the tub and hold the shower head over me. Then I found that the shower head was removable. I would remove it, turn over, belly down, squeeze the stream of water exiting the hose to make it stronger, and then direct this stream against the glans of my cock. This was astoundingly pleasurable.

Anal and Prostate Stimulation

The anus is highly sensitive to touch, and the prostate gland can be stimulated by inserting fingers or a toy into the rectum. Many men enjoy stimulation of this area during masturbation or partner sex play. You can experiment with your fingers or anal toys either by themselves or in conjunction with penile stimulation. Anal toys tend to come in two shapes. If you'll be inserting the toy and leaving it in, you'll want a "plug," which widens in the middle so that it stays put once inside. If you want to experiment with in-and-out sensations, get one that resembles a finger or small dildo, so that it slides in and out easily. Always choose a toy with a flared base if you'll be using it for anal play, to ensure that it doesn't slip out of reach.

My most memorable masturbation experiences actually involves some cross-dressing and anal "play." I will put on a tube dress and "mount" a dildo I have secured between the mattresses and ride it for a long time as I picture myself having sex with one of my partners.

Masturbation and Partners

Many of us may feel fine about masturbating in private, but when it comes to divulging this practice to a partner or—heaven forbid—actually masturbating in front of him or her, we'd sooner stop altogether. An interesting statistic comes from the Kinsey Institute citing a small study in which twenty-four couples were asked individually if they masturbated regularly. All forty-eight individuals responded yes. Some 92 percent of the husbands, however, did not know their wives masturbated, while only 6 percent of the wives thought their husbands did not. While we won't go into what this says about gender stereotypes, what's startling is how common it is to conceal one's masturbatory habits from a partner.

An overwhelming number of our survey respondents confessed to changing their masturbation habits when partnered versus single. Of those who elaborated, some explained that they got so much satisfaction from partner sex that they no longer wanted (or needed) to masturbate. Others cut down on masturbating because they didn't want their partners to know they did it. In either case, there seems to be a general belief that masturbation should not be part of partner sex.

These are some of the anxieties that were expressed, along with our suggestions for overcoming them:

When a lover walks in, I feel caught and have to work to overcome that feeling.

This may be triggered by your own ancient associations of masturbation with shame. If your partner is making you feel bad for masturbating, try to find out what's really causing his or her resentments. Only by discussing your anxieties about masturbation can you hope to overcome them. It may be a fear of rejection:

I once masturbated while kissing a woman, but when I finished she started crying. She took it as a personal rejection.

When I masturbate he asks plaintively, "Ain't I enough?" and seems to be in competition with my toys.

Try describing your solo sex as a complementary sexual activity, not a replacement for partner sex. Invite your partner to participate if you like. Perhaps simply sharing the act will supplant the feeling of rejection with one of adventurous experimentation.

People expressed concern that masturbation would reduce their desire to have sex with a partner:

I'm afraid if I masturbate too much, I won't get turned on by my partner.

If you're worried that you'll "spend" all your sexual energy masturbating and have little left for a partner, you should try it first. Many people find the opposite is true:

If I'm getting a lot of sex I tend to masturbate more— I get greedy.

Now that I'm married I sometimes masturbate when my sex drive is flagging—to get myself more in the mood.

You could also try to stop thinking of masturbation and partner sex as an either/or choice—"Either I have sex with myself, or I have it with a partner." As you probably surmised from the preceding section, we want you to have it both ways! If you enjoy masturbating, do it in front of or with your partner periodically. This both adds a new twist to partner sex and satisfies your lusty masturbatory urges.

Masturbation can also come in handy if you and your partner have different sexual schedules. Maybe your sex drive is strongest in the morning, but hers peaks at night. In fact, no two people will always be in the mood at the same time, so if you're both comfortable with masturbation you won't have to keep taking cold showers.

Sometimes I get so good at self-pleasuring, I worry that a partner will never be able to offer the same perfect stimulation.

Sometimes I think that if my sole sexual release is through masturbation, I will not be able to orgasm with other kinds of stimulation. I notice that I need a lot of stimulation on my cock to keep it hard.

If your partner aims to please, he or she will make a very attentive student. Masturbating is an excellent way to instruct a lover in the finer points of pleasure. We expect people to know intuitively how to please us, but unless we're willing to show them, we may indeed be disappointed.

Sometimes I'm afraid I will become a hermit and not look for partners anymore because reaching orgasm and enjoying self-stimulation is so satisfying and simple.

It's true that the beauty of masturbation is that it is an easy and extremely rewarding activity, but it doesn't satisfy our need for human interaction. Whispering "I love you" to yourself is a most respectable practice, but it won't necessarily have the same effect that it would coming from a lover's lips.

Mutual Masturbation

Watching him masturbate is just incredibly sexy because I can see what he's feeling in ways that I can't when I'm involved. It's so clear that he is intensely inside himself and his desire. It makes me jealous in this really neat way. I could swallow him whole, I think. Masturbating in front of him is great because I really enjoy my reactions—how wet I get, my sounds, my smell, how freely I can move—and I know that I am completely turning him on.

Throughout this chapter we've made references to the benefits of masturbating with a partner, otherwise known as mutual masturbation. In view of the difficulty people have sharing their masturbation practices with a partner, we'd like to summarize a few of the benefits of this practice, in the hopes that it will inspire you to give it a try:

- It is an ideal form of safe sex for new lovers.
- Seasoned lovers can enjoy incorporating their previously "secret practice" into sex play.
- You both don't have to be "in the mood" to enjoy this activity.
- It brings out the voyeur in you.
- It brings out the exhibitionist in you.
- It alleviates performance anxiety for your partner or for both of you.
- You get exactly the kind of stimulation you like best.
- Your lover learns first hand (no pun intended) what kind of stimulation you like best.
- It's a nice alternative to your usual sexual routine.
- It can help you through periods in life when your sexual responses may be changing.
- For young or new lovers, it's a great alternative to "going all the way."
- Try it during cybersex: It's the "next best thing to being there."

I was pregnant and the doctor had told me that I shouldn't have sex for a while because the penetration could be harmful to my cervix, so my partner and I sat on opposite ends of the bed and watched each other masturbate

I was being "faithful" to my boyfriend but met another man whom I found attractive. We decided it was only unfaithful if we touched each other/saw each other naked, so we both lay under covers—him on the floor, me in bed—and talked utter filth to each other while masturbating. A true "head-fuck" that lasted for about eight hours and still brings a smile to my face when I think about it.

Mutual masturbation can take any form you'd like. Although the term "mutual masturbation" implies that you're both jerking yourselves off at the same time, we encourage you to broaden the definition to include hand jobs (see below), fantasy, timing, and toys. Consider these variations:

SIMULTANEOUS: Masturbate yourselves at the same time while watching each other.

TIMING: Masturbate with your eyes closed and try to come when the other is ready. Try adding a little verbal sex play to stoke the other's fantasies.

TAKE TURNS: Flip a coin to see who goes first; if you're first, you masturbate while your partner attends to other parts of your body. Then trade off.

DOUBLE DUTY: Masturbate yourself with one hand and jerk your partner off with your other hand. Challenging, yes, but quite a turn-on.

POSITIONS: Try a variety of positions—use a low-key approach and take turns lying in each other's arms, or adopt any one of your favorite intercourse positions. Sixty-nine gives you a nice visual (great for learning a thing or two about a partner's preferred method) and an opportunity to add a little tongue play; doggie style gives the person in back nice access to both partners' genitals; sitting facing each other with legs entwined allows you to gaze lovingly into each other's eyes.

BODY PARTS: Rub your genitals along parts of your partner's body. You can simulate intercourse in the missionary position by rubbing the penis along the clitoral shaft; just remember that it is possible to get pregnant if any semen gets in the vagina.

TOYS, TOYS, TOYS: Take turns using your favorite vibrator on one another—either you or your partner can run the controls. Find a toy that provides direct stimulation to your genitals (vibrators, sleeves, etc), or accessorize with other items: nipple clamps, butt plugs, body paints, etc.

If that's not enough to inspire a little creative exploration, just read these testimonials from fans of mutual masturbation:

Mutual masturbation is my favorite sexual activity that does not involve penetration. My girlfriend and I sometimes still need to masturbate to reach orgasm. It is such a turn-on to see her touching herself, and she feels the same way. Sometimes I lie on top of her and touch myself while she is touching herself. I come when I feel her bucking under me when she comes. It is so steamy.

My lover and I discovered hot mutual masturbation when I was pregnant and wanted to try nonintercourse sex play. I was on my back (with lots of pillows) with a vibrator between my legs while he stood over me stroking his cock right in my line of vision.

My lover likes watching me when I masturbate. She'll pick up on my lead and soon we're rubbing our clits in synch!

When I masturbate with a partner I'm louder—for dramatic effect!

Mutual masturbation can be an incredibly intimate experience, as it requires you to let your guard down if it's to be highly pleasurable. It demands openness, trust, and caring.

Hand Jobs

Many people find masturbation to be one of the most satisfying aspects of their sexual repertoire—do you know why? Because we each know how to make ourselves come better than anyone else. Now imagine if your partner mastered your own special technique, and was able to get you off in the way you like best—

His and Hers Masturbation Sites

Jack and Jill may have gone up the hill, but their hands were too busy with other matters to fetch the pail of water. Don't ask us how these nursery rhyme characters got to be euphemisms for masturbation, ask the folks running the best websites on the subject:

Jackinworld.com
Launched in response to the firing of U.S. Surgeon General Joycelyn Elders for her promasturbation stance, Jackinworld is the ultimate male masturbation resource. Frank and nonjudgmental discussions of technique, penis size, foreskins, lube, and toys accompany excellent illustrations of male anatomy. Founder M. J. Ecker says that about half of Jackinworld's audience is made up of teenage boys whose favorite questions are about penis size and circle jerks. "The most tenacious myth I encounter is that 'only losers masturbate'," says M. J. "In their circle, if you masturbate it means you're not scoring with the chicks or you're queer. And yet, they're all masturbating, so this adds an element of guilt and shame to what should just be a pleasurable activity." This type of attitude inspires M. J.'s zeal in spreading Jackinworld's message: "I want to contribute to people's peace of mind, and help them experience guilt-free pleasure as much as possible!"

Clitical.com
Women can log on to Clitical, a site devoted largely to female masturbation. According to Jenne, Clitical's founder, "By creating a place where others can share their techniques, stories, and thoughts, we hope to dispel so many of the myths surrounding female sexuality." Clitical exists primarily to disprove the stereotype that women don't masturbate. "Many people still believe that it's okay for men to do it, but not women. We hope to get the message out that masturbation is the best and safest way to understand your body." Clitical visitors are treated to masturbation stories, detailed instructions about technique, lists of masturbation's benefits, and a photo gallery with diverse images of nude women. Clitical's upbeat writing and supportive community guarantee a satisfying visit.

---

that would be some gift! Hand jobs come in, well, handy, because you can give them anywhere, anytime, and they're incredibly gratifying when done right.

But giving a good hand job is a learned skill, a skill that will be refined to suit the particular needs of each partner. Not everyone likes a counterclockwise stroking of the clit with two fingers, or a hard and fast assault on the penis; the only way to learn your partner's favorite method is by watching closely and practicing. Keep in mind these tips when perfecting your hand job technique:

GET COMFORTABLE: A tired hand or awkward posture can kill the mood, so try out a few spots to see what works best. Lie beside a woman's body, so that your hand on her vulva approximates the angle that hers would have if she were masturbating while lying on her back. Sit by a man's side or kneel between his spread legs for a wider range of movement.

LUBE IT UP: Some people may prefer a "dry" rub, but most like the slippery sexiness of a wet hand job.

Your own juices may dry up and result in chafing, so keep a bottle of lube on hand and apply generously.

ASK FOR HELP: Have your partner place his or her hand over yours and direct the movement so that you can get a sense of the desired pacing and pressure. When you're on your own, check for visual or verbal cues from your partner to ensure that you're on the right track. If you're unsure, just ask.

KEEP BOTH HANDS BUSY: If both hands are free, use them unless it's too distracting. While one hand works the penis or vulva, the other can explore nipples, testicles, anus, perineum, or other sweet spots on the body.

FOLLOW THROUGH: A common instinct is to stop the stimulation once your partner starts coming, but most men and women find that continued stimulation through climax is ideal. You can always opt for this method, and can ask your partner to give you a sign, or can simply remove your hand when enough is enough.

Masturbators, Unite!

Although that may sound like a call for a circle jerk (and if it inspires you, go for it), it's actually our humble plea for all you masturbators to stand up and be counted. We know there are thousands of you happily engaged in this pursuit of pleasure, but public awareness of masturbation as a powerful and accessible source of sexual pleasure is fleeting at best. We've seen numerous TV sitcoms address the subject with humor, magazines pop up devoted to the subject, and celebrities admit to doing it. But we've also seen a Surgeon General dismissed for acknowledging its existence, and we wouldn't be surprised if public admission to the act was used to malign someone in an election year. As one TV dad tells his masturbating, adolescent son, "Everyone does it, but no one talks about it."

If you're like us, you're fed up with masturbation's bad reputation. Would you like to take matters into your own hands? Join in the celebration of National Masturbation Month, which Good Vibrations instituted in 1996. Every May, friends, customers, businesses, politicians, celebrities, and anyone who's ever twanged the wire or tiptoed through the two lips are invited to celebrate this popular pastime. We know many of you can't join us in San Francisco, but there are plenty of ways to pay tribute to masturbation, both publicly and privately, in your own hometown.

- *Choose one day to honor as National Masturbation Day by indulging in your own private celebration.* Call in late for work so that you can take an extra hour enjoying a bit of self-pleasure. Convince your coworkers to do the same, then fantasize about business as usual coming to a halt while everyone is home playing with themselves! We dare you to put a message on your answering machine telling callers why you're indisposed.

- *Send a proclamation to your mayor asking her or him to officially sanction May as National Masturbation Month.* Our mayor didn't endorse our proclamation—maybe he was too busy with a little one-handed business of his own.

- *Engage in a bit of healthy voyeurism—watch others masturbate.* We held a screening at a local theater and showed masturbation clips from X-rated videos to sold-out audiences. If you can't make it to San Francisco, and your local theater would rather show Disney movies, do a little at-home viewing. Check the videography section of this book for some notable masturbation movies and cue them up with your friends, with your partner, or by yourself. If porn doesn't inspire, try the real thing—dedicate an evening to watching your partner masturbate, and vice versa.

- *Home school.* There's no time like the present to improve your own technique. Check out one of the excellent books, videos, or websites in our resource listings to gain a few tips from your fellow masturbators.

- *Start a Masturbation Hall of Fame.* Know someone who has come out of the masturbators closet in a public way? Send them a note of appreciation and tell them they've been inducted into the Masturbation Hall of Fame. We wrote biographies of famous folks who've spoken publicly or written about masturbation and pioneers who've devoted their lives to its liberation. We displayed these in our store, much to our customers' delight.

- *Come up with your top ten reasons to masturbate.* We held a contest that drew hundreds of entries. Many participants said simply composing their lists was very empowering. Our favorite entry won the "most universal" prize: "fingers, freedom, fantasies, convenience, nostalgia, pleasure, love, hope, self-esteem, and fun."

- *Spread the word!* Phone your friends, family, and coworkers, or start your own letter-writing campaign. Announce it on your web page, post it to a newsgroup, or email all your acquaintances.

- *Start your own celebration.* We were tickled to discover the formation of The Masturbation Society at Miami University, whose stated purpose is to promote safer sex, to challenge stereotypes, and to "strive toward manual dexterity and hand–eye coordination!" We also learned we were not alone in hoping to honor masturbation with its own month; one men's group advocates creation of "Monkey Spank Month" on its web page.

The sky's the limit, depending on your imagination. A Good Vibrations customer wrote a letter to Hallmark chastising them for producing dozens of cards for Secretary's Day but not a single sentiment for Masturbation Day! With grassroots support like that, it won't be long before government employees get the day off.

Betty Dodson

"Masturbation is the ongoing love affair that each of us has with ourselves throughout our lifetime."

At 72, Betty Dodson is not your average grandmother. There are no biological offspring playing with Leggos and Barbies on her living room rug. No, Betty is affectionately known as "the grandmother of masturbation," and her charges come to her house to play with vibrators and vaginal barbells as part of her masturbation workshops.

The image of fifteen women lying nude in Betty's living room jerking off with Hitachi Wands may strike many as daring or risqué, but to the thousands of women who've learned how to orgasm this way, Betty is nothing less than a miracle worker. Her Bodysex workshops (which, after twenty-seven years, have now given way to private sessions) epitomize Betty's lifelong commitment to her self-proclaimed goal: liberating masturbation.

"Taking sex into your own hands is my credo," she says. "Masturbation is our first natural sexual activity. It is the ongoing love affair that each of us has with ourselves throughout our lifetime." Having witnessed tremendous numbers of women faking orgasm during group sex parties she attended in the sixties, Betty realized that cultural denial of masturbation underlies our sexual repression, so she decided to change that sad state of affairs, one orgasm at a time.

A classically trained fine artist, Betty dazzled the New York art world with an exhibition of her erotic nudes in the late sixties. In 1973, she wowed the attendees at a National Organization for Women conference with a slide show of female vulvas, or what she jokingly refers to as "split beaver for feminists." She received a standing ovation, which inspired her to take her show on the road, so that women everywhere could learn that their genitals were not "nasty, ugly, smelly or shameful. I wanted to show the world how beautiful they are."

Indeed, few have done more when it comes to teaching women to be "cunt positive" than Betty. Her descriptions of genital show-and-tell in her book *Sex for One* are positively lyrical: "we discovered when the hood was pulled back and each clitoris appeared that the variations were astounding—from tiny seed pearls to rather large protruding jewels." The accompanying pen-and-ink drawings of sixteen women's vulvas possess extraordinary detail and are downright rapturous. View one of Betty's video documentaries of her Bodysex workshops (*Selfloving, Celebrating Orgasm*), and you'll see a variety of real women's genitals (nothing airbrushed, no body makeup) in various stages of arousal.

Betty Dodson's most far-reaching contribution to women's masturbation emancipation, *Liberating Masturbation*, began as a slim, self-published book. "Between 1973 and 1986, I sold 150,000 copies of *Liberating Masturbation*. I stamped each one of them by hand (what I like to call a 'monumental hand job') and schlepped them to the post office each week in my old dilapidated grocery cart. I felt like I was mailing out an orgasm to every woman that ordered it."

Asked what she's found to be the most tenacious misconception about masturbation, Betty replied, "Women fear their partners will feel inadequate if they masturbate (which is often true) and men want to be the source of women's orgasms with penis/vagina sex. Both women and men are under the misconception that masturbation is not real sex and that partner sex is the best." Fortunately, Betty's newest book, *Orgasms for Two: Discovering the True Joy of Partnersex*, tackles this issue head on. Don't expect this grandma to rest on her laurels anytime soon!

Visit Betty Dodson's website at www.bettydodson.com.

CHAPTER 7

Lubrication

Who Needs a Lubricant?

At Good Vibrations, we consider lubricant one of life's more enjoyable essentials, right up there with bread, wine, and a decent cup of coffee. Every time a customer approaches the front counter at our store preparing to purchase a dildo, butt plug, or insertable vibrator, we ask politely, "Do you have some lubricant to go with that?" The responses we get can include blank looks or even hostile glares. A lot of people have been led to believe that their own bodies should generate enough lubrication to keep any sexual situation slippery, and they take the suggestion that this might not be the case as an insult to their sexual prowess. Of course, men are aware that their penises produce only a small amount of "pre-come" fluid when they're aroused, but many women and men believe that vaginal lubrication is an automatic physical result of a woman's sexual arousal and that lack of lubrication suggests a lack of sincere enthusiasm:

> I occasionally use lube when I have trouble getting wet. But I feel better when I get wet enough on my own—that usually means I'm into it more.

> I don't generally use lube—I want to do it on my own. It feels like admitting that my body is abnormal or dysfunctional. I don't know why. I'm trying to get over it.

In fact, vaginal lubrication doesn't automatically follow sexual arousal and doesn't automatically indicate sexual arousal. Lubricating is influenced by hormonal fluctuations and can vary dramatically, depending on where a woman is in her menstrual cycle. Women who have reached menopause, have had a hysterectomy, or have just given birth or are breast feeding will experience a decrease in their natural lubrication as well as a thinning of vaginal tissues as a result of reduced estrogen levels:

> I used lubricant following the birth of my child, when my tissues were tender and dry.

> I should use lube, but I'm ashamed to admit it. I know that decreased vaginal lubrication happens in middle-age, but it's a hard thing for me to accept and even harder to share with my partner.

Hormones aren't the sole influences on vaginal lubrication. Alcohol, marijuana, and over-the-counter cold medications dry up all mucous membranes—those in your head and those between your legs. The popular antidepressants known as SSRIs (selective serotonin reuptake inhibitors), such as Prozac, Paxil, and Zoloft, can negatively affect sexual response, which includes reducing vaginal lubrication. Certain medical conditions, such as diabetes, also reduce lubrication and blood flow to the genitals. And, of course, stress can throw almost any "natural" physical response off kilter.

> *Astroglide helped a lot when I was first on Prozac and had a hard time getting aroused or staying wet.*

Besides, even those situations in which a woman is lubricating heavily can be enhanced by the addition of artificial lubricants. Vaginal secretions don't necessarily make their way up to the clitoris, and most women enjoy direct stimulation of the clitoris far more when the touch is smooth and moist. Lubricant makes any kind of vaginal penetration more pleasurable—it's always more comfortable to have two wet surfaces sliding against each other—and is essential for anal penetration.

> *We use lube liberally. Sometimes friction is desirable, but most times "slipping and sliding" is better and allows us to play longer.*

> *My belief is that you can never have too much lube. The slipperier it is around my clit, the better.*

Whenever a customer returns from a first encounter with a new dildo or butt plug confessing that it was just "too big," we double-check that she or he took plenty of time to relax and used lots of lube. Lubes are a crucial accompaniment to anal insertion, as the anus and rectum don't produce any natural lubrication, and they're invaluable for vaginal insertion as well—many dildos have a sort of velvety surface texture that will absorb your natural juices, resulting in an unpleasant friction that only a lubricant can tame.

> *I didn't use lube for a long time. I thought it was kind of wussy. But now I've seen the light.... Lube is GREAT! I wish I'd had lube during some of my past experiences.*

What's in a Lube?

If all of life's minor inconveniences could be solved as cheaply, easily, and enjoyably as the insufficiency of natural lubrication, the world would be a wonderful place. There's a dazzling array of options when it comes to artificial lubricants. You can shop for lube in a bottle, or simply open the refrigerator—some folks swear that egg whites make a great organic lube.

Oils

For hundreds of years oils have been used as lubricants, but there are some facts you should bear in mind to have the best possible experience when anointing yourself for sex. Genital tissue is sensitive and easily irritated, so you should stay away from scented oils. Stick to pure, lightweight vegetable or mineral oils. Lotions and creams are absorbed into the skin too quickly to make very effective lubricants. Oils, which stay slippery indefinitely, are very popular for male genital massage, aka hand jobs. Men who enjoy using oils for masturbation often develop passionate preferences, from the classic Albolene hand cream, to coconut oil, to the latest and greatest Men's Cream. This petroleum- and Vitamin E–based formula boasts an enthusiastic fan club.

While women can also enjoy using oils for masturbation, we do entreat you not to use Vaseline or any petroleum product as a vaginal lubricant. This stuff is extremely hard to wash out of your body. Vaseline is likely to remain coating the walls of your or your loved one's vagina for days, welcoming all kinds of bacteria and creating an environment that promotes yeast infections. In fact, all oils will linger in your vagina longer than you might wish, as there is no way for them to be flushed out of your body. And oils of any kind will destroy latex condoms, dental dams, gloves, or diaphragms, so oils are completely incompatible with practicing safer sex. Your best bet would be to restrict your genital use of oils to solo sex activities. (But keep in mind that oils will also ruin the surface of any sex toys that contain latex—which includes those made from jelly rubber and cyberskin.)

Water-Based Lubricants

The safest type of all-purpose lubricant is the water-based lubricant. This kind of lube is especially formulated to be taste-free, nonstaining, nonirritating to genital tissue, and easy to wash out of your body. Water-based lubes contain deionized (that is, purified) water, long-chain polymers (biologically inert plastics commonly found in foods and cosmetics), and a preservative (such as methyl paraben or propyl paraben) to prevent contamination by viruses or bacteria. Many water-based lubes also contain glycerin, a syrupy-sweet byproduct of fats, which adds a slippery quality. Like many fine things in life, water-based lubes are an acquired taste, and people's initial responses to them can be less than positive:

Using lubricant makes me feel like a frog swimming in a pond.

I don't use lube if I can help it—I hate it. Sticky, messy, yuck!

The sticky quality folks find disturbing about lube results when the friction of your activities causes water to evaporate, leaving only the polymer and glycerin ingredients on the surface of your skin. Customers frequently complain that water-based lube gets used up too quickly and that they have to keep applying more. Actually, you can reconstitute and reactivate the lube by simply adding some water or saliva to your genitals. We recommend keeping a glass of water or, for the playful, a water gun, by the bed. One good squirt with a plant mister, and your lube will be flowing again. Lubricant is specifically designed for use on moist membranes, where it should stay slippery. When applied to the rest of your body, it will dry, leaving a sticky residue, which makes it completely undesirable as a massage product. Glycerin-free lubes tend to be less sticky and are more likely to just absorb into the skin like a lotion. Lots of people like to wipe the lube off themselves with a warm washcloth after sex, to avoid the experience of hopping into the shower the next morning only to slide off their feet when water hits skin and reactivates the lube residue. (Keep this in mind if you're romping around a hot tub, and watch your step!)

For some people, the problem with lubricants is that they generate not too little but too *much* moisture:

Sometimes I don't want lubricant because it takes away a certain friction that is good when I have my vulva touched/rubbed. Without that friction, it doesn't feel as good.

GV Tale: Space-Age Serendipity

A revolutionary lube formula can have its genesis in the most unexpected places. Slippery Stuff was originally designed to make it easier for surfers and divers to slide in and out of their rubber wet suits. The manufacturers didn't take long to figure out that any liquid that remained slippery under water could be equally handy on dry land. Astroglide, an enduringly popular lube, was developed by a gentleman who had worked at NASA. When a female relative complained about postmenopausal loss of lubrication, he turned his attention to cooking up a useful aid. His final recipe was inspired by the fluid used to lubricate O-rings on space shuttles.

I hate when I can't get the traction I need. I also hate the cat-hair factor.

If you too crave more friction, by all means scrub that lubricant off your genitals with a washcloth, and you'll be back to your natural state in seconds. Whenever you feel "too wet," you should consider incorporating safer-sex supplies such as condoms, latex gloves, or dental dams into your activities—latex requires a lot of lubrication before it will get slippery.

As for the argument that water-based lubricants are too "messy," we have to wonder why anyone would want a sexual encounter to be tidy. Nobody refuses a massage on the grounds that it is "messy," and in fact water-based lubes are much easier to wash off both your body and your bed sheets than massage oils. It's true that some water-based lubricants are stringier than others and may form long, sticky strands that land on your sheets or in your hair on their journey from the bottle to your genitals, but a little practice will enable you to show the lube who's boss. The decision whether to apply a discreet dab or a big, sloppy handful is entirely yours.

I like the feeling of lube—that it is increasing the sexy wetness/messiness of sex.

Lube is the greatest thing to happen to sex right after the pill and the condom. You have to be very wet and relaxed to enjoy penetration—need I say more?

Silicone-Based Lubricants

Perhaps the hottest new lubes on the market are silicone-based—look for the brand names Eros Bodyglide and Wet Platinum. While they have a sleek, oily consistency, these lubes aren't greasy and are completely safe to use with latex (in fact, most prelubricated condoms are actually coated with silicone). Since silicone lubes contain no water or glycerin, they stay slippery almost indefinitely—so if you want to indulge your underwater sex fantasies, these are the lubes for you. Furthermore, they're taste-free. And if your thoughts are straying to leaky breast implants, fear not; silicone lubes are completely nontoxic, as the silicone molecules are too large to be absorbed into your system in any way.

Note a couple of downsides to silicone lubes: They're far pricier than water-based lubes. They require more effort in the clean-up department—you'll need soap and water to get them off your skin. Finally, silicone lubes don't interact well with silicone toys. While the effect is not as thoroughly destructive as the effect of oils on latex, a silicone lube can ruin the smooth surface of your silicone dildo, and we don't recommend combining the two.

Buying a Lubricant

Name-brand and generic water-based lubricants produced by major pharmaceutical companies can be found in drugstores across the country. These lubricants, such as KY Jelly, were originally formulated for use during medical exams, so they don't have the slippery properties of lubes specifically designed for sex. They tend to get tacky and "pill up" with extended use. For low cost and wide distribution, however, these over-the-counter lubricants can't be beat. Thanks to public health campaigns stressing the importance of using latex barriers in conjunction with water-based lubes to prevent disease transmission, mainstream companies are cooking up more sensual lubes. Johnson and Johnson have produced a sleeker KY Liquid, which is marketed explicitly as a sexual lubricant in women's magazines with ads promising "another good night's sleep, lost."

By and large, sexual lubricants are produced by small manufacturers and sold through adult bookstores, Internet retailers, and sex boutiques. Here in San Francisco, brands such as Astroglide, ForPlay,

---

Lube Shopping Checklist

✓ *Purpose*. Will you be using the lube with latex or for vaginal intercourse? Then look for water- or silicone-based lubes. Anal sex? Try a thicker lube. Oral sex? Avoid lubes containing nonoxynol-9. Want a lube with staying power? Try Liquid Silk or any silicone lube.

✓ *Sensitivities*. Do you have sensitive skin? Check that your lube doesn't contain methyl or propyl paraben or nonoxynol-9. Are you prone to yeast infections? You may want to avoid lubes containing glycerin.

✓ *Taste*. Do you want a lube with the least possible taste? Avoid lubes containing nonoxynol-9. Try Probe, Slippery Stuff, or silicone lubes.

✓ *Texture*. If you'd prefer a thinner lube, try Astroglide, ID Lube, or Slippery Stuff. If you'd prefer a thicker lube, try Embrace, ForPlay, or Probe. If you're looking for a creamy lube that won't get sticky, try Liquid Silk or silicone lubes.

✓ *Compatibility*. Don't combine a silicone lube with a silicone toy.

Probe, and Slippery Stuff share space on drugstore shelves with KY Jelly. Our mail-order lubricant sales, however, suggest that sensual lubes aren't as readily available in the rest of the country. So what's the advantage of these lubes? They tend to stay slippery longer than pharmaceutical lubes, and they come in user-friendly flip-top bottles or pump dispensers, rather than fiddly little tube containers. You can expect to pay anywhere from fifty cents to six dollars per ounce of lube, depending on how concentrated a brand you're buying.

Lubricants are a "personal care" product about which folks can develop almost fanatical brand loyalty. This loyalty can result from specific preferences regarding texture or from purely sentimental associations.

I always use Wet Light. I like the slipperiness—it feels natural and isn't sticky or gummy like KY or some other lubes Also, I have very sensitive skin and this brand never gives me a rash.

My first girlfriend turned me on to Probe, and now I can't imagine using any other brand.

Liquid Silk is the best. Period. Nothing else feels as much like the real thing.

To me, Astroglide is liquid gold for the sex gods. I won't use anything else!

For every customer who turns trustingly to one of our store clerks and asks which one of our lubricants is "the best," there are always two or three customers clustered around the lube shelf ready to jump into the discussion with conflicting advice:

"Get Astroglide. A little bit goes a long way, and it's not stringy, like Probe."

"Probe is the best: It isn't too sticky, it doesn't irritate me, and it's similar to human lubrication."

"I like ForPlay because it's nice and thick."

"Good old KY Jelly works fine for me."

"Silicone lube rocks my world."

So what's a lube novice to do? If possible, get sample packs or small bottles of several different brands and experiment to determine your own preference. Water-based lubes all have basically the same ingredients, the main distinction between them being their consistency. Some folks prefer thin and watery lubes—close to saliva in texture—while others prefer thick and jelly-like lubes.

People with highly sensitive skin should try applying the lube to the insides of their wrists and waiting a day to see if any irritation develops before trying the lube on their genitals. Individual reactions can vary greatly. If you have environmental or dermatological sensitivities, you might want to avoid lubes that contain the preservatives methyl paraben or propyl paraben—some folks report allergic reactions to parabens. Probe is a good paraben-free options. Some women look for lubes that are glycerin-free, out of concern that the sweetness of the glycerin promotes yeast or bladder infections. Glycerin is, however, completely nonirritating to the vast majority of people and is used widely in everything from lubes to liquid soaps to cosmetics. You may choose to avoid glycerin because you object to its stickiness—so try Liquid Silk; this glycerin-free lube with a creamy texture is one of the most popular lubes on the market.

If you expect to encounter the lube during oral sex, its taste will matter to you. All water-based lubes are advertised as being taste-free; most containing glycerin, though, have a slightly sweet taste. Some will have a slight citrus flavor due to natural acids (like grapefruit seed extract) added as preservatives. Some will have a slight bitter taste. And any lubricant containing spermicidal ingredients such as nonoxynol-9 will have a somewhat soapy, medicinal flavor and may even briefly numb your tongue.

I prefer nonflavored and nonspermicidal lubes because if we want to engage in oral sex after penetration, there's less in the lube to irritate the tongue and other mucous membranes. I can't stand the taste of spermicides, and they always leave my mouth feeling incredibly nasty.

Since the preservative ingredients in lubricants are all capable of killing sperm, you should be cautious in your use of lube if you're attempting to get pregnant. For instance, use lube only on the shaft of the penis, not the glans, and forego the lube entirely if you're inseminating. We hasten to add that lubricants, in and of themselves, are *not* effective contraceptives.

Lubes and Anal Play

There aren't many places in this book where you'll find us making an absolute statement or insisting that there's only one way to go about sexual play, but this is one of them: Never try any anal penetration without using a lubricant. While the anal canal produces some protective mucus, the anus and the rectum produce no natural lubrication. Please don't ever insert so much as a finger inside your anus without the aid of some form of lubricant. Anal tissue is thinner and more delicate than vaginal tissue and can be easily damaged by a rough, dry approach. You do have plenty of options as to what kind of lube you can use anally. Since your anus naturally flushes itself out during defecation, it's not as problematic to use heavy oils anally as vaginally. Many people prefer oils for extended anal play, as they don't dry up the way that water-based lubes do. However, for the vast majority of people who should be observing safer-sex precautions, oils are out of the question for partner play, because any type of oil will destroy latex barriers. Instead, consider using the thicker varieties of water-based lubricant such as Embrace, ForPlay, and Maximus. While until recently lubes containing nonoxynol-9 had been frequently recommended for safer sex, there's considerable support for the idea that detergents are too harsh for tender anal and rectal tissue and may do more damage than good.

If you've shopped in adult bookstores or with adult mail-order or Internet companies, you may have come across products marketed as "anal lubes." These products usually contain desensitizing ingredients such as lidocaine or benzocaine, and their existence is based on the false premise that anal play always hurts and that you need to anesthetize yourself before you can be receptive to anal penetration. In fact, with sufficient relaxation and patience, anal play need never be the slightest bit uncomfortable. If you experience pain upon penetration, your body is warning you to stop what you're doing. Rather than anesthetizing yourself to deaden sensation, you should be learning to voluntarily relax your anal sphincter muscles and to bring a heightened awareness to bear on all the sensations you're experiencing. You'll learn specific techniques in the Penetration chapter.

Lubes and Safer Sex

We have one more absolute statement to make in this chapter that is critical for your health and safety: Never use any oil whatsoever with latex products. Oils destroy latex—this means that even the lightest-weight massage oil, Albolene cream, hand lotion, baby oil, or Vaseline will eat into a condom or diaphragm and produce microscopic holes in the latex within sixty seconds of contact. Although many condom manufacturers have begun labeling condoms with warnings against using them with oils, we need consumer education on an even broader scale. Please take the time to read the label on any lubricant you are considering for purchase. Don't be taken in by lubes that advertise themselves as "water-soluble"— these frequently contain oils.

On the bright side, water-based lubes and latex make ideal companions. Lube helps transform latex gloves and dental dams into sleek, slippery instruments of pleasure, and complements condoms beautifully. A dab of lubricant on the inside tip of a condom increases sensation for the wearer—just be careful to use only a drop or two, so that the condom doesn't slide off the wearer's penis. Lube on the outside of a condom minimizes uncomfortable friction for the receptive partner while it reduces stress on the condom. Even if you've purchased a lubricated condom, adding more from your own bottle is often an excellent idea.

Since I use condoms and gloves, I always use lubricant, and why not? It feels nice, and it kinda adds to the whole experience.

Increased safer-sex awareness has inspired a lubricant boom. Lubes are now available in a variety of textures, sizes, prices, and flavors. Several companies manufacture flavored lubricants and edible gels as oral sex accessories—these are great for those who don't relish the taste of latex. If you'd like to experiment with transforming that condom-covered penis or those dental-dam-clad labia into a fruity taste treat, check out ForPlay Succulents, ID Juicy Lube, and others. We wouldn't recommend these lubes for internal use—since the artificial colors and flavors could be irritating to mucous membranes—but they are fun safer-sex enhancers.

Nonoxynol-9, as noted above, is frequently added to lubricants as a safer-sex precaution; it is a detergent that has been shown to kill viruses (including the HIV and herpes viruses) in a laboratory setting. While nonoxynol-9 is a common ingredient found in everything from contraceptive foams to baby wipes, it can be irritating to people with sensitive skin. Genital tissue is nothing if not sensitive, and repeated, regular use of nonoxynol-9 has been found to irritate mucous membranes to such an extent that it can produce vaginal or rectal lesions. In fact, recent international public health studies have determined that the use of nonoxynol-9 lubricants not only failed to prevent disease transmission, they actually *increased* STD infection rates—presumably due to the higher rate of lesions, which could have facilitated transmission. Consequently, Good Vibrations does not carry lubricants that contain nonoxynol-9.

Health organizations continue to search for a safe and effective microbicide (a product preventing transmission of viruses and bacteria) that could be incorporated into lubricants and other safer-sex products. A study performed at the University of Texas in 2001 found that certain Astroglide ingredients actually killed HIV in a laboratory setting. As of this writing, the researchers haven't identified the ingredients by name, but describe them as common, widely used, and inexpensive compounds. If further clinical field trials prove that these ingredients are equally effective outside the lab, the public health benefits could be huge.

Last Lube Words

We'll close this chapter with the following enthusiastic endorsements from *our* kind of lube fans:

Once I started using lube, my sex life improved one million percent. It just makes everything easier and feels better all around.

Lube changed my life! Not being able to get wet enough to have sex felt like being impotent—but that first tube of KY Jelly improved my sex life (and relationship and sex esteem) forever.

┌─ GV Tale: Anne Learns That Lube Makes the World Go Round ─┐

Several years ago, a friend and I were traveling through Egypt. Tired of self-guided tours, we decided to splurge and hire a tour guide for our day trip to the Valley of the Kings, the burial ground for ancient royalty. Much to our delight, our guide was a woman.

She reminded me of an Egyptian Oprah Winfrey—full of confidence, style, humor, and showmanship. During a pause in the tour, while she and I waited for the rest of the group to catch up, our guide asked me what I did for a living. Without thinking, I blurted out that I worked for a women-run sex shop in San Francisco. She looked puzzled but before we could talk further the rest of the group arrived and she slipped back into her routine. Since all of the treasures from King Tut's tomb are now in museums, I stayed behind with her while the others went off to explore the tomb.

As soon as we were alone, the guide began to discuss her sexual problems with me! She said sex with her husband was very painful because there was too much dryness and friction. Her doctor, who was uncomfortable discussing sex, simply told her to get used to the pain. As a result, she was losing interest in sex. I told her all about lubricant and asked whether she could get some in Egypt; she said it would be difficult. I asked for her business card and told her I'd send some lube along with a catalog. She specifically requested that I send the package to her office so that her husband wouldn't open it first! Too soon our group returned, and the two of us reverted to a conversation about the unbearable heat.

I hope that bottle of Astroglide reached its destination and that my wonderful guide was able to slip back into a happy sex life. As for me, nothing inside Tut's tomb could have thrilled me as much as our conversation that day.

CHAPTER

Creative Touching

Sometimes an accidental touch by a stranger can hold a sexual charge. Maybe because I'm tuned into the eroticism of my whole body, I adore overall body stimulation with hands, tongues, lips, toys—you name it!

In our touch-deprived culture, even the most casual physical contact communicates a message of intimacy. When you extend your hand in greeting to a new acquaintance, touch a coworker's shoulder, or brush up against someone in a crowded subway, you're establishing familiarity (whether acknowledged or not) with the physical contact. If you stop to think about it, that's some powerful stimulus.

Many people do not take full advantage of the erotic potential of touch. Sure, you can wax ecstatic about the first time you pressed your naked body against your lover's, but can you describe the sensations evoked when the back of the knee or the small of the back is lovingly caressed? Your entire body is capable of being aroused—not just the buttons you push "down there." Awakening your body to its pleasure potential can boost your self-esteem, expand your definition of sex, and improve your intimacy with a partner. In this chapter, we encourage you to explore the tactile delights of the entire body, not just the genital area, through activities we've dubbed "creative touching." This includes the basics of massage as well as our suggestions for other activities and toys with which to experiment.

I like a lot of stimulation and find that in "real" life people get fixated on one body part or activity (oral or anal sex, for example) and don't have the imagination to view the entire body as an erogenous zone. So many of my fantasies involve getting and giving whole-body stimulation with at least one partner—preferably stimulating a number of body parts at any one time.

Erotic Massage

Massages are the best, especially if you have massage oil. They are so intimate and relaxing, filled with so much caring and love.

Massage can be used for many different reasons: to soothe aches and pains, to reduce stress or relieve tension, to improve circulation, to heighten physical sensations. All of these can positively affect your sex life. Many people discover the erotic possibilities of massage by accident. Have you ever been turned on during a professional massage? Or been surprised when a friendly massage given by someone you had no sexual interest in left you aroused? It's perfectly natural for the body to respond this way—after all, the skin, like the brain, is also a sex organ.

I get off on giving my partner massage—great foreplay.

I love just holding and being held, caressing, and spending long hours in bed.

Many folks enjoy massage as a warm-up to a sexual encounter, while others experience the eroticism of the massage as an end in itself. Whatever your preference, you can benefit from going slowly and learning how to give and receive pleasure. Too often we're in a hurry to move on to some other activity and don't take enough time to appreciate the subtle pleasures of a lingering touch. Pregnant women (who should be sure to see someone trained in massages for pregnant women) and people with chronic pain or disabilities are among those who speak enthusiastically of the rewards of massage:

I have partial feeling from my waist down, but my face and head have become incredibly sensitized to any form of touch—a kiss, a caress, a cheek upon mine is incredibly exciting.

During pregnancy, massage helped alleviate some of my back pain, but also helped me stay in touch with my ever-changing body. The massage was sometimes relaxing and at other times profoundly erotic.

You don't necessarily have to be aroused to want a massage—many folks find that the massage itself is what triggers their excitement:

Nude massage often gets her in the mood, and will help get me in the mood too if I am not feeling real horny to begin with.

Although massage professionals may describe their specialties differently, we've chosen to include any type of touching in this category. Whether it be a light touch, a tickle, or a firmer stroke, the goal is to discover new sensations. And massage by no means has to involve a partner—you can incorporate many of these techniques and toys into your solo sex play.

Your attitude about giving and receiving pleasure can affect performance, often to the detriment of your own satisfaction. To enjoy a massage, both the partners need to let go of expectations and simply enjoy the physical sensations. Embrace the concept of selfishness and indulgence when it comes to giving and receiving pleasure. If it's not clearly understood beforehand, you might want to discuss the nature of the massage. Are you both interested in an erotic massage? Is the massage meant to ease tension and induce sleep, or to arouse? Are orgasms expected? Will you explore heightened sensation by prolonging the build-up to orgasm?

I enjoy giving body massage without actually touching any sexual organs. The movement of our hands on each other's bodies is intended to be erotic but not explicitly sexual.

I like massage that moves into mutual masturbation.

The person giving the massage should try to be as comfortable as possible. Anticipate what positions you'd like to avoid and set up your massage area accordingly. If you prefer standing, set up a foam pad or cushion on a sturdy table. During the massage, remember to change positions often so that you don't get sore—try kneeling, sitting, or straddling your partner. It's just as important for you to enjoy the massage as it is for your lover. The receiver's job is simply to relax, breathe deeply, and focus on tactile pleasures.

Try to avoid conversation during the massage. This allows both of you to keep your attention on the physical sensations and eliminates any distractions. It's fine to communicate what does and doesn't feel good, but remember, you can convey pleasure or satisfaction with a moan or a smile!

The most important thing to consider when preparing your space for massage is temperature. We live in chilly San Francisco, where the flat's only heater may not be in the bedroom. Buy a portable heater and turn it on well in advance! The surest recipe for disaster is to try to give a massage to a lover covered in goose bumps. An excellent way to warm up prior to the massage is to take a hot bath. Not only does it raise your body temperature, but it's exceptionally relaxing.

- If it helps your partner feel warmer and more secure, cover her or his body (except for the portion you're massaging) with a sheet, light blanket, or towel.
- If you've got a dryer, throw in some bath towels. Your lover can lie on these during the massage or be wrapped in them upon emerging from the bath.
- Use a bed, a padded table, or thick blankets on the floor. If you're using a bed, position your partner diagonally so that you have a bit more room. If you're using oil or lubricant, place easily-washable towels or sheets under your partner.
- Find out if your partner has specific physical needs or special requests, and prepare your massage area accordingly. A pregnant women might find lying on her side most comfortable, or she might like to use cushions to help support her stomach and breasts.
- Warm oils ahead of time. Microwave your bottle, or immerse it for a few minutes in warm water.
- If you're planning to use other toys, have them nearby.
- Unplug the phone, put the kids and the pets to bed, play some music if you like. Your goal is to relax as much as possible.
- Remove any jewelry and make sure your nails are trimmed.

Tips and Techniques

With the preparations completed, you now have your delectable, nude lover awaiting your ministrations.

If you've agreed on a genital massage, consider saving the genital area for last to heighten the anticipation. You may want to experiment with avoiding the genitals altogether to see how it affects your experience of other body parts.

If you're giving a full-body massage, here's a suggested itinerary. With your lover face down, start with the back, shoulders, arms, and hands, then move on to the butt, legs, and feet. Turn your partner over. Begin with a scalp and face massage; move on to the abdomen, chest, arms, legs, and feet; and end with the genitals.

There are numerous books and videos about sensual massage, offering detailed descriptions and illustrations of dozens of strokes. Since most folks just want to know where and how to begin, we'll explain some very simple strokes that can be adapted to suit your needs. Let your imagination run wild. Take any one of the following strokes and modify it slightly, using your fingertips, fingernails, palms, back of your hands, knuckles, heels of your hands, and thumbs; or try varying the pressure, speed, or direction of your stroke—each will evoke a different sensation. The point is to discover what movements feel best so that you can use them to please your partner in the future. And by all means start with a little massage oil; it adds a pleasant smoothness to your strokes, and the warmth and aroma can be a subtle aphrodisiac.

Full Body

I find gentle strokes and gentle kisses all over my body very enjoyable. It's all about lying back and being pampered. Some areas of my skin, like my neck, back, and sides, are very sensitive.

Here is a superb way to begin and end your massage: With your partner face down, arms at her or his sides, position yourself at your partner's feet. Place one of your hands on each of your partner's hands and travel lightly up the arms, around the shoulders, and then straight down the body all the way to the feet, ending at the toes. Don't remove your hands, but follow the same path now in the opposite direction. Try this stroke several times, gradually adding more pressure. When it's time for your partner to turn over, repeat the same stroke on her or his front side.

Fanning

Place palms side by side on the skin. Simultaneously fan each hand out about ninety degrees, then slide them gently up or down; bring hands back together and repeat the motion. The pressure should come from the heel of each hand or the thumbs (or both), while your fingers will feel great grazing over the skin on the back, butt, abdomen, thighs, and breasts. This stroke feels particularly good if you stand at the head, start low on the spine, and move upward. When your hands reach the top of the spine, separate them and apply pressure from the palms as you travel outward along the shoulders.

Pulling

Stand (or sit) on one side of your partner and place your hands next to each other along your partner's opposite side (fingers pointing toward bed) and pull them up toward your partner's spine (or belly, if partner is on back), alternating each hand. As one hand pulls, the other slides back down. Try this on a woman who's on her back; you're moving up from the stomach toward the armpit. As your hands approach the breast, slide lightly over the nipple with your palm. This is also an excellent stroke for the thighs, starting at the knees and moving away from the feet. As you work up the inside of the thigh, approaching the butt, the pulling motion tugs on the genitals, which can be quite arousing.

Kneading

Work your hands as if you were gently kneading bread dough (a kind of push/pull motion) and continue as you move up along a large stretch of skin. This stroke feels great along more sensitive areas, particularly the backs of legs, inner thighs, arms, and butt.

Thumbs

With your thumb at a right angle to your fingers, place your hands at the base of the spine with your thumbs pointing at each other. Press down with your thumbs and glide slowly up the spine. Try this on the arms and legs as well. Modify this stroke by pressing each thumb in turn, or by rotating them in a circular motion. The focused, direct pressure afforded by thumbs makes them ideal for hand, foot, and face massages. When massaging the face, apply gentle pressure, starting in the middle of the face and sliding toward the outside. For example, place your thumbs where your partner's eyebrows connect and move toward the temples, or start on the nose bridge and travel down under the eyes toward the ears.

I love massage that includes having my hair and face stroked.

Butt

Seated at your partner's feet, place one hand on each butt cheek and slide your hands up and down in opposite directions. Kneading or dragging your fingers lightly across the butt can also feel good, as can light slapping.

Breasts

Don't ignore the breasts if you are doing a full-body massage (unless, of course, your partner asks you to avoid them). If you're seated at your partner's head, place your hands next to each other on the stomach and slide them up between the breasts. Circle the breasts with your hands, then draw them back down the outside. Repeat this motion several times, allowing your palms or thumbs to cover more of the breast area each time.

Place a hand over each breast so that the nipple touches the center of your palm. Spread your fingers as if they were the spokes of a wheel, and as you pull your hand up and off the breast, let your fingers graze the skin until they approach the nipple. You may want to finish the stroke with a light pinch.

I think massage is great as long as I get my nipples played with.

I enjoy stroking my partner all over her belly, breasts, ass, and mons. I love fat women and enjoy kneading and sucking my lover's heavy, soft breasts and large belly.

This is one of the most wonderful sexual experiences I've had in my life. I had stupidly gone without a bra all day and my nipples were sore by the time my lover and I got home. He massaged them with moisturizer and then moved on to a full-body massage. It was great because it was much slower and more gentle than usual.

Genitals

If you've ever watched closely when your partner masturbates, you've had the best possible instruction for genital massage. You've seen what kind of stimulation feels good on certain areas. Use this as the starting point from which to further explore other pleasurable sensations.

While you may wish to continue using oil during genital massage, please note that some oils, particularly scented ones, can cause an allergic reaction when they come into contact with mucous membranes. If you are sensitive, try testing a small amount first, or consider using a water-based lubricant instead. Also, a note about safer-sex massage: While massage in general is considered a very low risk activity, the risk increases if there's a chance that blood, vaginal secretions, or semen will come in contact with broken skin or mucous membranes. You may want to use a rubber glove during a genital massage along with a water-based lubricant (oil will break down rubber), or to place a condom over the penis.

Here are a few areas you'd do well to include:

ON WOMEN

The labia: With your partner on her back, place a well-oiled (or -lubed) hand over her labia, fingers pointing toward her anus. Pull up toward the navel and alternate hands, always keeping one hand on the body.

Explore the inner and outer lips with your fingers. Pull gently on one and then the other and work your way down the right side, then switch to the left. Rub the outer lips gently between your forefinger and thumb, then the inner lips while applying varying degrees of pressure and asking your partner which feels the best. Starting at the perineum, place your forefinger between the inner and outer labia and trace a clockwise pattern up and around the clitoris.

The clitoris: Encircle the head of the clitoris during a stroke that takes you up the length of the inner lip and around the head of the clitoris. Try not to touch the clitoris directly (as most women find this too

intense), but run your fingers over the clitoral hood. Remember to maintain a fluid, continuous motion and repeat these strokes several times.

The vagina: Circle the outer edge of the vagina several times and then pop in a finger or two and let it rest a moment. Then explore the vaginal walls by stroking or applying pressure, asking for your partner's feedback.

The anus: Lightly circle the rim of the anus.

The perineum: Lightly massage or apply pressure to the area between the anus and the vagina with one hand while you explore her vulva with the other.

My boyfriend gives the most awesome PUSSY MASSAGES *with lube! It gets me so* HOT!

ON MEN

The penis and scrotum: With your partner on his back, place a well-oiled (or -lubed) hand over his penis and scrotum, fingers pointing toward the anus. Work your palm up toward the navel, sliding along the penis and gently pressing the penis against his stomach. Try alternating hands with each stroke and slowly massaging the penis around the body in a clockwise motion. Another technique involves forming a ring around the scrotum with your forefinger and thumb and gently pulling his balls away from the body while stroking the penis in an upward motion. You can also leave the penis for a while and gently massage the testicles in this position.

The shaft: Try anchoring the skin at the base of the penis with two fingers of one hand and stroking upward with the other hand. Or cup one hand around the base of the penis and begin to slowly slide upward. When you reach the head, finish the stroke with a twisting motion. As your hand gets near the head of the penis, place your other hand at the base of the penis and begin the same motion. You can also reverse the direction of this stroke. Another stroke often referred to as "the twister" involves cupping both hands around the penis and then gently twisting in opposite directions. If you think your partner would like spot stimulation of the frenulum, clasp the penis between both hands and interlock your fingers together with the thumbs pointing toward the glans and massage using your thumbs.

The glans: In a move known as "the juicer," wrap one hand around the penis while you place your palm on top of the glans and rotate, repeating this motion just as if you were juicing an orange. Another version of this utilizes just your fingers in a motion similar to unscrewing a jar.

The anus: Lightly circle the rim of the anus.

The perineum: Apply firm pressure or stroke the section of skin between the base of the scrotum and the penis. Many men find stimulation of this area particularly pleasurable when they're approaching orgasm, as it puts pressure on the prostate.

Variations

So far we've discussed just one way of tickling someone's tactile fancy—with your hands—but there are other, playful, and just-as-pleasurable means to this end.

Other Body Parts

Your mouth is an incredibly versatile and intimate sex toy. Think of all the possibilities—trace a path on your lover's body with your tongue; kiss, suck, nibble, bite, or blow on the skin. All of these can evoke pleasurable sensations.

> *I love when my boyfriend bites my neck. Not hella hard or anything, but definitely with some force. When he's lying on my back, without penetrating me, I like him to bite the back of my neck.*

If kissing isn't very erotic for you, you and your partner may need to practice your lip chemistry. You may prefer deep kisses while she or he prefers soft, light ones. You don't need to assume there's only one way to kiss—experiment so that you can find kisses that work for both of you.

> *Kissing turns me on—my neck, shoulders, and arms especially. I love to be sucked and licked all over from fingers to nipples.*

You've got quite a number of nerve endings under your arms, which is why many folks find that area

---

Massage Basics

Never given a massage before? Feeling a little intimidated? Not to worry, you're certain to meet with undying gratitude if you remember these basic tips:

- *Go slowly.* You know that feeling of disappointment you have when you race through a delicious meal and then realize you've devoured it so fast you've barely tasted it? Don't race through the massage! Linger over each part of your lover's body so that she or he can savor the sensations.
- *Repeat strokes.* The consistency of repetition soothes, relaxes, and allows your lover to luxuriate in the skin contact with one area. Repeat each stroke anywhere from several to a dozen times.
- *Don't break contact with the skin.* Once you've started the massage, stay connected. If you're using oil, squeeze some into your hands before applying it, to avoid shocking the skin. When you need to apply more oil during the massage, turn your hand over while it's still resting on your lover's skin, cup it, and pour some more oil into it.
- *Practice symmetry.* If you massage one hand, don't forget to do the other one. A neglected body part will feel odd if its mate has been well cared for.
- *Pay attention to your partner's reactions.* If you see goose bumps, turn up the heat. If you see a grimace, don't press so hard, or ask what caused the reaction. If you see a smile, continue with that stroke. If you're uncertain, ask. You might both agree on some signs beforehand to communicate pleasure or discomfort.

---

erotic as well as ticklish. Try different strokes to see what elicits the best response.

> *I really like to have my armpits licked.*

The nipples are particularly responsive to stimulation; some folks claim to orgasm from nipple stimulation alone. Sadly, men's nipples are often overlooked as an erogenous zone.

*I adore being blindfolded and sensually kissed, my
nipples and my neck bitten.*

Experiment with sucking, licking, and blowing on
the nipples, or try pinching, flicking, or tickling them.
Women's breasts are very responsive to stimulation,
though you should check in with your partner since
tenderness can vary depending on where she is in her
menstrual cycle. Try some of the massage techniques
we described earlier.

A woman's breasts can also be a wonderful tactile
tool for her *and* her partner. Try dragging your breasts
over your partner's body. Vary the pressure from just
lightly grazing your nipples over the skin, to pressing
firmly against it. Rub your breasts against your partner's
genitals.

Hair can create a pleasing sensation when dragged
across the skin, and certainly holds a fetishistic appeal
for many. Running your hand through someone's hair,
gently tugging on it, or giving someone a scalp massage or an erotic shampoo can also be pleasant.

*I like dragging my hair over skin and listening to
the sighs.*

*I always find my visits to the hair salon slightly
embarrassing because the shampoo sequence is s
uch a turn-on. I love having a stranger's hands
gently scrubbing my scalp, and pulling on my hair
slightly during the rinse.*

We encourage you to linger over every part of
your lover's body, but there are some particular
places you may want to give special attention. Your
hands can be skilled instruments of pleasure, but
don't forget they should be worshiped as well. We
use our hands so much we usually take their sensitivity for granted. Whether you're giving a massage
or sitting next to your sweetheart in front of the TV,
take the time to gently and lightly explore the intri-
cacies of your lover's hands. Explore the surface of
the skin, each finger, the nails, and the knuckles.
Apply pressure with your thumbs to the palms, and
slide up each finger, finishing off with a gentle tug at
the tip.

*Out of the blue, my girlfriend will take my hand and
start running her fingers along it while we're chatting
away. Sometimes it gets me really excited.*

The feet are also tremendously sensitive—toe
sucking did not originate as an alternative to bathing!
The toes and soles of the feet are full of nerve endings,
so take some time to discover them. Bathing your
partner's feet in warm water and toweling them off
can be a sensual experience. Applying powder or
oiling the feet can evoke a range of pleasant sensations. If your partner is ticklish, try applying a firmer
stroke. If that doesn't work, move to another part of
the foot.

Even playing with a partner's ears can be arousing
and intimate. Those who orgasm from ear play can
thank a phenomenon known as "auriculogenital
reflex," which traces your orgasm to a nerve found in
the ear canal. You might try lightly exploring the ear's
folds and creases with a finger or lips. Touch or nibble
on the lobe. Don't probe too deeply into the ear
cavity, and remember how loud this sounds to your
partner if you're sucking, blowing, or smacking your
lips. Some folks find ear play incredibly erotic and
others find it a sure-fire turn-off, so attend to your
partner's desires and responses.

*I like to initiate sex with a little gentle touching, neck
kissing, and ear blowing.*

The nape of the neck lends itself to continuous
smooth strokes, kisses, and licks. Try blowing on it.
You may want to continue up the scalp and stroke
the hair.

Pour me wine, kiss my neck, and finger me.

*I love to be touched everywhere with her fingertips as
gently as possible. I especially love to be caressed from
my shoulder to the nape of my neck. My hot spots
include my ass, feet, hands, and breasts.*

The backs of the knees and inner thighs can be
highly pleasurable spots in both men and women. Try
a light licking on the back of the knee, then vary a
soft caress of the hand with a firmer stroke on the
inner thighs.

Food

Folks are endlessly creative about what they like to
lick off another's body—you can turn yourself into an
ice-cream sundae or a tropical fruit platter.

My girlfriend and I love licking small dabs of yogurt off each other's nipples. The shock of the coldness on my nipple sends ripples to my cunt, and when her warm, wet mouth starts to suck it off, I nearly lose consciousness.

Food can be a creative way to camouflage the taste of bodily fluids, if you're not fond of them. Chocolate, whipped cream, jellies, spreads, and honey are all popular.

Water

I really like mutual masturbation in the shower.

Baths, Jacuzzis, saunas, and hot springs not only relax mind and body, they can also awaken desire. There's no denying that warm water feels exquisite on skin, so immerse yourself in it! The Romans had this pastime down to an art form; their bathhouses were luxurious and ornate—the epitome of sensual decadence. While those grand days may be gone, most people do have a bathtub at home. If you don't, hot tub places are usually as close as the nearest phone book. You might also enjoy late-night skinny-dipping in a cool lake, pool, or ocean, or sharing a Jacuzzi with friends or a lover. Bath accessories like shower massagers, sponges, and brushes can also enhance bath time.

Toys and Accessories

FEATHERS: Try lightly running a feather over your partner's body for a sensation that even the lightest fingertips can't approximate. Ostrich feathers, which are about two feet long and exquisitely soft, are harvested from farms where the birds shed them. If you aren't up for hunting down your own feather, you can sometimes find these in sex toy or lotion stores. Be careful not to let massage oil gum up your feather!

FUR: It may be a cliché today, but sex on the bear-skin rug originated somewhere! Soft fur on naked skin is luxurious, but if you're short on rugs or fireplaces, you can invest in a fur mitt for a similar feel. Fake fur has made it possible for everyone to appreciate this sensation.

FABRICS: Satin, velvet, silk, suede, latex, and who-knows-how-many other fabrics feel terrific against the skin. While satin sheets have been commercially available (and popular) for decades, other fabrics may be a little harder to play with, unless you're willing to do a bit of sewing ahead of time or to shop around in sex boutiques. Blindfolds, fur-lined restraints, and a variety of other leather and latex accessories can be found at specialty shops or on the Web.

TEXTURED MITTS: These are usually large rectangular gloves that fit over the hand so that you can use them on a lover's body. Mitts can be made out of any of the fabrics listed above. The adult industry's version is made out of soft rubber with tiny nubs on the glove. Some also have a small pouch that will hold a vibrator.

WHIPS, PADDLES, AND BONDS: Whips and paddles can offer you a range of sensations—from a light slap to a hair-raising sting. Bonds can add an element of restraint to your massage.

POWDERS, GELS, AND EDIBLE ITEMS: Rub 'em on and lick 'em off. These appeal to folks' desire to eat something off a lover. Flavor selections rival that of ice cream these days—passion fruit, cappuccino, hot chocolate, for just a few examples—but beware: These products run the gamut from sweet-as-honey to tasty-as-motor-oil. Almost all have some kind of preservative in them, though a few boast natural ingredients and really do taste authentic. We polled our survey respondents about their most disappointing toys, and a large percentage cited some kind of edible lotion. Most shops have samples open for you to taste—it's definitely worth the time to try them before you buy.

These edible gels do not double as massage lotions since they won't spread easily—imagine using grape jelly for a full body massage. However, many of these contain no oil and they're safe to use with latex, so next time you complain about the taste of latex, flavor it with strawberry. Some of these gels heat up upon application or when you blow on them, which can be a nice sensation and which can produce some interesting possibilities for oral sex.

Kama Sutra brand products are available nationwide and continuously earn the most fans. Some favorites are Honey Dust, an edible powder perfect for after-bath dusting, or Oil of Love (in six flavors), which heats up when you blow on it—ideal for an after-dinner treat. The manufacturer also makes a minty gel called Pleasure Balm. Its main ingredient, benzocaine, has a numbing effect, but when placed on nipples or genitals it can feel pleasantly cool, especially when you blow on it.

BODY PAINTS: That's right, your canvas is your lover's body and you can "express yourself" with these colorful, washable paints. They tickle when applied, and the edible variety offers you the unique opportunity to eat your work of art and your lover at the same time. You can even find edible finger paints in the finest Belgian chocolate these days!

OILS: Massage oils are intended for external use, but can be used for genital lubrication, as long as you don't combine them with latex. Remember that oil destroys latex, rendering any safer-sex barrier completely useless. If you intend to practice safer sex during your erotic massage, use water-based lubricant for genital massage.

Massage oils come in several textures and dozens of scents; if smelling like a flower or citrus doesn't appeal to you, you can find unscented oils. It's nice to have a variety on hand, but bear in mind that vegetable oils will go bad after a period of time. To maximize their life span, store them in the refrigerator (just make sure to warm them before applying to skin). It's easy to find massage oils that are made exclusively from natural ingredients, most commonly almond and safflower vegetable oils. Be advised, however, that if you have a nut allergy you should avoid almond oils. Unless you're allergic, these oils are safe to ingest, though they're not intended as edible treats. Some women are allergic to scented oils if used on the genitals, so experiment first with a small amount or use water-based lubricant instead.

VIBRATORS: Since vibrators are usually packaged as "massagers," why not try them during your next massage? They provide an intense stimulation that can work wonders on sore muscles or merely offer a pleasant alternative to hands. If you're trying a variety of sensations on your partner's body, a vibrator—especially one with several attachments like the coil vibrator—is a must. Experiment on the scalp, the feet, the inner thighs, the neck, and face.

LATEX AND LUBE: The smoothness of a lubricated latex glove or condom can offer a unique sensation for both the giver and the receiver during a genital massage. Lubricants are an especially appealing option for genital massage since you'll get the slipperiness of oil without getting any oil inside your vagina or rectum (oils linger in your body and jeopardize any latex condoms you may introduce later). If your lubricant starts to dry out, reactivate it by spraying on a bit of water.

Sensate Focus

If you find you don't enjoy these activities because you're easily distracted or anxious, you might want to pursue something known as "sensate focus" exercises. Sensate focus teaches an expanded awareness of the entire body and its surrounding environment, and involves coordinating your breathing and mental state with your body's physical responses to a variety of caresses. Several good books outline self-help programs of this nature, and many sex therapists prescribe these exercises to individuals who experience performance or desire problems.

The Universal Language

The massage techniques presented in this chapter complement many sexual activities, and we encourage you to experiment with your own pleasurable combinations. But before we leave the subject we want to remind you that not all touch is sexual, and that nonsexual touch has the power to improve our quality of life from infancy to old age. Touch allows us to heal, to communicate emotion, to show friendship, and to offer comfort. The right kinds of touch can make us feel loved, appreciated, at home.

If you're a parent or an adult who enjoys spending time with children, you've probably gained insight into how we compartmentalize touch in our culture. As adults, many of us have come to associate intimate touching only with lovers, yet children provide a liberating reminder that nonsexual touch is a universal source of physical and emotional pleasure. Infants need to be held, babies have skin so soft it begs to be touched, and children are unselfconscious about demanding cuddles or back rubs.

Of course, one source of our culture's touch-phobia is a growing awareness of the very real problem of child sexual abuse, which has created a diffuse anxiety about touch, with unfortunate consequences for both children and adults. Adults such as teachers, who are in positions to provide the affection that can foster a child's social development, are forbidden from displays of physical affection. How sad that such caretakers feel constrained from embracing a hurting, needy, or happy child. Even parents may come to fear that the joy they derive from touching their children is somehow inappropriate, which can lead them to withhold physical affection. Ultimately, both children and parents lose out. (See Noelle Oxenhandler's *Eros of Parenthood* for an excellent discussion of this subject.)

It's no surprise that studies have shown that infants who are held often, massaged, or breast-fed are more likely to grow up with a sense of well-being and belonging. Parents are taught that infant massage is vital to a child's healthy development, but almost as soon as kids start walking, the emphasis (both at home and at school) shifts to protecting them from inappropriate touching. Of course it's important to teach kids to distinguish between wanted and unwanted touch, but it's just as important that they learn—through example and word—that there are many kinds of good touch.

If we don't get to experience what "good touch" is all about when we're young, how do we develop a healthy body image and sexual self-esteem? If physical contact with others is perceived as awkward and difficult, how can we enjoy dating, courtship, or sex without a great deal of trauma and shame?

We encourage you to seek ways to include touch in your daily life. Certainly you should respect each individual's preferences regarding personal space, but we can all benefit by appreciating how vital the simple act of touch is to our health. Pat a coworker on the back (literally), give your family members hugs, take a toddler's pudgy hands in yours. Remember, touch is a universal language—so go out there and improve your vocabulary!

CHAPTER

Oral Sex

When we asked our questionnaire respondents to describe their favorite sexual activities, oral sex topped the list. Oral sexperts are upbeat, enthusiastic cheerleaders for this art form.

Oral sex is the sine qua non of sexual play for me. Any sex date that doesn't include oral sex is a missed opportunity as far as I'm concerned. My fantasies and my porn almost all concentrate on fellatio and cunnilingus. Oh! I can't get enough.

I love giving blow jobs! It's like an extremely intimate kiss that I'm in total control of. Feeling his whole body tremble as I take him in my mouth is an immense turn-on—a totally sensuous experience.

I feel much more coordinated with my mouth than with my hands.

There is nothing so intimate, so erotic, so mind-blowingly in your face as stroking a sweet thing's labia with your tongue.

I love cunnilingus, especially receiving. I could do it all day (well, I wish I could, anyway). It's so warm.

Oral–genital sex is legally defined as "sodomy" in many parts of the United States. Some states prohibit unmarried consenting adults from engaging in oral sex, while others prohibit consensual oral sex between married people, even in the privacy of their homes. In this country, nonprocreative sex acts tend to get classified as "crimes against nature." Is it any wonder that Americans—even presidents—find it hard to shake the notion that oral sex somehow doesn't qualify as "real" or "normal" sex?

I actually enjoy oral sex more than normal sex. It seems more personal, like a gift from the lady involved.

Although the majority of sexually active adults engage in oral sex, many people are embarrassed, uncomfortable, or downright repulsed by the idea of mouth-to-genital contact. What makes oral sex so simultaneously arousing and unnerving? Perhaps it's that oral sex, by definition, brings you face to face with your partner's genitals and the sights, smells, and sounds of his or her sexual arousal. The arms-length detachment of manual stimulation or the lights-out decorum of intercourse can't be maintained when you've got your nose, lips, and tongue soaked in your partner's juices. There's a unique intimacy and vulnerability involved, whether you're exposing yourself to your partner's tongue or savoring your partner's genitals. Since sucking is a powerfully infantile pleasure with an unavoidably primal appeal, with oral sex you've got a potent blend of physiological, emotional, and mental stimulants.

I could suck cock twenty-four hours a day. I love the feeling of it in my mouth, the smell, the taste. And I love to make men writhe in ecstasy.

I go down on my wife every chance I can get. I enjoy observing her enjoyment and the intensity and volume of her response to my pleasuring her.

Many people build a versatile and satisfying sex life around oral sex. Oral sex is a gratifying technique for women and men, old and young, disabled and able-bodied alike. It's a time-honored activity for adolescents who want to be sexual without grappling with the risks and complications of intercourse. Both women who find that the physiological changes of menopause make penetration less appealing, and men who find that their erections are less predictable with age, often rediscover the joys of oral sex. People with spinal-cord injuries that limit physical mobility or sensation frequently develop a rich sexuality based on oral play:

I'm spinal-cord injured and have limited sensation below my nipples. I can still get erections, but I get a lot more pleasure from my hands and tongue than from my penis.

I'm in my late seventies and still active sexually, especially orally, which is beautiful.

Inhibitors
Body Odor

Probably the most common factor inhibiting people from experimenting with oral sex is the fear that their own or their partner's genitals will smell or taste bad. After all, in our culture, an entire industry exists to mask, erase, or transmute natural body odors into scented wonderlands of "spring rain" or "pine forest." Yet, there's nothing inherently "dirty" or unpleasant about genital odors and secretions (except in the case of certain vaginal infections, which can result in an unpleasant smell). Plenty of people find natural body odors much more arousing than the smells of soaps and deodorants.

I've always delighted in female scents, especially when a woman is aroused.

It's exciting to kiss someone who tastes like my pussy.

I like immersing my face in someone's cunt, getting her juice all over my mouth and face and her scent up my nose.

I love the way penises taste and feel in my mouth. I like to masturbate while taking a man in my mouth.

However, if you feel that a little body odor goes a long way, you might be more comfortable bathing or showering with your partner before sex. When it comes to oral sex, cleanliness is next to confidence for a lot of people.

I love performing oral sex on my partner…especially in the shower. With the water running over his body it is almost like my own personal water fountain.

Another option is to experiment with flavored latex and lubricants. You may consider a penis clad in a mint condom irresistible, or enjoy tonguing your partner's labia through a berry-flavored dam.

We don't want to drop the topic of hygiene without encouraging everyone who hasn't already done so to try tasting and smelling their own sexual secretions. To enjoy sex, you have to enjoy your sex organs—this means appreciating everything about them. Take the time while masturbating to raise your fingers from your genitals to your lips and nose. Women can compare how the odor and consistency of their vaginal secretions change with different phases of their cycle or with different levels of arousal. Men can compare the taste of pre-ejaculate with that of ejaculate. The natural salty, musky tastes and smells of sexual secretions are biochemically designed to arouse, delight, and inspire us to sex. Why not take conscious pleasure in them?

I let a little cum drip into my hand and lick a little bit, just enough for a powerful taste. Believe me, this is an aphrodisiac, even for a heterosexual. I don't do this all the time, but when I do it's a real turn-on.

The Gag Reflex

The fear of gagging or choking during oral sex is generally more an issue for those performing oral sex on men than on women. The gag reflex is a natural one, and it takes a bit of practice to get to the point where the sensation of a penis at the back of your throat won't make you gag a bit. Your best recourse is to wrap your hand around your partner's penis while you suck—not only will this enhance sensation for your partner, but also it will let you control the depth of his thrusting. We've read that the military once claimed it was easy to identify gay recruits by applying a "Gay Reflex Test." Any man who didn't gag when a large tongue depressor was inserted in his mouth was considered unfit for military service. If, by some chance, you're worried about gagging or choking while performing oral sex on a woman, just remember to breathe through your nose, and you'll be fine.

Sexual Fluids

Sexually transmitted diseases can certainly be transmitted through oral sex, and we'll discuss safer oral sex and risk management in depth below. However, there's nothing inherently harmful in semen, female ejaculate, or vaginal secretions, and if your partners are not carrying sexually transmissible diseases, there's no reason to feel you shouldn't swallow their sexual fluids. Swallowing semen cannot make you pregnant, nor is it fattening. According to the Kinsey Institute, the average amount of semen a man ejaculates contains about five calories. Not surprisingly, no one seems to have calculated the calories in female ejaculate or vaginal secretions.

By the same token, there's no reason to feel you should swallow your partner's fluids if you don't want to. Plenty of sincerely enthusiastic lovers simply may not find the taste or texture of male ejaculate pleasing enough to go that extra mile. If you don't want to swallow semen, you can ask your partner to let you know when he's about to come. At this point you can

remove your mouth from his penis and continue stimulating him by hand. Or your partner can wear a condom during oral sex, in which case his ejaculate will be contained and swallowing won't be an issue.

I don't much like swallowing sperm, so I reserve it as a treat. More often I'll ask my husband to withdraw or we'll use a flavored condom (strawberry and mint are my favorites). When he does come in my mouth, I use my tongue so he spurts onto the roof of my mouth— that way I don't choke.

If your partner is an ejaculating female and you don't particularly want to be flooded by her fluids, you can arrange some sort of signal for when you should move your mouth away and continue stimulating her by hand.

Boundaries

The same intimacy and sense of vulnerability that make oral sex so arousing to some make it frightening to others. Respect your partner's feelings, and let her or him set the pace of your explorations.

I like fellatio, but I've never felt comfortable with cunnilingus. I was sexually abused for ten years, and that seems to be one lingering aftereffect. I've not had the opportunity to surmount that fear with a partner yet, but I look forward to it.

Oral sex may offer a kind of physical stimulation not to everyone's taste. Some men find that fellatio doesn't provide sufficiently intense stimulation to reach orgasm, while some women find cunnilingus more irritating than pleasurable.

The truth is, I don't really care for blow jobs. I believe I give good ones, but I rarely ever come close to ejaculating when I'm being blown.

Cunnilingus doesn't arouse me as much as I'd like it to. It makes me tense. Sometimes a lover puts too much pressure on my clit that way (I'm sensitive).

If oral sex makes you anxious or uncomfortable, you can certainly enjoy a satisfying sex life without it. But if you've never explored this simple sexual technique, we do hope you'll give it a chance—many people find oral sex a uniquely pleasurable and fulfilling activity.

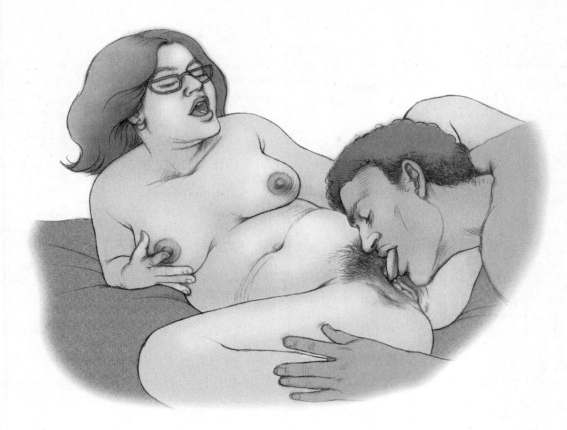

Cunnilingus

Cunnilingus

Techniques

The word "cunnilingus" comes from the Latin *cunnus* meaning "vulva" and *lingere* meaning "to lick." But licking is only one of the many delights involved in cunnilingus. Your moist lips and mouth are capable of creating a uniquely subtle range of sensations. Sucking your partner's clitoris, nuzzling her labia, and penetrating her vagina with your tongue or fingers can all enhance the experience of oral sex. As with any sexual activity, the same strokes won't work for all folks, and the same woman might prefer different types of stimulation depending on how aroused she is. Start by finding out what kind of clitoral stimulation your partner prefers: She might like you to lick or suck directly on the tip of her clitoris, to approach it from the underside, or to concentrate on the less-sensitive hooded side. She might favor a slow, gentle tonguing, or she might crave a ferocious licking. She might prefer feeling the tip of your tongue, the flat of your tongue, a circular motion, a lapping motion, even a slight scraping of teeth.

Tongues are usually soft enough and slick enough to feel good directly on my clit.

I found that I simply needed the courage to grind into him, to get a more forceful touch from his tongue, in order to come completely. I overcame my shyness and really got off!

The softness and delicacy of a tongue on my clitoris is heavenly. I love an indirect approach with lots of teasing—coming close, backing off, returning, etc.

If I'm being eaten-out, it's a total turn-on to have him pull me against him by wrapping his arms around my thighs and holding me tight as he licks me hard and fast.

Many women enjoy having the whole vulva licked, from pubic bone to perineum. Pay attention to the sensitive area around the urethra. You can insert your tongue in your partner's vagina, though obviously the average tongue will only go so deep. Most women would much rather have their external genitalia tongued. Generally, it's easier to use a finger or a dildo for penetration during oral sex.

I enjoy the combined effect of sitting on my girlfriend's face while she has her finger inside me stimulating my G-spot and is licking my clit.

Bear in mind that as your partner approaches orgasm, she'll probably appreciate it if you maintain a steady stimulation up to and through her orgasm. Many women need consistent, reliable stimulation to put them "over the top," and if you test-drive a brand-new tongue stroke right before she's about to come, it may not go over too well.

I like cunnilingus because it calls on me to be more subtle and adventurous in determining where the locations of pleasure could be for my lover. The searching and ingesting quality is very exciting— especially if she comes.

You may have read or heard mysterious warnings that you can actually kill a woman during cunnilingus by blowing too forcefully into her vagina. In fact, there is medical literature describing cases in which oral sex has resulted in potentially fatal air embolisms. However, in every one of these unusual cases, there had been some damage to the uterine wall that allowed air to pass from the uterus into the bloodstream—for instance, the woman's uterine lining was disrupted by an IUD or (in the majority of cases) she was pregnant. During pregnancy, the placenta produces enzymes that eat away part of the uterine wall, creating a pool of blood between the placenta and uterine wall. Therefore, an air embolism could result if a forceful blast of air makes its way through the cervix, beneath the edge of the placenta, and into the bloodstream. These embolisms have, on occasion, proven fatal. However, they are exceedingly rare events. If you are going down on a pregnant partner, please rest assured that, as one doctor we spoke with put it, "It would take a lot of air and a lot of force. Plain oral sex and 'Whoops, I accidentally breathed on her!' wouldn't be a problem."

Positions

Experiment with different positions to see which are most comfortable and pleasurable for the two of you. You may enjoy simply lying between your partner's legs, facing her vagina, while she lies on her back— this position also allows you to reach her upper body with your hands. You can try kneeling on the floor between her legs while she lies back on the bed (or the sofa or the kitchen table) or stands over you. Or you can lie on your back while your partner straddles your face—she'll be free to move her pelvis and control the rhythm of movement. This straddling position is popular both with those women whose arousal is enhanced by watching their partner perform oral sex and those cunnilinguists who enjoy the sensation of being surrounded by their partner's vulva:

I love having my lover sit over my face, feeling her lose control.

In any event, there are more possible positions for cunnilingus than we could ever name—you're limited only by your imagination.

My fondest oral sex memory is of the time I made my girlfriend go down on me while I was standing in a phone booth in our hotel lobby. No one passing by could see her kneeling between my legs, but I must have looked like I was having the most exciting phone call of my life!

Enhancers

There's truly no limit to the variations you can come up with when you're eye-level with your partner's vulva. Your hands are free to wield a dildo on your partner and/or on yourself. You can slip a finger in her vagina or anus, or both. Women who find their orgasms are more intense when the vagina is full may particularly enjoy having a dildo inserted during oral sex.

My fantasy involves having my partner give me oral sex while his penis is inside me—but that seems impossible. My partner surprised me once by inserting a vibrator in my vagina and his fingers in my anus while licking my clitoris. This gave me one of the most memorable orgasms I've had, and I think this is as close to my fantasy as I will be able to get.

Try playing a vibrator across her labia while you suck on her clitoris. Or hold a battery vibrator against the underside of your tongue while you're licking, thus transforming your mouth into a sex toy. If that last idea makes your teeth hurt to even think about, bear in mind that sound creates vibration, so you can create a similar, slightly less dramatic effect by humming and purring while you lick. An innovative oral sex toy is a harness designed to strap over the head and hold a dildo over the wearer's mouth or over the wearer's chin. Anyone willing to transform themselves into a cross between a sex toy and a unicorn is rewarded with a whole new perspective on penetrating their partner.

Before we leave this topic, we should admit to a bit of a bias. We like to think that every woman and every lover of women should experience the pleasure of cunnilingus. That women's genitals are more hidden than men's has led to an exaggerated sense of mystery and, in some cases, a certain fear and disgust toward what's "down there" between a woman's legs. When you go down on a woman, you're bringing all your senses to bear on an appreciation and admiration of her genitals. When you invite someone to go down on you, you're affirming that your entire body is worthy of tender attention.

I'm a huge fan of cunnilingus. Sometimes it takes a while for me to really let go and get into it, but wow! It's so cool to feel like someone's worshipping my cunt.

Fellatio

The word "fellatio" derives from the Latin verb *fellare,* "to suck." Where would our sex vocabulary be without Latin? However, "sucking" barely begins to describe the pleasurable possibilities of going down on a man. Take your cues from your partner's body language, and respect that different men will have different preferences when it comes to oral stimulation. Find out whether your partner prefers firm or gentle pressure, attention lavished on the head of his penis or the base, a vacuum-style suck or a rhythmic flicking of the tongue. Of course, your partner might be perfectly happy with a variety of approaches:

I love fellatio, from teasing licks to deep sucking.

My favorite kind of orgasm these days is squatting over another man's face and having him kiss and chew my nuts with his snorting nose tickling my asshole.

The one rule of thumb that you can safely apply to most men is: no teeth. Do make sure not to scrape your teeth across your partner's genitals, as this could be quite antierotic. If your partner happens to enjoy a little nibbling on his penis, he'll probably let you know.

What I don't like is if I'm sore, or a woman nicks me with her teeth or uses too much pressure.

Techniques

Generally speaking, there's more to giving head than bobbing your mouth up and down over the shaft of the penis. Of course, you can simply open your mouth and let it be a passive receptacle for a thrusting penis. There's even a specific term for this technique, *irrumation,* but this kind of fellatio is not as popular—or as fun for the fellator—as that in which the sucking partner is in charge of the action. As with cunnilingus, your best bet is to put your mouth to work on those areas of greatest sensitivity: namely the glans, or head, of the penis; the coronal ridge around the base of the glans; and the raphe, which is the seam running down the underside of the penis. With the exception of the raphe, the shaft of the penis is not particularly sensitive, so licking away at the shaft as though it were a popsicle won't necessarily generate a great deal of sensation. Instead, concentrate on working your mouth around the glans and coronal ridge—you can wrap your hand around the shaft as a sort of continuation of your mouth. Your partner may enjoy your sucking the head of his penis while stroking up and down on the shaft.

She would move very slowly, taking me in her mouth and using very soft, light touches with her lips and tongue. What I liked best about her technique, besides the slow and deliberate use of her mouth, was that she always kept her hand on my body, stroking the lower part of my shaft. As I got closer to orgasm, she would pick up a steady rhythm, moving her whole head up and down in a long then short, slow then fast, milking motion.

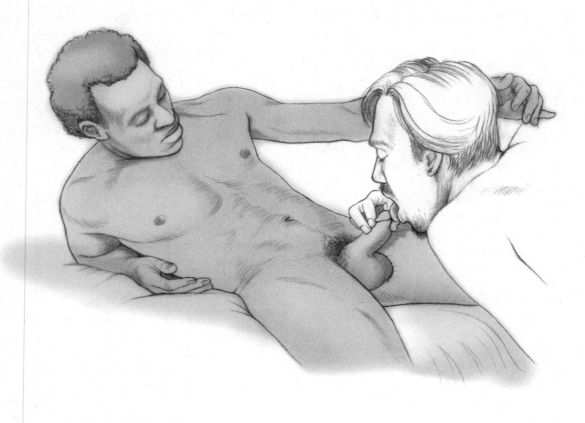

Fellatio

I run a fingertip lightly around the rim of the glans or brush very gently across the tip—this always results in signs of ecstasy and a satisfying wetness. I push my tongue into the slit at the tip of his glans and swirl it round the head. When he's close to coming I just suck him as the final trigger.

One technique I very much enjoy is when my partner opens her mouth and, with her hand on the base of my shaft, rapidly shakes or wiggles my cock about in her mouth. It makes a wonderful sound, which I find exciting.

Positions

Frequently, a man will lie on his back to receive oral sex while his partner lies, crouches, or kneels between his legs. If you're sucking your partner's penis while facing his head, you'll be able to rub your chest against his penis and scrotum and to reach your hands up to stroke his body. If you're facing his feet, you'll be at a better angle to take more of his penis in your mouth, though you won't be as well-positioned to lick the sensitive underside of his penis. You may want to kneel on the floor to suck his penis while he stands or lies back on a bed. Or you may prefer to lie on your back with your head well supported by pillows while your partner kneels over you, straddles your face, and penetrates your mouth from above. Basically, any position in which you both feel comfortable is a good position.

With one woman, we would gaze into each other's eyes when we were doing one another. I found that really mesmerizing and erotic. I think it can be easy to lose eye contact during oral sex, but she would lie down on her back and have me straddle her. This is a great position for fellatio and prostate massage.

Enhancers

In your attentiveness to your partner's penis, don't forget the rest of his body. You can reach a hand up to play with his nipples, or massage his butt and thighs while you suck. Many men enjoy anal stimulation—with a tongue, finger, dildo, or vibrating butt plug—as an accompaniment to oral sex.

Gentle prostate simulation complements cocksucking. I like to have my nipples bitten and sucked. Simple thumbing of my anal opening is nice.

You may want to hold a vibrator against your partner's perineum, or you may want to play with a vibrator yourself. There's no law that says only one of you at a time is entitled to sexual stimulation. Many heterosexual couples enjoy incorporating breast play into fellatio—tit-fucking is a popular alternative to intercourse, and it can easily be combined with oral sex.

I used a vibrator once while performing fellatio—it was great! It's the only toy experience I've had with a partner.

I like fellatio if it's preceded by my partner alternately fucking my breasts and then my mouth while doing a lot of sex talk. When he's at the point of coming, I like him to take control of his cock with one hand and move my head with the other. This frees up my hands so I can start rubbing my breasts and touching myself so that we can come together.

Giving head provides you with a great opportunity to explore your partner's genitals. You can massage his perineum with your fingers, gather his scrotum together using your hand as a cock ring, lick or mouth his testicles, and otherwise lavish attention on his entire genitals. As with cunnilingus, fellatio allows you an intimate view of your partner's arousal and an almost unparalleled sense of control over his sexual pleasure.

Actually performing fellatio on my partner is one of the most wonderful pleasures. I've gotten it down to such an art of sweet torture, ending in an outrageous orgasm for him and an inability for him to move for the next thirty minutes or so. The most recent time, I almost came just from going down on him.

What I like about fellatio is feeling the slow approach to orgasm. Often I'm just lying there, maybe moving slowly,

just feeling the nerve stimulation building and building and knowing it's going to keep building until I come.

Deep Throat

This is the term commonly used for the technique of taking an entire penis into your mouth and throat. What this technique lacks in finesse—you won't be able to lick, suck, or do anything more than hold your lips around his shaft—it makes up for in terms of impressing your lovers. Relaxation and positioning are both key to performing this technique. Either you have to be kneeling over your partner's penis facing his feet, so that your mouth and throat will be at the right angle to accommodate a whole penis, or you should be lying on your back with your head off the side of a bed so that your mouth and throat are in a line. Basically, you'll be taking his penis all the way into your throat, which means you need to work on relaxing your gag reflex. Keep your hand at the base of his penis with the understanding that you can push the penis out of your mouth in a hurry without any hard feelings between you. Gagging is a natural response to having any object blocking your throat. Practice and trust will make it easier to relax this reflex. Of course, you can be an excellent fellator without ever swallowing more than a couple of inches of penis.

We always use a condom if I'm going to deep-throat him because I found that his sperm spurting into the back of my throat made me choke. His ejaculations are usually quite powerful and prolific.

Sixty-Nine

This is the popular term for simultaneous mutual oral sex. The term derives from the fact that a six looks like an upside-down nine and vice versa. In a sixty-nine position, you and your partner lie side by side facing each other's feet, or one of you lies on your back with the other kneeling above facing the prone partner's feet. The notion of arranging yourself in an unbroken circle with your mouth on your partner's genitals and his or her mouth on yours is unquestionably an appealing one.

I like to fantasize about sixty-nine a lot if a particular guy has hold of my heartstrings...that always seems so loving and mutually giving and incredibly intimate.

It's wonderful to be falling into someone else's cunt while my own is also being stimulated.

Sixty-nine is my absolute favorite. Being eaten while returning the favor with two naked bodies touching is the most intimate and intense experience.

Sixty-nine all the way—mmm-mm-mmm. I prefer it over just having my man go down on me. My partner is most often on top of me, and I am underneath with his luscious dick in my mouth. It makes me twitch even thinking about it.

My number-one favorite activity is sixty-nine—it fills a lot of cravings all at once, i.e., to suck cock, to be sucked, and to be in close physical coupling with my partner. It's wonderful as a mutually narcissistic circuit of oral nurturing and trusting masculinity.

For every individual who swears by sixty-nine, there's one who finds this technique overrated. It's difficult to concentrate on orally teasing and tantalizing your partner while your own genitals are flooded with pleasurable sensations. Most of us find that sexual arousal is accompanied by a certain amount of heavy breathing and increased muscle tension. It's hard to maintain a rhythmic tonguing of your partner's clitoris or to refrain from scraping your teeth across your partner's penis if you're trembling on the brink of orgasm yourself.

Sixty-nine is too confusing for me...I forget to hold up my end of the bargain.

Sixty-nine is, for me, overrated, since one or the other partner is distracted.

Sixty-nine is all right once in a while for variety, but I like taking turns better than doing oral sex simultaneously. I like to focus either on pleasing my partner or on being pleased.

But by all means, don't let this discourage you from experimenting with mutual oral pleasuring. You may well wish to incorporate sixty-nine as part of your sex play without focusing on it as a means of reaching orgasm.

I prefer to either receive or give oral sex, not both simultaneously, but I also don't turn down an offer of sixty-nine!

Tips and Techniques

Playing with temperature is a tried-and-true method of enhancing oral sex. You might want to try holding a small ice cube in your mouth while you run your tongue up and down your partner's penis. Or you could apply ice to your partner's clitoris and then warm her back up with your mouth. Similarly, some folks drink hot fluids before wrapping their mouths around their partner's penis or clitoris. Blowing on your partner's genitals up close creates a warm rush of sensation, while blowing or fanning the genitals from six inches away creates a cool, tingling sensation. Another popular way to play with temperature—which got an unprecedented publicity boost from coverage of Bill Clinton and Monica Lewinsky's affair—is to suck on breath mints or mentholated cough drops while going down on your partner.

When giving head, an Altoid works wonders. It gives him a totally new sensation and it helps keeps my mouth "juicy."

Many sex toy businesses sell a variety of flavored gels for enhancing oral sex. These gels usually come in two varieties: those that generate heat and those that numb sensation. The former usually contain either glycerin or essential oils such as cinnamon, peppermint, or clove oil. When you apply these gels to the surface of your skin and blow softly, warmth spreads over the skin. The latter frequently contain benzocaine or other mild anesthetics. The pleasure of using these numbing gels lies in feeling sensation flood back into your genitals as the anesthetic wears off. While these gels can be safely applied and licked off a penis or clitoris, women should be careful not to get these products inside the vagina. Essential oils and anesthetics are potentially irritating to delicate mucous membranes. The licker should also bear in mind that his or her mouth will get quite numb.

Those people who'd rather stick to food and drink, which don't contain artificial ingredients, may enjoy licking whipped cream, chocolate sauce, or berries off each other's bodies. (If you're using latex barriers for safer sex, do abstain from using food products containing oils, which destroy latex.) Whether you prefer your oral sex au natural or à la mode is entirely up to you.

I once had a banana inserted and eaten out of me—fabulous!

We use chocolate sauce quite a lot on his naked penis—it makes sperm swallowing more palatable, as the taste of the chocolate does mask the taste of the sperm. We also squeeze chocolate sauce over my clitoris so he can lick it off.

One of my best lovemaking memories is of the time I had jam licked off my clit, a full wine bottle inserted in my cunt, wine poured in, and then my lover drank the wine out of my cunt.

Rimming

This is the popular term for oral–anal stimulation. Licking, kissing, and tonguing the anus are also referred to as "analingus." The whole notion of rimming is highly charged for many people, and even those who are comfortable with oral–genital sex can find themselves repelled by oral–anal sex. The opposing points of view about rimming can basically be summed up as: "Why would I want to lick the orifice that feces come out of?" and "Why wouldn't I want my anus to get the same loving attention as any other erogenous zone?" After all, the anus is highly sensitive and loaded with nerve endings, and there is no question that, physiologically speaking, it feels as good to have your anus kissed as to have your mouth kissed.

Rimming is a special treat and only happens once in a while by "accident." My current partner thought it was disgusting until I did her and she came big time. She refuses to talk about it.

If you follow basic hygienic precautions, you should feel free to enjoy the pleasures of rimming. The risks involved in ingesting feces include contracting hepatitis A or intestinal parasites. While early AIDS researchers grouped rimming under high-risk activities for transmission of HIV, this classification is now considered debatable. Given that feces are stored in the colon, and do not pass through the rectum or anus until just before defecation, it's unlikely you'd encounter more than traces of feces in your partner's anus. You may be inspired to bathe together before embarking on a rimming episode, but bath or no bath, you should seriously consider using a barrier of some sort between the mouth and anus. Dental dams (small squares of latex), cut-open condoms or latex gloves,

and Saran Wrap are all considered acceptable barriers. If you aren't using a barrier, you should never lick your partner's anus and then move to kiss her vagina or his mouth. Licking from the anus to the vagina or from the anus to the mouth can transmit feces—and therefore infection—from one orifice to another.

Once you've taken the hygienic precautions you feel necessary, and your tongue is poised over your partner's anus, what shall you do? You can circle the anus with your tongue; flutter your tongue against the anal opening; lick, suck, or slip your tongue into the anus. Our anuses are the seat of so much tension that any kind of tender tonguing will doubtless feel extremely relaxing and pleasurable to your partner.

I love being on my knees, ass held high, while she works my ass with her tongue. Not so much thrusting, but teasing, flicking, licking. Luckily all of my girlfriends, save for one, liked to eat my ass.

Safer Sex

While we've made several mentions of safer-sex precautions throughout this chapter, we'll close with a more detailed summary of current findings and opinions regarding risk management in oral sex.

Hepatitis

As noted above, it's possible to transmit hepatitis A through unprotected oral–anal contact, and we highly recommend that rimming fans get vaccinated against hepatitis A. Hepatitis B, a far more serious illness, can certainly be transmitted through unprotected oral sex, as the virus is contained in saliva, semen, vaginal secretions, and blood. If you are infected with hepatitis B, please use a barrier for oral sex. If you've never been infected, consider getting vaccinated. While hepatitis C is transmitted via blood-to-blood contact and is therefore not generally classified as an STD, oral sex could provide opportunities for blood contact, and folks with hepatitis C should practice safer sex.

Herpes

This is a virus that's easily transmitted via unprotected oral–genital contact. Oral herpes (cold sores) can be transmitted to the genitals, and genital herpes can be transmitted to the mouth. You should never have unprotected oral sex if you or your partner are having an outbreak. Furthermore, it's possible to transmit herpes asymptomatically, that is to say, even when you aren't experiencing an active outbreak. Consider using a dental dam, a cut-open condom or latex glove, or Saran Wrap as a barrier during oral–vaginal or oral–anal sex. And use condoms during fellatio. It's a good idea to forego fellatio during a herpes outbreak, as herpes sores can cluster at the base of the penis or on the testicles, where a condom would not cover them.

Bacterial STDs

Chlamydia, gonorrhea, and syphilis are bacterial sexually transmitted diseases that can all be treated with antibiotics. It's unlikely for chlamydia to be transmitted during oral sex, but both gonorrhea and syphilis can be transmitted via oral–genital contact. Folks being treated for these infections should not have unprotected oral sex until the infection is resolved.

HIV

Currently, oral sex is considered to be a fairly low-risk activity with regard to the transmission of HIV, as there have only been a handful of cases in which oral sex was the proven means of transmission. There is, however, simply no such thing as "absolutely safe sex," and we hope you will weigh all the relevant information to decide what precautions are appropriate to take.

HIV is contained in the semen, blood, and vaginal fluids of those infected with the virus. While it's present in trace quantities in sweat, saliva, urine, and tears, there's no evidence that it can be transmitted by these fluids (unfortunately, we don't know of any studies of whether HIV is present in female ejaculate). Blood, including menstrual blood, contains HIV in much higher concentration than vaginal fluids, and therefore it is riskier to come into contact with your female partner's menstrual blood than it is to contact her vaginal secretions. There's some debate as to whether an HIV-infected woman has ever transmitted the virus to a partner through oral sex alone. Enzymes in the mouth of healthy people are known to kill viruses as delicate as HIV. However, if you have open sores in your mouth or even tiny cuts in your gums from brushing your teeth or flossing, and you go down

on a person with HIV, it's conceivable that the virus could enter your bloodstream. So save your dental hygiene routine for *after* sex. Allowing your male partner to ejaculate in your mouth is a higher-risk activity than his withdrawing before ejaculating. However, the risk that an HIV-infected individual could transmit the virus by going down on a partner is slight.

What to Do

None of the above information need stop you from enjoying safe and pleasurable oral sex. A variety of latex and plastic barriers are available to protect the mucous membranes of one partner's mouth from contacting the mucous membranes of the other partner's genitals. Dental dams are one type of latex barrier that can be used during oral–vaginal or oral–anal sex. On the plus side, dams are available in different scents: bubble gum, vanilla, or wintergreen, for example, and creative people have been known to wear them in place over their genitals by using a leather harness or a garter belt. On the minus side, dams are only six inches square, thick, and unwieldy—after all, they were designed for use during oral surgery, not for use in the bedroom.

Fortunately, sex-positive entrepreneurs have stepped into the breach to devise alternatives: Glyde brand dams are larger (about six by ten inches) and thinner than dental dams, yet equally strong—and they come in vanilla and berry scents. Lixx dams (about six by eight inches) are also designed especially for oral sex and come in vanilla and strawberry scents. Good Vibrations sells large sheets of thin latex (about eight by twelve inches) as well as disposable latex panties. Other options include cutting open a condom or latex glove or using large sheets of Saran Wrap. Condoms, gloves, and Saran Wrap are thinner and transmit sensation better than dental dams do. In 1993, the FDA tested Saran Wrap for its permeability and found that it was effective in halting the transmission of virus-sized particles. Synthetic latex, or Nitrile, dams are also available for the estimated 2 to 4 percent of the population with latex allergies.

Whatever barrier method you use, be sure to put some lubricant on the side of the barrier pressed against your partner's genitals. This will enhance the sensations received through the latex or plastic. Using barriers during oral sex can add a whole new array of tricks to your repertoire. If you stretch a dam tightly across your partner's genitals, pucker your lips, and suck in a little bubble of rubber directly over her clit, you can create a stimulating vacuum-suction effect. Needless to say, it's also extremely liberating to lick freely back and forth between your partner's vagina and anus without feeling restricted by hygienic considerations.

Many people have already made the adjustment to using condoms during oral sex. Several flavored condoms are on the market, including mint, banana, chocolate, and cola flavors, or you can flavor an unlubricated condom with a water-based edible gel. Then again, you may be someone who prefers plain latex flavor to disguised latex flavor. The condoms manufactured these days are so thin as to be almost like a second skin. You may be surprised to find that latex transmits sensation and temperature with arousing intensity and that being sucked through latex can feel just as good as being sucked without.

The Avanti polyurethane condom hit the U.S. market with great fanfare in 1995. Polyurethane is a clear, odorless plastic that is considerably stronger than latex, so polyurethane condoms can be made thinner to allow for greater sensitivity than latex condoms. It has the further advantage of not breaking down upon exposure to oil and not smelling or tasting like latex. But it has the disadvantage of being considerably more expensive and less elastic than latex. The Avanti's lack of elasticity initially resulted in high slippage and breakage rates, though its quality has improved. If you're someone who is allergic to latex or who wants to experiment with a thinner condom for oral sex, you may want to check out polyurethane.

Nina Hartley

"Once I saw my first adult movie, I knew that the world of sexual performance was where I'd find myself and my greatest happiness, and it's been true!"

For over fifteen years, feminist porn star Nina Hartley has been putting her beautiful butt on the line to create a more sex-positive world. She's appeared in countless adult videos, and she's the star and director of her own line of educational videos—on topics from oral sex to anal sex to erotic dancing. In her best-selling videos *Nina Hartley's Guide to Cunnilingus* and *Nina Hartley's Guide to Fellatio* Nina (who's also a registered nurse) dishes out detailed anatomical information and calls on her porn star pals to help her demonstrate sexual technique in scenes that are filled with affection, humor, and heat.

Raised in Berkeley during the sixties and seventies, Nina grew up "understanding that I had a right and responsibility to my sexuality. Once I saw my first adult movie, I knew that the world of sexual performance was where I'd find myself and my greatest happiness, and it's been true!" Always a feminist, her proudest achievement is "to have been part of the group that has spread the word about sex-positive feminism as a viable, honest, authentic point of view—to be peers and friends with people like Kat Sunlove, Annie Sprinkle, Betty Dodson, Susie Bright, and Carol Queen."

Nina sees her work as a way to give back to the community through education. "People engage in sex without knowing what they're doing. I think it's sort of sad that we teach people how to drive, we teach people how to do all kinds of things, but we don't teach people how to have sex because it's considered embarrassing or private. Sex isn't so private for me, so if you can take what I've learned and apply it to your private life, take the information and use it, please!"

She's also deeply influenced by her Buddhist faith. "Compassionate awareness is crucial to my work. I've had to work through my own fears and issues in order to be a help to other people. Our culture makes people sexually sick. Everyone's born sexually healthy—before we beat or molest or shame or terrorize it out of them, children love their bodies! Sex and massage and dance are wonderful ways to bring yourself back into your body so that you live in the present moment—so that you can live presently, as opposed to absently."

Nina's greatest hope for the future is that "we'll learn to recognize and respect children and young adults as sexual beings, and find an appropriate way to acknowledge that sexuality is an inherent inborn right." But the woman once called porn's "Bowl of Sunshine" is predictably cheerful about how far we've already come: "You know, it's been thirty years now of unremitting, unrelenting, over-all forward progress with sex and pornography. I know that a lot of people don't believe this because of the Religious Right, but the fact is that now the average person with a little bit of gumption can log on to goodvibes.com in Podunk. Now people who are growing up gay or kinky and feeling bad can connect to a wider group of people like themselves and see that they're not alone. It's just wonderful to see the slowly changing attitudes. Our kids have a much better chance of sexual happiness!"

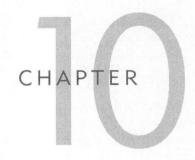

CHAPTER 10

Vibrators

*I love waking up in the morning with a jolting orgasm from my beloved vibrator. Better than a
cup of coffee!*

Vibrators may well go down in history as the best-kept secret of the twentieth century. We
have waited on hundreds of people curious about vibrators who, until their first visit to
Good Vibrations, were unable to find out much about them. If you've ever gotten up the
nerve to visit an adult toy store, you probably encountered piles of vibrating novelties but
received little assistance or information from the clerk. Not surprisingly, many of our
survey respondents described disappointing experiences with toys like the Throbbing Ten-
Inch or the Fantasy Joystick purchased on such trips.

Trying to find answers in sex books used to be hit or miss. In recent years, manuals
have begun to endorse vibrator use, but old myths die hard. Many mainstream sex manuals still treat the vibrator as a woman's masturbatory tool at best, an evil and addictive
device at worst. Vibrators often are given little more than a paragraph with a not altogether accurate description of one or two models, and perhaps a few words reinforcing or
dismissing the anxiety they generate. (Will I get addicted? Electrocuted? Will it replace
my partner?) Take this classic example from *The New Joy of Sex*:

> *Vibrators are no substitute for a penis—some women prefer them to a finger for
> masturbation, or put one in the vagina while working manually on the clitoris....
> Careful vibratory massage of the whole body surface is a better bet than over-
> concentration on the penis or clitoris.*

Let's dissect what's wrong with this paragraph. Rather than clearly explaining that
vibrators aren't intended for vaginal stimulation, author Dr. Alex Comfort defensively
states that they are "no substitutes" for penises—we detect a bit of insecurity here, Doc.
He then correctly relates that women enjoy them both clitorally and vaginally. However,
he ends with a mysterious warning against using vibrators solely for genital stimulation—
never mind that that's what they were invented for!

This lack of accurate information about vibrators prompted Good Vibrations' founder
Joani Blank to write her how-to manual *Good Vibrations: The Complete Guide to Vibrators*

in 1977 (revised in 2000). This remains the only book devoted exclusively to the subject.

In this chapter we enthusiastically bring vibrators out into the light of day. There are thousands of people out there plugging in and turning on, and it's not because they're dysfunctional, single, man-hating, sex-crazed, sex-starved, frustrated, preorgasmic, or disappointed with a partner—it's because vibrators feel great. There are a million ways to have fun with a vibrator—you're limited only by your imagination. We'll give you the who, what, when, where, and why of vibrators, but it's up to you to play with your toys to discover what brings *you* the most pleasure.

We're happy to report that in recent years, vibrators have begun to come into their own. They're more accessible: Mainstream retailers have begun carrying them, they're available on the Web, and more stores modeled on Good Vibrations have popped up around the world. They're also better made; technological innovations have improved sex toy quality, and consumer expectations have risen, so manufacturers can't get away with producing so much junk. Finally, more and more women are coming to view their sexual gratification as a right, so they're less inhibited about demanding the resources, tools, and partners that will get them what they want sexually. We truly believe that in *this* century vibrators will come proudly out of the closet to receive the respect (and use!) they so richly deserve.

A Brief History of Vibrators

The illustrious history of the electric vibrator begins in 1869 with the invention of a steam-powered massager, patented by an American doctor. This device was designed as a labor-saving medical tool for use in the treatment of "female disorders." Within twenty years, a British doctor followed up with a more portable battery-operated model, and by 1900 dozens of styles of electric vibrators were available to discriminating medical professional.

Treating Hysteria

What, you must ask, were these esteemed physicians doing with their vibrators? They were treating hysteria—the most common health complaint among women of the day. While the existence of hysteria as a disease was debunked in the 1950s, medical experts from the time of Hippocrates up to the twentieth century believed that hysteria expressed the womb's revolt against sexual deprivation. A woman's display of mental or emotional distress, the theory went, was a clear indication of her need for sexual release. Genital massage was a standard treatment for hysteria, its objective being to induce "hysterical paroxysm" (better known today as orgasm) in the patient. Since then (as now), vaginal intercourse was considered the only *real* sexual activity, Victorian doctors who would have blanched at the impropriety of performing a pelvic exam had no qualms about manipulating women's external genitals. Obviously, genital massage demanded both manual dexterity and a fair amount of time, so turn-of-the-century physicians were delighted with the efficiency, convenience, and reliability of portable vibrators.

Health, Vigor, and Beauty

Ours being a consumer society, the vibrator was soon marketed as a home appliance in women's magazines and mail-order catalogs. Ads proffering "health, vigor, and beauty" promoted the vibrator as an aid to health. By the 1920s, doctors had abandoned hands-on physical treatments for hysteria in favor of psychotherapeutic techniques. But vibrators continued to have an active commercial life in which they were marketed, much like patent medicines, as cure-alls for illnesses ranging from headaches and asthma to "fading beauty" and even tuberculosis!

Ad copy for these vibrators was coy and ambiguous. "Be a glow getter," one package insert suggests. And who wouldn't be tempted to experience "that delicious, thrilling health-restoring sensation called vibration," when assured that "it makes you fairly tingle with the joy of living!" The vibrator's usefulness for masturbation was never acknowledged; however, as vibrators began appearing in stag films of the 1920s, it became difficult to ignore their sexual function. Probably as a result, advertisements for vibrators gradually disappeared from respectable publications.

A Superior Sex Toy

To this day, electric vibrators are marketed solely as massagers, and their sexual benefits are steadfastly ignored by manufacturers. Vibrators are a big business;

they are sold through drugstores, department stores, general catalogs, and the Internet, yet their true talents remain unsung. We dream of the day when electric vibrators are proudly promoted as the superior sex toys they are. After all, as an early advertisement points out, "almost like a miracle is the healing force of massage when rightly applied."

When I first got my vibrator and learned how to incorporate it into my self-loving, I found it to be the best thing for a girl to have in her house.

This history of the vibrator was first uncovered by Rachel Maines and is detailed in depth in her excellent book *The Technology of Orgasm.*

Why Would I Use a Vibrator?

If you're asking this question, you might be inclined to skip the entire vibrator section. Perhaps you're thinking "I'm a man and vibrators are only for women," or "My orgasms are perfect and I don't need additional stimulation," or "I'm in a relationship where I'm completely satisfied," or "Vibrators just seem so unnatural." If any of these rings a bell, or if you're deterred by any reason short of "I've tried them all and none please me," we encourage you to read on. Just about anyone can enjoy a vibrator, but the charms of these versatile instruments of pleasure are often obscured by a cloud of misconception, stereotypes, and sex negativity.

Allow us to clarify a few main areas of confusion.

Vibrators Can Be Enjoyed by Everyone

Vibrators have traditionally been associated with women because so many learned how to orgasm—or how to orgasm more easily—using a vibrator. Most women require consistent, intense stimulation of the clitoris to achieve orgasm, which a hand or a tongue isn't always able to give:

I used to masturbate with my hand, but it would get so tired. Just as I was about to come, my hand would start to cramp up and sometimes it just froze before those crucial last strokes.

Since most men learn how to masturbate to orgasm during adolescence, they're less likely to seek "outside"

assistance. This shouldn't mean, however, that vibrators are exclusively girls' toys. As Joani Blank points out in *Good Vibrations:* "If men, like women, enjoy a wide range of stimuli (and we know they do), then why shouldn't a vibrator be another potential source of sexually arousing stimulation?"

In fact, many men are happily discovering vibrating sleeves, cock rings, and anal toys, as well as inventing ways to adapt and enjoy more traditional massagers:

I remember one time staying at a hotel in Aspen, and there was a powerful foot massager in the room. I used it on my dick and balls at the same time and had a memorably intense orgasm.

People with disabilities have also discovered the sexual appeal of vibrators. If you're experiencing reduced sensitivity, you may find that the intense stimulation offered by a vibrator can be felt when the stimulation offered by a hand cannot. If your mobility is impaired, you may enjoy lying on top of some of the larger vibrators, or wearing styles that don't require the use of your hands. If you have difficulty grasping smaller toys, slip the battery vibrator inside a cloth mitt or insert the base into a Nerf ball with a hole cut out of the center to give you a greater surface area to grasp. Velcro, adhesive tape, and certain types of everyday hardware can assist you in modifying your toys. See our resource listings for referrals to retailers and websites that offer more tips.

During the later stages of pregnancy you may find that vibrators help alleviate soreness or pain and provide convenient genital stimulation if your mobility is reduced. In *Susie Bright's Sexual Reality,* Susie describes using her vibrator as her focus object during labor: "I have a great photograph of me, dilated to six centimeters, with a blissful look on my face and my vibrator nestled against my pubic bone. I had no thought of climaxing, but the pleasure of the sweet rhythm on my clit was like sweet icing on the deep, thick contractions in my womb."

In *Good Vibrations,* Joani Blank offers this additional tip for new parents: "Keep a battery vibrator handy for the first few months of your baby's life. Parents report that some fussy babies can be calmed with a gentle back massage à la vibrator, or by placing the vibrator, wrapped, in the crib." And more than a few nursing moms have found that applying a small vibrator to a painfully clogged milk duct in their breasts will loosen it right up.

Finally, for those of you who eschew vibrators because you're completely satisfied with your orgasms, we'd like to remind you that variety is the spice of life! Just as your taste in food can change, so can your experience of orgasm. Many women report vibrators make them come more quickly as well as make their orgasms feel more intense. Others find vibrator orgasms less intense. Some men claim vibrators allow them to orgasm quickly, while others find the stimulation too overwhelming. Some use vibrators to create a powerful buildup for an orgasm that they then finish by some other method.

Vibrators Can Enhance Partner Sex

The belief that masturbation and vibrators are merely temporary substitutes until a real live body comes along is a prevalent one. As you read through this book we hope you're struck by the number of both men and women who reject this notion by happily incorporating masturbation and sex toys into their partner sex play. Remember Mom telling you to share your toys? Take her advice—sharing your sex toys can add an exciting new dimension to your sex life. Chances are, if your partner discovers that an erotic accessory is bringing you pleasure, she or he will want in on the action.

Seize the opportunity to expand your sexual repertoire, rather than confine it. Instead of assuming that your partner will be threatened or disinterested, take the time to find out how she or he feels. Vibrators may be just the thing to help you break out of a dull routine. You can enjoy the added visual charge, the new sensations, and the undeniable fantasy component that come with playing with all kinds of toys. We hope to both pique your curiosity and spur you into action with our suggestions, later in this chapter, for how to introduce toys into partner sex.

Vibrators Come in All Sizes and Shapes

The penis-shaped, plastic vibrator is probably the most well-known model, yet it is also the source of endless confusion and frustration for women hoping to use one to vibrate to orgasm. The dildo shape suggests insertion, but most women orgasm from pressing a vibrator against the clitoris, not thrusting it in and out of the vagina. We could weep for the scores of misled women who have pumped and thrusted in vain—searching for that elusive orgasm they heard came so easily with a vibrator. By learning about various vibrator sizes, shapes, and uses, as well as experimenting to find out what kind of stimulation you personally like, you're bound to find a vibrator (or several) with your name on it.

Vibrators Are Natural Pleasers

Many people feel sex should only involve the body parts we were born with, but *why*? We could make the argument that humans were put on this earth naked, therefore we should have no need for clothing. But none would disagree that we have adapted to our environment, donning clothes in the process. We maintain that we've also evolved sexually, earning the right to play with toys.

Vibrators complement our natural sexual impulses by allowing us to explore a variety of sensations. If vibrators are too artificial to incorporate into "natural" sex, what sensual pleasers aren't? What about lingerie, satin sheets, massage oils, furry mitts, and feathers? The enjoyment of tactile stimulation is as natural as it gets, and we object to anyone's drawing an arbitrary line in the sand over vibrators simply because they're powered by electricity.

If you're in a relationship with someone who has an ingrained aversion to the artificial aspect of sex toys, you can try offering some of the arguments we just proposed. Be flexible—you may work out a compromise where you both agree to use the vibrator some of the time. Perhaps in time, after watching it bring you so much pleasure, your partner will grant your toy a place in his or her heart (or between his or her sheets!).

Playing with Vibrators
How To

Both women and men can enjoy vibrators in a number of ways. Although vibrators are most commonly associated with women seeking vaginal and clitoral stimulation, many men rhapsodize over the penile or testicular stimulation they afford, and both sexes can use vibrators to tap into anal eroticism. Whatever your preference, take a tip from the many people who employ more than one toy, and try out several different models, either singly or in unison. You never know what pleasures await you behind door number three! Here are some basic tips for anyone interested in playing with a vibrator:

- Get yourself in the mood. Read a dirty book, walk around the house naked, explore a favorite fantasy.
- Monitor your arousal level and experiment with deep breathing to see how this affects your sexual response.
- Try different positions. Lie on top of the vibrator, lie on your back with the vibrator on top of you, grasp it between your thighs. Run the vibrator over different parts of your body.
- Try moving the vibrator around to touch different parts of your genitals. If you're a woman, you can press it against your clitoris, the clitoral hood, the mons, labia, vaginal opening, and anus, or you can insert it into your vagina or anus. If you're a man, you can run the vibrator along the shaft of your penis, or press it against the base, the scrotum, the perineum, and around or into your anus. Try pressing below the glans on the bottom side of your penis. You can also press your penis against your abdomen with the vibrator to disseminate the vibrations through your pelvis.
- Vary the pressure and speed. Experiment with a steady, direct pressure; alternate between a hard and light pressure; or try stopping and starting. Many vibrators come with more than one speed or a variable-speed control, so that you can switch gears any time.
- If the vibration is too intense, don't place the vibrator directly against your genitals, but move it slightly, diffusing the vibration. Or place your hand, clothing, or a towel between the vibrator and your genitals to absorb some of the vibration.
- Enhance your vibrator play by teasing yourself. Pay attention to your arousal level and turn your vibrator off intermittently.
- Incorporate other types of stimulation—touch other parts of your body, use some other toys, watch a porn movie, or talk nasty to yourself.
- If the vibrator doesn't make you come, don't worry—for now, just play with it for fun. It might make you come too fast, or it might numb you out so that you're unable to come. Only by experimenting can you figure out how to maximize your own pleasure.

First Timers

If You've Never Had an Orgasm... For the woman who has never had an orgasm, a vibrator can literally be the key to the kingdom. Because vibrators provide consistent, reliable clitoral stimulation, many therapists recommend them to preorgasmic clients; masturbating with a vibrator can be an excellent way to explore your own patterns of arousal. As you read through this chapter you'll find descriptions of many different styles of vibrators along with advice on how to choose between them. If you find the sheer number of options overwhelming, it might help to know that the Wahl Coil and the Hitachi Wand, both of which offer strong, steady vibration, are among the most common vibrators recommended to preorgasmic women.

If You've Never Played with a Vibrator... You might be surprised by the results. Many people claim to orgasm more quickly, and sometimes more intensely, from vibrators. Even if you're perfectly content with your masturbation habits, you might be inspired to incorporate vibrators into your repertoire for the sheer novelty—and thrill—of it:

The first time I used a vibrator, I had no idea, absolutely none, about how stimulating it was compared to my fingers or how quickly I would come. I think I lasted maybe ten seconds. After that, I experimented and learned to control myself better.

The very first time I used a vibrator just blew me away. I came within seconds and it lasted forever! After that experience I figured that life without a partner might not be so bad!

The first time I used a vibrator was when I was 45. I thought it was sinful how much ecstasy one of those things can bring!

And once you discover the possibilities, you'll probably be back for more:

I will not forget my first experience using a vibrator. The feeling on my body and the sound was different. Then I felt my clitoris respond...oh my! I thought I was going to fly off the bed. My body would not stop having orgasms. I wanted to shut off the vibrator, but turned it on the higher speed! The vibrator flew across the bed and I curled up enjoying the experience.

One day when I was 15 and my parents were out, I found a vibrator under their bed. I knew immediately that I needed to try it. I started to masturbate using my hand, just rubbing and getting wet, and then when I knew I was getting to the point of coming, I turned on the vibrator and held it on the top of my vaginal opening by my clit. I came and let loose with a cry that probably echoed 'round the neighborhood. It was a rolling orgasm and I couldn't stop using the vibrator. I kept coming, my clit throbbing, and I think I came five times.

We hope that if you have a less than satisfying experience your first time playing with a vibrator you won't give up. You may just need to experiment in the ways described in the How To section above, or you may need to try a different style. There really is no one perfect vibrator—we've heard from just as many women disappointed that a toy was too weak as from those who thought it too strong. Only you can decide what pleases you sexually, and this will be an ongoing process of self-discovery. Good resources are Betty Dodson's book *Sex for One* and her video *Selfloving; For Yourself* by Lonnie Barbach; and *Good Vibrations: The Complete Guide to Vibrators* by Joani Blank.

Minimize Disappointment

Anybody who plays with sex toys regularly has at least one disappointing experience to relate, and some people have more than their fair share. As one survey respondent reminds us:

One problem with sex toys is that you generally can't take them for a test drive before purchase!

True enough, but unlike with a car, there aren't too many people who'd want to take a vibrator out for a spin once another customer's done with it! If you're dubious about the orgasmic payoff, you'll think twice about plunking down a bunch of cash for a toy you can't necessarily return (many sex toy retailers accept returns only on unused or defective toys).

It's truly unfortunate to anticipate a great erotic adventure, only to be let down. For those new to vibrators, this can be enough to discourage further use. Because the adult industry has traditionally exploited consumer fears and embarrassment around sex toys,

many have gotten away with selling low-quality merchandise at inflated prices. We've heard from more than one person who bought a fifty-dollar toy only to have it break down in three days. By contrast, we've heard from countless others who described their most disappointing toy experience as having their batteries die. Yes, that's unpleasant, particularly if it happens at a crucial moment, but—duh!—there is a simple remedy: Keep a supply of batteries on hand! We can't spare all of you the pain of a poorly made toy, but we can give you some tips that will help you keep your expectations in check and minimize disappointment:

- Keep spare batteries on hand.
- If you have a favorite toy, consider stocking a backup, in case your beloved dies.
- Take care of the toy—check the Vibrator Care and Cleaning sidebar for details.
- Think about what you want the toy to do before you buy it: Refer to the Vibrator Shopping Checklist sidebar for advice.
- Wear a skeptic's hat: If the sales hype on a toy sounds too good to be true, it probably is.
- Shop at places you trust or look for brand-name toys reputed to be higher quality.
- Get advice from others. Shop at webites that post customer product reviews, ask friends about their favorites, look for best-sellers.
- Check the returns policy. Some retailers will let you return any toy for any reason within a certain time frame.
- Give the vibrator a second chance. You might've been too nervous the first time, or your expectations were too high.
- If at first you don't succeed....

Keep Your Sense of Humor

Sex can be a nerve-wracking business. There's the performance anxiety, the communication issues, the awkwardness. It's no Hollywood movie, that's for sure—though sometimes it qualifies as a romantic comedy. If you're playing with sex toys, you'll have a lot more fun, and a better chance of meeting with success, if you keep your sense of humor. Bear in mind that sex is supposed to be fun!

Just pulling out my vibrator, turning in on to waggle, and demonstrating the five speeds usually puts my partners into hysterics.

Trends and Innovations

The more people discover what powerful tools of pleasure vibrators can be, the more they crave new and different types. Fortunately, many toy manufacturers and entrepreneurs are listening. Thanks to technological advancements and more-demanding consumers, vibrators have reached new heights of quality and variety. As in the fashion world, there will always be vibrator trends that come and go, but among these latest innovations, more than a few are here to stay.

MICROCHIPS. The microchip didn't just revolutionize computers, it literally transformed vibrators—they're smaller, they run faster, and they offer more options when it comes to playing with speeds. Some vibrators come with push-button controls that let you program the desired speed, pulse, rhythm, or rotation of the toy. One of our manufacturers thinks this is overkill and that consumers will eventually want to "return to the days of the simple variable speed control, just like they want the knobs back on their car radios." We tend to agree, but find the microchip's other effects quite pleasing—tinier but more powerful toys, remote-controlled toys, and vibrators needing no battery packs.

WATCH BATTERIES. Vibrators have typically been on the bulky side because they needed to house a battery pack large enough for a AA or C battery. One ingenious inventor discovered that a watch battery could provide ample power and fit in a much smaller toy. The result: the first-ever fingertip vibrator, called the Fukuoku 9000. A small pad fits over your fingertip, giving that ordinary hand job a buzzing boost (wear five of them, and your hand becomes a vibrating machine). It's a great toy for hands that tire easily, or when you want to retain the feel of skin on skin but need a little extra stimulation. We expect to see more products that take advantage of watch batteries.

WATERPROOF. It took a while, but the adult industry finally figured out that if you insert an ordinary washer into the base of a battery-operated vibrator, voilà, it's waterproof. What no one anticipated was the popularity of this innovation, but when you think about the endless possibilities for sex in the tub, the shower, the pool, the hot tub, the lake, the ocean (um, you get the idea), it makes a lot of sense. Plus, waterproof vibrators are so much easier to clean. Today many styles come in a waterproof version; just check the packaging.

NEW MATERIALS. For years, vibrator lovers have contented themselves with certain basic materials: rubber, vinyl, or hard plastic. But the emergence of two new materials, used first in dildos, gives consumers more options in insertable vibrators:

- *Silicone*. The recent marriage of vibrators with silicone—a premium-grade material used for dildos—elevates the quality of insertable vibrators tremendously. Silicone is easy to clean, retains body heat, and transmits vibrations extremely well. Look for silicone dildos and plugs with vibrators built in, or with hollowed-out cores that accommodate battery vibes.
- *Cyberskin*. The most recent breakthrough in sex toy material, cyberskin feels more like skin than anything else on the market. It warms quickly, is pliable and soft, and stretches easily but will "remember" its original shape. It is porous, however, so remember to clean it after each use with mild soap and water, or use it with a condom.

COLOR. Long gone are the days when vibrators came in a just a couple of colors—usually some hideous attempt at Caucasian flesh tones. Nowadays, vibrators come in as many colors as fashion will permit. Depending on what's currently trendy, your vibrator might be translucent lime to match your iMac or leopard-skin print to match your hand bag. We've seen many color trends come and go: One year primary colors are in while pastels are out, then the next year metallics make a splash while glitter, swirl, or jewel colors take a back seat. But one thing is clear: You'll never have to worry about too few choices again!

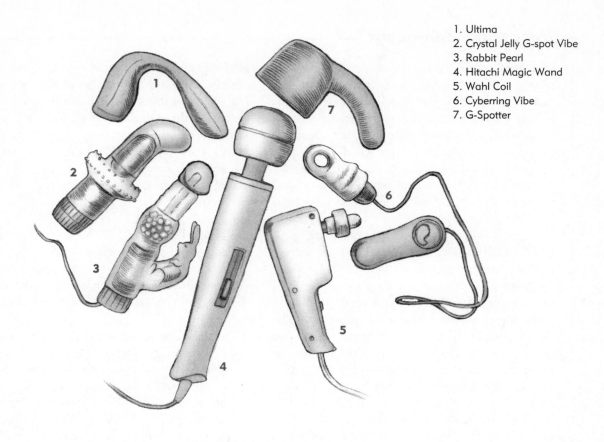

1. Ultima
2. Crystal Jelly G-spot Vibe
3. Rabbit Pearl
4. Hitachi Magic Wand
5. Wahl Coil
6. Cyberring Vibe
7. G-Spotter

Various styles of vibrators

Shop Around

Vibrators—also commonly referred to as "massagers"—come in all sizes and shapes. Some look like eggs, some like hand-held mixers, some like, well, penises. Depending on what kind of stimulation you like, you might find one style, or a combination of several styles, to be your favorite. In this chapter we'll describe a multitude of different models and offer suggestions for incorporating them into your sex play. Keep in mind that while this may look like an exhaustive list, it isn't—there are enough different vibrators on the market to fill a dozen toy chests. Since we don't want to overload your circuits with too much information, we've limited our selection to the most popular, well-made, and best-known. Also keep in mind that sex toys come and go. We'll list the latest trends and styles, but today's hot ticket might end up in tomorrow's waste bin.

Many people confuse vibrators and dildos. What distinguishes a vibrator from a dildo or another type of sex toy is that it vibrates. The vibrator is powered either by electricity or batteries (no solar-powered toys yet!). Phallic-shaped vibrators can be used as vibrating dildos (that is, they can be inserted vaginally or anally), but if you want something penis-like that does not vibrate, you're looking for a dildo or plug.

We debated whether to list prices for the different models in this book. Obviously, any prices we list today will be outdated next year, one reason why we chose not to include them. And depending on where you buy them, the prices vary drastically. We used to tell people that, in general, electric vibrators are more expensive than battery vibrators. But these days you can buy an inexpensive electric vibrator at most department stores, then turn around and pay twice as much for a novelty battery vibrator purchased from an adult bookstore or catalog. We have included the names and addresses of our favorite sex boutiques, catalogs, and websites in our resource listings and we encourage you to shop around!

Electric Vibrators

These vibrators run off the standard 110 volts. The body of the vibrator is attached to a plug-in cord. Most commonly marketed by major appliance manufacturers like Panasonic and Hitachi as "personal massagers," electric vibrators are well-made (most have a one-year warranty) and are widely available—you can almost always find a brand or two in drugstores or department stores, shelved as beauty-care products or sports massagers. Because they are not marketed as sex toys, you are less likely to find electric massagers in adult bookstores.

Besides being well-made with long life expectancies, electric vibrators are great for other reasons. Most feature a couple of different speeds or a rheostat so that you can adjust the vibration to your liking. Because they run on electricity, you won't experience the frustration of your batteries running out at the crucial climax. (Although there is the chance of a power outage or a blown fuse!) Electric vibrators tend to be more powerful than their battery brethren, something you may or may not appreciate for sexual massage, but which makes them far superior for full-body massage.

In countries with different electric currents, it is possible to use your electric vibrator with an adapter. Pay careful attention—the vibrator may heat up more quickly than usual.

Wand Vibrators

To celebrate my 50th birthday. I stayed home alone, put on a wonderful silk gown, laid out candles and incense, listened to my favorite music, got a little stoned, and spent the evening with my Hitachi Magic Wand, on a quilt spread on the living room floor. I must have come twenty or thirty times in the course of that evening.

WHAT THEY LOOK LIKE: Dubbed "wand" vibrators because the long shape resembles a magic wand, this type of vibrator has always been popular at Good Vibrations. Wand vibrators are usually about a foot long, with a soft, rubber, tennis ball-sized head attached to one end. Before your mouth drops open, let us just say: *Wands are not designed for insertion, but for external clitoral stimulation.* You grip the long plastic handle and place the vibrating head against the clit. Most wands have either a high and a low speed or a rheostat. When the vibrator is on it emits a low whirring noise. The Hitachi Magic Wand is by far the best-known.

VARIATIONS: The length of the body, the size of the head, the weight, the noise, and the intensity of the vibrations vary somewhat between brands. Some also have angled bodies for "hard to reach" places. Rechargeable versions of some wand vibrators are on the market, so you don't have to be connected to an outlet. The charge usually lasts from thirty to sixty minutes, then takes eight to twelve hours to recharge.

HOW TO USE: Women can try pressing the side of the head against or near the clitoris. The shape of the wand lends itself well to numerous positions—lie down on top of it, prop it up against your clit while on your side, hold it between your legs while on your back.

I like to lie on my side with the head of the wand gripped firmly between my thighs—keeping it snug against my clit. This frees up my hands to do other things.

I prop my Hitachi up on a pillow and lean forward onto it while I'm squatting on a vibrating dildo (the kind that rotates and vibrates). I orgasm to my heart's content.

The large head spreads the vibrations out over a greater surface area when it's pressed against the skin, which many experience as a more penetrating vibration. Because the vibrations are diffused by the large head, the intensity is not all focused solely on one spot.

Where was I before my Magic Wand? The level of stimulation is just great.

Men can try pressing the wand directly against the base of the penis, running it along the shaft, touching the head, or resting the penis on top of the head. If this is too intense, try cupping the penis with one hand and holding the vibrator against the back of your hand. You may also enjoy the indirect vibrations provided when your penis is inside the vagina of a woman using the wand on her clitoris:

The first time she turned on her wand when I was inside her, I came in thirty seconds. Once I got used to the stimulation of the vibrator, I would often use it on myself, resting my soft penis on top of the vibrator head. I found the vibration was more numbing than stimulating though, once I got hard.

The straight body and large head allow the wand to be easily positioned between face-to-face partners, offering dual stimulation:

During intercourse my wand vibrates the base of his penis and my clit at the same time, which gets us both off.

Because the vibrating head is fairly large, people with limited mobility may find it easier to lie on top of the wand or to clutch it between their thighs. Finally, wand vibrators can't be beat for full-body massage—they feel particularly good run along either side of the spine, across the shoulders, or on the lower back.

ATTACHMENTS: To date, there are only a few specifically sexual attachments designed to fit over the head of a wand (and they will only fit over a head shaped like the Hitachi's). The Wonder Wand and G-Spotter are two lightweight, vinyl caps that can be pushed all the way down over the head of the vibrator. The Wonder Wand has a seamless, four-inch, straight tip and is about three-quarters of an inch in diameter. The G-Spotter is the same size, but curved to vibrate against the G-spot area in the front wall of the vagina. When you insert the tip, the area of the cap below the tip will vibrate against your clitoris, offering you glorious simultaneous clitoral and vaginal vibrations! More recently, silicone manufacturer Vixen Creations has created the Gee Whiz—similar to the G-Spotter, but with a larger dildo portion, and a raised bump on the cap for clit stimulation—all fashioned out of supremely comfortable silicone. These attachments also provide more focused clitoral stimulation if you place the tip against your clit.

The G-spot stimulator on the Hitachi Wand is my favorite sex toy. Wow! Now there's an intense orgasm. It also makes the vibration against my clit less intense, which is better for me since my clit is very sensitive.

These attachments are also ideal for anal insertion, since the insertable portion has no chance of slipping off and getting lost in the rectum.

The third attachment, called the Magic Connection, fits over the head of a wand vibrator like the other two. It has a small black protrusion, which is used to adapt attachments from coil vibrators to a wand. The Magic Connection is used most commonly to adapt the Come Cup, a tulip-shaped attachment designed to stimulate the head of the penis (see the discussion of attachments in the following section).

Coil-Operated Vibrators

WHAT THEY LOOK LIKE: These vibrators resemble small hand-held mixers or hair brushes. They're usually about six or seven inches long with a handle; the attachments fit over a small round metal nub (about one-half inch) that sticks out at a right angle from the body. The term "coil-operated" refers to the electromagnetic coil inside the body that creates the vibration (and is also responsible for the relative heaviness of this type of vibrator). These vibrators are practically silent, making them very appealing to folks who don't want to hear a motor running while they masturbate. They are always packaged with a variety of attachments (see below). Most models have a high and a low speed, but never an adjustable speed. This type of vibrator has been on the market the longest, which is why you may recognize one that looks like your grandmother's! Wahl is the most famous name brand—but there are plenty of other good-quality models as well.

I own a Wahl Coil. I have nicknamed it "Wally," and haven't had a dull night (or day) with it.

VARIATIONS: The shape of the handle, color, attachments, weight, and speed vary only slightly between models. Most are packaged with numerous attachments, whose shape and size may vary by manufacturer.

HOW TO USE: Place the desired attachment over the metal nub on the body. When you turn it on, it should be practically inaudible (without an attachment, the vibrator may make a loud rattling noise). Grasp the handle and place the vibrating tip on your genitals.

Because the attachment is relatively small, the vibrations are quite focused when placed against the skin, creating a very intense, localized vibration. It is a markedly different sensation than that produced by the larger-headed wand vibrators, and the reason why some people remain true to one type or the other for their entire lives. Remember that you can experiment—stop and start the motor, switch the speeds, or place a towel between you and the vibrator.

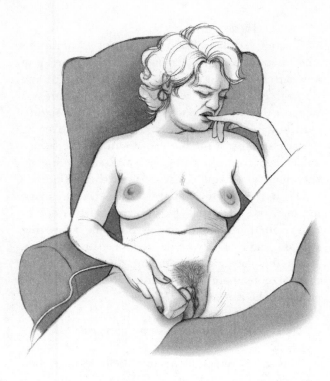

Masturbating with coil vibrator

I've had the coil massager for four years. I enjoy the stimulation through cotton or something like a sheet or underwear.

ATTACHMENTS: Coil-operated vibrators are usually packaged with multiple attachments. For clitoral stimulation, most women prefer the small, rounded attachment we call a Clitickler (sometimes referred to on the box as the "spot massager"). Some models come with a modified version of this that resembles three concentric rings in the shape of a small pyramid. Try different attachments; one woman told us her favorite attachment was the spiky one advertised as the "scalp massager." Another intrepid customer discovered that the concave attachment will form a tight seal when pressed against the base of a silicone dildo or plug, thus creating a powerful vibrating dildo.

I love my plug-in Wahl vibrator with clit attachment. I use it as much on myself as I do on my partner (on his butt, or during intercourse so that it hits the base of his penis and also my clit).

I've gotten off from holding the vibrator with the scalp massager attachment gently against the underside of my testicles. Also lightly running the clit attachment along either side of my penis.

Other attachments designed specifically for sexual purposes can be purchased separately. These are long, insertable attachments, but, as in the case of the wand attachments, they're usually only available in one size (about four inches long by about one-half inch in diameter). You can choose between a straight or curved attachment—the straight one will maneuver more comfortably inside your vagina if you're using the vibrator in different positions, while the curved one is designed to stimulate the G-spot. These are *not* safe for anal use.

An attachment we call the Twig with two, finger-width branches set at a forty-five degree angle provides both clitoral and vaginal vibrations. If the angle isn't perfect for you, try pressing down on the clitoral branch with your free hand. Vixen Creations has designed a silicone G-spot attachment similar to the Twig called the Wally, which sports a clitoral branch. Both these attachments are safe to use anally, because the branch prevents them from disappearing into the rectum, should they pop off the short shaft of the vibrator.

The Come Cup, an attachment just for men, is designed to vibrate the head of the penis. The attachment is tulip-shaped (about one and a half inches deep) and is expandable, though we do recommend placing ample lube inside the attachment to prevent pinching.

I have to be in the right mood for it because the vibration on the head of the penis is pretty intense, but when I am, that Come Cup attachment feels great. I alternate stroking my penis and vibrating the tip.

Double-Headed

WHAT THEY LOOK LIKE: These powerful vibrators boast two tennis-ball-sized heads that protrude several inches apart at an angle from the vibrator body. They are motor-driven, usually have a high and a low speed, and are fairly loud and quite heavy.

VARIATIONS: Not too many of these are on the market, but the couple we've seen vary in size—of both the body and the two heads—and subsequently in weight. The speed of the vibrations can vary noticeably between models.

HOW TO USE: The heads on these personal massagers are placed just far enough apart so that you can enjoy simultaneous vibrations on the genitals and the anus. The Hitachi heads will accommodate the wand attachments described above, enabling you to experiment with multiple vibration and penetration. A penis will fit nicely between the two vibrating heads—but hold on to your hat, for this is one powerful vibration. The angle of two heads makes this perfect for two people who want simultaneous vibrations. You may have to argue over which of you has to hold it in place, as some models are heavy and cumbersome. Don't forget to use this for massage—moving the double heads slowly down the spine has turned scores of our customers into jelly.

Eroscillator

This vibrator resembles an electric toothbrush and creates a sensation somewhat like a subdued coil vibrator. Why then, at a retail price of over one hundred dollars, does it cost more than three times as much as a coil vibrator? According to the product packaging, seven years of research and state-of-the-art Swiss engineering have gone into the design of the "oscillating" Eroscillator head, which moves side to side "thirty-six hundred times per minute" with "pinpoint intensity" that "provides easier, faster, better orgasms." It's great that a decent quality toy is finally being openly promoted for sexual use, but it's depressing to us that the toy comes with an inflated price tag and irresponsible hype.

Battery Vibrators

If we conducted a poll asking people to name the portable toys that give them the most pleasure, we know battery vibrators would rate right up there with cell phones and digital cameras.

Battery vibrators come in a mind-boggling variety of shapes, sizes, and colors. Most run on the common C or AA batteries, though some run on other kinds. You insert the batteries either into the body of the vibrator or into a battery pack that is attached to the body by a cord.

Overall, battery vibrators emit gentler vibrations than electric vibrators. However, the intensity of any battery vibrator can vary based on the type and number of batteries required. In other words, a vibrator that runs on one AA battery will be significantly weaker than one that runs on three C batteries. Many of the battery vibrators have a variable speed control at the base and, depending on the quality of the construction, the difference between the "high" and the "low" speeds can be minimal or substantial. New microchip technology has resulted in control panels on some vibes that will let you program your desired speed and rotation. While this may appeal to techno-lovers, we find we expend more energy programming the machine than enjoying the ride!

Battery-operated vibrators are my only deities!

This survey respondent is not alone; battery vibrators boast a large and faithful following. Their charm lies primarily in their portability, versatility, and low cost. Because it does not rely on an electric outlet, your battery vibrator can accompany you anywhere—on a trek through the woods, across international borders, or to a play party. In general, battery vibrators are usually fairly lightweight and compact, making them ideal for tucking into an overnight bag or a purse.

I like my tiny battery vibrator, which I use in traffic (only in still traffic). Because I have so much time, it usually does really get me going and I have come occasionally on the road.

I like to be prepared for any sexual encounter, and along with condoms, battery vibrators are a key item in my portable bag of tricks.

The adult industry has flooded the market with a million variations on a couple of themes. A typical cylindrical vibrator can be used externally to stimulate the clitoris, or internally for vaginal or anal vibrations. There are vibrating sleeves for the penis, gadgets to simultaneously vibrate the penis and the clitoris during intercourse, vibrators you can sit on, strap on, clip on, and so on.

While battery vibrators are generally fairly inexpensive, expect the price to go up for every new and unusual feature. It bears repeating that it's worth shopping around; prices can fluctuate as much as twenty dollars for similar models sold by different companies.

Of course, the flip side of their relatively low price (and you knew there was one) is that quality is not usually a consideration in the manufacturing of these toys. If there is a warranty at all, it's for one month, tops. Many battery vibrators are poorly made; they can break easily or poop out for no apparent reason. We'll give you some tips on how to take the best care of your battery toy, but even with proper care and a supply of fresh batteries, history has proven their life span to be as unpredictable as the timing of the next earthquake:

> My battery-operated vibrator broke at the screw-on part and every time I use it, it loses its contact with the battery and dies. I end up having to whack it to get it to work. Sometimes it stops tragically right before I come.

That said, it's worth noting that toy quality has improved greatly over the years. Yes, there are still plenty of shoddy vibrators out there, but as consumer expectations have risen, so too has the number of better-made sex toys. Periodically, appliance makers like Hitachi will release a battery vibe, and more recently entrepreneurs like Candida Royalle (see sidebar) have come out with high-quality models like the Natural Contours. You can expect to pay more, but in the long run it's worth it if you get more bang for your buck.

Finally, keep in mind that many of the vibrators we're about to describe are packaged and sold under a variety of different names. We're using the names we're familiar with, but in general, you're usually better off trying to hunt down a battery vibrator by description (size, shape, color, and any special features) rather than by name.

Cylindrical Vibrators

WHAT THEY LOOK LIKE: These are the toys that come to most people's minds when you say the word "vibrator." There are two basic versions: one designed to resemble a penis, the other smooth and usually straight. They are ordinarily made of hard plastic, pliable vinyl, or jelly rubber, with a few made of silicone or cyberskin. In general, vibrations from vinyl, rubber, and cyberskin models are not as strong as their hard plastic counterparts, primarily because the thicker material absorbs a lot of the vibration. At the other end of the spectrum is silicone, which transmits vibrations very well.

They range in size from about four to eight inches, an average size being about seven inches long by one-and-a-quarter inches wide. Most of them have a variable speed control at the base, though some are attached to a battery pack by a cord. These vibrators are available individually or can be found packaged as kits, with an assortment of attachments (see below).

VARIATIONS: Design, size, color, texture, and type of battery vary. Here are four common versions of this type of vibrator.

- *Realistic:* Designed to look and feel like a real penis. While the mold attempts to capture the look of an actual penis (veins and all), no one has ever mistaken the color or texture for actual flesh. Usually about seven inches long and available in multiple colors, the most common being peach—the color the adult industry thinks resembles Caucasian skin tone.

- *Smoothie:* Cylindrical, smooth, and made of hard plastic, Smoothies are usually about seven inches long and have the strongest vibrations of the cylindrical vibrators. They come in a mind-boggling array of colors, from pastel to metallic to pearlescent hues, as well in waterproof versions—which makes them the ideal choice for someone who wants a vibrator to match every outfit, every room, every car, not to mention a spare for the swimming pool!

- *Softer Smoothie:* These versions of the Smoothie (made from rubber, cyberskin, or silicone) produce gentler vibrations. They too are available in assorted colors. Some jelly rubber models are also slightly rippled or textured, and are attached to a battery pack by a cord.

- *Mini Smoothie:* Simply a smaller version of the Smoothie, usually about five inches long by one inch wide, also available in many different colors. A slight variation on the Mini, called the Twig, features a short branch at the base that can be used for clitoral stimulation when the dildo portion is inserted. This model can also be used safely for anal insertion.

HOW TO USE: We can't reiterate enough that, despite the myth and marketing of cylindrical vibrators as "penis substitutes," most women don't orgasm from inserting them without accompanying clitoral stimulation. These can, however, be easily pressed into service as effective clitoral stimulators:

I come using a dildoesque battery-operated vibrator. It was only six dollars when I bought it, but it's brought me tons of pleasure. I like to read erotica while I place it on my clit.

Since they offer fairly gentle vibrations, these vibrators can be ideal for men who find electric vibrators overwhelming and for women who prefer mild stimulation. But if power is what you seek, they may not do the trick. If you enjoy the feeling of fullness in your vagina combined with vibration, try placing one vibrator on your clitoris and another in your vagina. Or you can use this style to explore prostate or G-spot stimulation.

I like to steal my girlfriend's jelly jewel while she's on business trips and give my prostate a little buzz. I prefer the kind attached to a battery pack because I can easily reach and manipulate the speed control.

I like sex with a vibrator inside me while rubbing my clit on a pillow, which I've mounted. I love it while being held by my lover cooing in my ear and saying, "Oh yes, oh yes, uh-huh...."

I stuck my battery vibrator in the freezer once and got an intense thrill masturbating with a vibrating popsicle!

ATTACHMENTS: Most of the standard cylindrical vibrators (about one-and-a-half inches in diameter) will accommodate a variety of attachments, or "sleeves," that allow you to change the shape and texture of the vibrator. Among the more functional is the "anal sleeve," a four-inch-long, finger-width attachment. For the most part, these attachments feature a range of rubbery nubs or spikes, rather like French ticklers, that evoke little sensation when inserted vaginally, but might be worth experimenting with on the more sensitive clitoris.

G-Spot Vibrators

WHAT THEY LOOK LIKE: In reality, you can use any insertable toy to stimulate the G-spot, yet many women find that these modified cylindrical vibes get more to the point. They sport a curve or a strategically placed bump toward the end of the shaft, which is designed to vibrate against the front wall of the vagina. G-spot vibrators are made of plastic, soft vinyl, or jelly rubber. Some women prefer G-spot toys made from firmer materials (since the G-spot responds more to pressure than vibration), while others find those made from softer materials more comfortable for insertion.

VARIATIONS: We've seen a large (eight inches long by one-and-a-half inches in diameter) and a small (five-and-a-half by one-and-five-eighths) version of this vibrator, as well as a waterproof model and one shaped like a banana. Some sport external ridges or branches designed to simultaneously stimulate the clitoris.

HOW TO USE: Some women can orgasm through stimulation of the G-spot, though not all women respond to this type of stimulation. If you're trying to locate your G-spot, you may want to explore it manually first and then experiment with G-spot vibrators. The most popular positions for G-spot stimulation are squatting or rear entry. Insert the vibrator and angle it so that the tip is pressing firmly against the front wall of the vagina. Sometimes arousal or orgasm triggered from G-spot stimulation will result in ejaculation of fluid through the urethra—this fluid is female ejaculate, not urine (see the Sexual Anatomy 101 chapter for more on the G-spot).

The curve on a G-spot vibrator also makes it a handy tool for stimulating a man's prostate gland. Insert the vibrator about three inches into the rectum, angling the tip toward the front of your body. Experiment to find out what feels the most pleasurable—steady pressure or gentle movement.

Dual Vibrators

WHAT THEY LOOK LIKE: Another variation on the cylindrical model, these have a branch protruding from the shaft of the vibrator, intended to stimulate the clitoris while the swiveling dildo portion is inserted into the vagina. Each function has separate variable-speed controls; the swiveling motion of the dildo can be adjusted independently of the strength of the vibrating attachment. You decide whether you want to experience rotation, vibration, or both together.

This style originally hails from Japan, where it used to be against the law to make sex toys that resemble genitals. Consequently, manufacturers there launched a tradition of creative alternatives. The vibrating dildo portion of these toys often resembles a person or totem, while the vibrating clitoral branch resembles an animal—usually the animal's tongue or nose flicks the clitoris. If you've ever fantasized about an animal's tongue on your private parts, this is probably as close as you'll get. The sheer versatility and novelty of these toys renders them slightly more expensive than your typical battery toy. As microchip technology has gained in popularity, more American novelty companies are producing these vibrators. Choosing a style can be somewhat daunting, but we'd caution you not to base your choice on price alone—for the cheaper the vibrator, the cheaper the parts. Japanese-made vibrators, particularly those distributed by Vibratex, tend to be of better quality.

My favorite vibrator is black rubber with two controls, one for the part that you insert and the other for the part that flicks at the clitoris, anus, or whatever's handy. On mine, the flicking part is attached to this fetching little beaver. I really like masturbating with something that has a distinct personality.

VARIATIONS: The size of the dildo varies; a common size is about seven inches long by one-and-a-half inches in diameter (though the insertable portion is only about four inches long). The dildo portion on several models, such as the Rabbit Pearl, features rotating plastic balls in the center, adding yet another dimension to an already extraordinary experience! We've peddled a veritable menagerie of animals over the years—beavers, bears, cats, and kangaroos, many of which are available in a range of colors. On some versions, the vibrator is attached to a battery pack by a cord, while others have a self-contained battery pack in their base. Manufacturers are always coming up with new twists on this toy; we've seen models that sport a flashing light at the tip, some that are waterproof, and some that offer an illuminated LED control panel. Many of these features come and go, but the basic design remains a classic.

Some models have no clitoral attachment, which you may prefer if you like the size and vibration of the dildo, but prefer your own hand or another vibrator to

the gentler clitoral vibrations offered by the animal tongue. Another variation is the dual vaginal/anal vibrator, which is outfitted with two insertable branches.

HOW TO USE: You've probably figured it out by now, but the beauty of this style is the explosive combination of internal and external vibrations. If you're using the vibrator vaginally and need more external stimulation, apply pressure to the clitoral branch to increase the vibrations against the clitoris. Whether you're using the vibrator vaginally or anally, try inserting the dildo portion while the vibrator is off and then turning the power up slowly. The swiveling dildo alone may offer just the right stimulation of the G-spot or prostate gland. You may have to hold on to the base of the dildo with one hand to prevent it from sliding out, or from swiveling only at the protruding end. Another way to enjoy this toy is by kneeling or squatting and moving up and down on the dildo.

The Rabbit Pearl vibrator is my favorite because I can fuck it to death and no one is there to see what a slut a nice lady can turn into.

Vibrating Eggs or Bullets

WHAT THEY LOOK LIKE: Vibrating eggs are slightly smaller than a real egg and come attached to a battery pack by a cord; they are made of hard plastic or plastic covered in soft vinyl, jelly rubber, or cyberskin. Eggs are designed to be inserted vaginally, but they can certainly be pressed against the clitoris. If the egg is less robust in the middle, it is often referred to as a "pearl" or a "bullet." You can find these in almost any adult store, but one Japanese model stands above the rest. It's often called the Pink Pearl (as it's pink and shaped like a bullet), and while it's a little more expensive than other bullets it's much better quality.

Variations: The dimensions and girth of the egg/bullet vary as do the color choices. Thanks to technological innovations, you can now find remote-controlled eggs, cordless bullet vibes the size of peanuts, or models with settings that include "vibrate," "pulsate," "escalate," and "surge!"

HOW TO USE: Grasp the egg between your fingers and insert it into the vagina as you would a tampon.

The cord keeps the egg attached to the battery pack outside the body. Because the egg will nestle securely inside the vagina, you can literally wear this vibrator underneath your clothing and turn it on and off as you please! Just tuck the battery pack under your belt. When you're ready to remove the egg from your vagina, do not pull on the cord. Reach up inside your vagina and pull on the bottom of the egg. If you concentrate on relaxing your vaginal muscles and bear down a little, the egg will slide right out. Use your cordless egg externally unless you are comfortable reaching into the vagina and retrieving it.

A vibrating egg is a great clitoral stimulator as well, as you can nestle it comfortably against the clitoris or folds of the labia, focusing the vibrations right where you want them. This type of vibrator lends itself well to erotic combinations with other toys.

I recently had great orgasms with a nubby silicone dildo and an "egg" clit vibrator, working simultaneously. Wow! The only thing I would like when using these two toys is a third hand!

The first time I ever had what I call my Whole Body Orgasm, I was eight months pregnant, on my knees with a dildo up my butt and a pillow behind me to keep it there, another dildo in my vagina and a bullet vibe on my clit. It started in my toes and went clear up my whole body. I lay there shaking, thinking "What the hell was that?"

I bought a remote vibrating egg for a friend of mine and she wore it in her panties at several meetings. I had the control and sat at another table. She's very sensitive, and we both enjoyed the game of my "buzzing" her almost to the point of orgasm and then backing off over and over during the meetings. The looks on her face as she attempted to not have orgasms were wonderful, and she thoroughly enjoyed the titillation.

Women have different reactions to vibrating eggs when used vaginally. Some find the sensation of vaginal vibrations riveting, others find it downright annoying, while still others can barely feel anything. You might want to try combining vibrating eggs with a clitoral vibrator to achieve sensations similar to those offered by the dual vibrators described above.

Many toys are designed to accommodate vibrating eggs. You can wear them in panties—offering endless possibilities for no-hands clitoral stimulation (see the next description). Or you can insert them into a hollowed-out dildo or anal plug to create a vibrating toy. Their compact size also makes them a convenient masturbatory device for men; you can easily place a vibrating egg between your palm and your penis or rest your penis on top of it:

My favorite masturbation method involves placing a vibrating egg underneath the tip of my penis and fantasizing. Although this tends to take longer to be successful, the orgasms are usually more powerful than with other methods.

Many customers have inquired about using these vibrators anally. We discourage folks from this practice because the cord can become detached from the egg once it's inside the anus, thus making it difficult to remove.

No-Hands Vibrators

WHAT THEY LOOK LIKE: Leg and waist straps attach to a vibrator (powered by a battery pack) and strategically position the vibrator over the clitoris. This model is often requested by women who desire a vibrator that can offer clitoral stimulation during intercourse, yet doesn't require a hand to hold it in place. While the concept is ingenious, many models suffer certain shortcomings: flimsy elastic straps fail to hold the vibrator in place, the vibrations are weak, or the clitoral stimulator is poorly designed.

It was disappointing that the harness straps for the Venus Butterfly are designed for someone with far tinier thighs than mine. To use it, I had to figure out some way to hook the straps together to make them longer. It was fun to use, but it is easier just to hold it in place than to try to put it on, and part of the fun was that it was a hands-free toy.

There have been significant improvements in design and motor-strength, but expect some degree of confusion when donning one of these (so many straps), and prepare for the likelihood that you'll want to press on the vibe to get the desired stimulation (thus defeating the "no-hands" feature!).

VARIATIONS:

- *Butterfly:* The original, and probably the best-known, models are Joni's Butterfly and the Venus Butterfly, but hummingbirds, dolphins, and bunnies have all been pressed into service as clit vibes. Thanks to our friend the microchip, these vibrators are substantially more compact than the original bulky models, and offer up stronger vibrations.
- *Panty/G-string and egg combination:* A more secure panty or G-string sports a small internal pouch, into which you insert a small vibrator. Look for leg and waist straps that are adjustable. In general you'll find that this ensemble sits more firmly on the clitoris than do vibrators attached to elastic straps.
- *Remote:* You wear one of the above versions of the toy, and your partner operates the controls.

HOW TO USE: Regardless of which model you use, the idea is to adjust the straps around your thighs or waist, and position the vibrator directly over your clitoris. If there's a battery pack, it can be tucked underneath one of the straps. This toy combination is particularly ideal for folks whose hands tire holding vibrators, or who have limited mobility. An adventurous few report wearing no-hands vibrators underneath clothing to a nightclub or loud party where no one can hear the buzz!

Because the vibrator is small and covers only the clitoris, you can wear these toys during penetration (if yours has a single, thong-style strap, simply move the strap aside).

Vibrating Sleeves

WHAT THEY LOOK LIKE: These are basically male masturbation sleeves with a vibrating egg tucked inside to create vibration. They're made of vinyl, jelly rubber, or cyberskin, and some have little nubs inside, for additional stimulation. Outwardly, these vibrators take on all manner of appearance. Some are plain tubes, others are sculpted to look like a pair of sucking lips or a vagina.

VARIATIONS: Some simply vibrate; others also move up and down in a simulated sucking motion. Some are attached to pumps (similar to blood pressure pumps), which add suction; some vibrate just the tip of the penis; and some are waterproof.

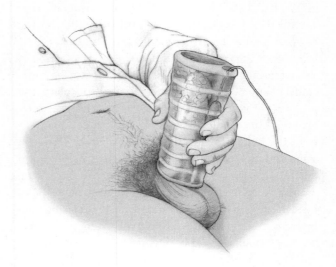

Masturbating with vibrating sleeve

HOW TO USE: You can squirt a bit of lube inside to make the sleeve more comfortable, particularly if you'll be thrusting in and out. Insert your penis and turn on the vibrator; most have a variable speed, so that you can control the intensity of the vibrations.

Vibrating Cock Ring with Clitoral Stimulator

WHAT IT LOOKS LIKE: These are cock rings with a small bullet vibrator mounted on one end. The vibrator is attached to a battery pack by a cord. Originally these were only made in hard plastic (necessitating the use of ample lube), but you can now find more comfortable versions made of stretchy rubber or cyberskin.

VARIATIONS:

- *Removable bullets:* Instead of the vibrator being fused to the cock ring, there's a loop or pouch into which a vibrator is inserted. This gives you the option of choosing from a wider variety of vibrating eggs, including cordless models.
- *Anal attachment:* This version features a vibrating anal plug attached by a separate cord to the same battery pack as the cock ring and bullet vibrator.
- *Latex:* A pouch for the scrotum is attached to the base of the cock ring.

HOW TO USE: For solo sex, place the cock ring around the base of your penis with the bullet on the bottom to enjoy testicular vibrations. The latex model is designed especially for solo play; the snug feeling of the latex combined with the vibrations can be especially pleasurable. For vaginal intercourse, place the cock ring around the base of your penis with the bullet on top. This vibrates the penis, and in certain positions the bullet vibrates the woman's clitoris—though some find problematic the fleeting, start/stop vibration during thrusting. You can also flip the cock ring around to make the vibrator stimulate the testicles instead of the clitoris during partner sex. During anal intercourse in certain positions, the vibrator can also provide stimulation for both partners.

My husband bought a clip-on vibrator that went on his penis (near the base) that had a cylindrical bit that rested against my clitoris (you could turn it around for front or rear entry). It had a hand control that one or the other of us could use to vary the intensity of the vibrations. This was amazingly effective. Because of the speed control it was brilliant for controlling my progress toward orgasm. If I operated the control I could push the intensity of my sensations higher and higher, just holding myself short of orgasm each time (by alternating between slow and fast) until eventually I'd have a blinding climax.

Love the cock ring vibrator—I swear I'm having a whipped cream ejaculation!

I have a hard time experiencing clitoral stimulation during intercourse, so my partner and I tried cock rings with vibrator attachments. Unfortunately, those vibrators are still too big/awkward to be pleasurable. If you're doing a lot of close, hard fucking, that vibrator ends up being more painful than pleasurable.

This type of toy can also be adapted quite nicely for use with a dildo and harness. You can try it the same way (placing the cock ring around the dildo on the outside of the harness) so that the receptive partner gets her clit stimulated. Or for direct self-stimulation the harness-wearer can place the cock ring around the dildo, between the harness and her own clit. Either way, you end up with a vibrating dildo!

Vibrating Strap-on Dildos

WHAT THEY LOOK LIKE: This is a vinyl or jelly rubber vibrating dildo (attached to a battery pack), which can be strapped on with elastic leg straps, enabling the wearer to penetrate a partner. There are usually nubby bits, on the bottom of the dildo portion, that the wearer is supposed to enjoy.

VARIATIONS: A slightly more secure variation has the vibrating dildo (attached to a battery pack) built into some latex briefs, but sizes can be problematic. Neither all-in-one toy holds a candle to the combination of a harness with a hollowed-out silicone dildo and a egg/bullet vibrator. You'll end up with a secure fit, a quality dildo, and a stronger vibration.

HOW TO USE: If you don your strap-on correctly, you can penetrate your partner with a vibrating dildo—definitely a unique sensation. However, if your lover has a tight grip on the vibrating dildo, the flimsy elastic leg straps will end up being mercilessly pulled out like a rubber band waiting to snap! The vibrations are also focused primarily in the base of the vibrator, which is nice for the wearer, but essentially defeats the purpose for the receptive partner. Using a vibrating dildo in a harness ensures the wearer a secure fit and allows for much more control over the action. In addition, a silicone dildo will transmit vibrations far better than vinyl or jelly rubber do.

One variation in this product line combines a strap-on dildo with a vibrating cock ring and clitoral stimulator. A man can slip his penis through the cock ring, clitorally stimulate his partner, and penetrate her both vaginally and anally—all at the same time! Similarly, a woman could wear this toy in a dildo harness to double-penetrate a female partner. The dildo portion of this toy is made of jelly rubber with a highly flexible spine, allowing you to mold it into the perfect position. Such ingenuity leaves us breathless!

Vibrating Double Dildos

WHAT THEY LOOK LIKE: Two dildos joined at the base are attached by a cord to a battery pack. There are usually two controls, one for each dildo, enabling you to vibrate the dildos separately or simultaneously.

VARIATIONS: Length (typically fourteen inches) and diameter (one-and-a-quarter inches) may vary.

HOW TO USE: Lying in a scissors position, two women can accommodate each end of the dildo vaginally, or a coupling of either sex can play with anal/anal or vaginal/anal penetration. Once the dildo is inserted, you can grasp its center and move it in and out, or you can leave it in one place and focus solely on the vibrations. We recommend using lots of lube for anal play, and remember, don't switch ends or move your toy from anus to vagina unless you're using fresh condoms. If you find this model unsatisfactory, you may want to consider using a first-rate double dildo, called the Nexus (see the Dildos chapter) and slipping a cock ring vibe around the center to add vibration.

Vibrating Nipple Toys

WHAT THEY LOOK LIKE: These tend to fall into two camps: nipple clamps or suction toys. With the clamps, two little bullets attach to your nipples with adjustable, vinyl-padded clamps, and are connected to a variable-speed battery pack. Suction toys are usually shaped like small cups and are attached to a hand pump (which provides suction) and a battery pack vibrator.

HOW TO USE: Use these for nipple stimulation if you want to free up your hands or if you wish to experiment with a new sensation.

I orgasm by just touching my nipples, so nipple teasers are the best!

"Personal Massagers"

A number of other battery-powered toys have appeared in mainstream stores recently. These are marketed, much like their electric counterparts, as "personal massagers." You won't find any that are phallic-shaped, but you will find them in almost every other imaginable size and shape. We've see some resembling paperweights and pens—the perfect desk accessory for the overworked executive! The smallest one we've seen looks like a spark plug—you've probably seen this advertised as the "Pocket Rocket."

The good news is, these are often better made than adult novelties, and many can't be beat for portable clitoral stimulation. Most are quite small and innocuous-looking (though they pack a punch), so you won't be embarrassed when the X-ray machine picks them up at the airport. The bad news is, styles tend to come

and go, so the toy you purchase today may not be around tomorrow. One exception is the Natural Contours vibrator line. Candida Royalle (see sidebar) designed this line specifically for women, and her most popular vibrator, the Ultime, offers simultaneous clitoral and G-spot vibrations.

Anal Vibrators

A vibrating butt plug has brought the most enjoyable intensity to sex.

I was lying on my back. She put a well-lubed battery vibrator in me while stimulating my penis. I got instantly hard, approached orgasm very quickly, and sprayed come all the way up my chest—which was common at 16, but not at 47!

Anal vibrators are popular sex toys for masturbation as well as partner sex; they can stimulate the anal opening and rectum in men and women, in addition to the prostate in men. You can use an anal vibrator to penetrate a partner, or an individual can "wear" one. As you probably noticed in the previous sections, many vibrators come with anal attachments—anal stimulation is a popular complement to other types of stimulation. Anal vibrators come in a variety of sizes and shapes. They tend to be either long and slender, or slightly diamond-shaped. Some models have a flexible spine, which allows you to mold the plug into any angle you desire. Others are set on handles, so that you can reach yourself or a partner with ease. To date, there are no electric toys designed specifically for anal use (though you can adapt a coil vibrator—use suction to affix the concave attachment to the base of a plug). Most anal vibrators run on AA or C batteries, are attached to a battery pack, and are made of vinyl or jelly rubber. Silicone manufacturers have started producing hollowed-out anal plugs, which usually hold a bullet vibrator.

If you'd prefer to be free of the cord and battery pack, you can use a variety of cylindrical battery toys as anal vibrators, or can slip slender sleeve attachments over them. If you're going to use one of the vibrators described in the previous section anally, make sure it has a flared base or a branch on it so that it won't slip into the rectum. If it lacks some kind of base, make sure it is at least seven inches long and keep a good grip on it. Also remember to change condoms on toys that go from anus to vagina.

Vibrator Shopping Checklist

✓ *Purpose:* What part (or parts) of your body do you want to stimulate? Is it for solo play, partner sex, or both?

✓ *Intensity:* Electric vibrators offer stronger vibrations than battery ones.

✓ *Durability:* Electric vibrators and brand-name battery vibrators last the longest.

✓ *Portability:* Battery vibrators or rechargeable electric models travel well.

✓ *Texture:* If you'll be inserting the toy, do you want hard plastic, pliable vinyl or rubber, or realistic cyberskin or silicone? Nonporous surfaces are easier to clean.

✓ *Shape:* Smooth? Rippled? Curved? Resembling a penis?

✓ *Color:* Flesh tones? Pastels? Metallics? Jewel tones? Glow-in-the-dark?

✓ *Noise:* Coil-operated electric vibes are the quietest, hard plastic battery vibrators and some large wand vibrators are the loudest.

✓ *Price:* You get what you pay for: Electric vibrators and dual-battery vibrators are on the high end, basic battery vibrators are on the low end.

Buying a Vibrator

You've made the decision to buy a vibrator, but you're not sure what the next step is. We suggest you answer the following questions to help ensure the success of your shopping expedition:

Do you want to stimulate the clitoris, vagina, G-spot, anus, prostate, or penis? If you have masturbated before, you probably have some idea which areas you'd like to try your vibrator on. If you have never masturbated before, you might want a vibrator that's a bit more versatile so that you can experiment. You might try a cylindrical model for insertion as well as external genital stimulation. Or you could test a massager with a variety of attachments, which would offer the same options in addition to a good full-body massage.

Are you looking for one vibrator that will do it all, or a variety of vibrators? Maybe you'd like to stimulate several areas simultaneously. It's usually a better

investment to combine a few different vibrators, each successfully stimulating one area, than to purchase some gizmo with lots of appendages. The other advantage to this is that you can pick and choose what to stimulate when, for those times when you'd rather not have everything going at once.

I love my Great King battery-operated dildo—using this with while I wear tit clamps is the best. A butt plug makes it absolutely beyond description.

Will you be inserting the vibrator? If you plan to insert a vibrator vaginally or anally, you will be concerned with size. Like Cinderella and that glass slipper, there's nothing better than the perfect fit. You can get a fair approximation of size if you know how many fingers fit comfortably in your vagina. Or, for even more accuracy, pare a cucumber down to a size you find accommodating and measure the length and diameter. If you're planning to insert the vibrator anally, you can use the finger test to judge size. When purchasing an anal vibrator, make sure to invest in one with a flared base.

Do you want gentle vibrations or strong vibrations? If your clitoris or penis is very sensitive to touch and responds to light stimulation, you might be content with the gentler vibrations offered by a battery vibrator that runs on a single AA battery. If you prefer more intense stimulation, consider an electric vibrator or a stronger battery vibrator (one that runs on two C batteries). If you want a vibrator that offers a range, invest in one with a rheostat, a variable-speed control, or programmable button controls.

Is durability important? If you want a vibrator that will last for years, you'll want an electric vibrator by a name-brand manufacturer. Their life span far outlasts the time limit specified in their warranties. If you're fond of battery vibrators, stick to the Japanese imports like the Rabbit Pearl or the Pink Pearl.

Is portability important? If you travel a lot, or like sex in the great outdoors, you'll want a battery vibrator. You can use a rechargeable electric vibrator outdoors, but you still need to be near a 110 volt outlet to recharge it when it runs out of steam.

I already have a longtime plug-in vibrator but I needed a portable companion on my marathon treks along beaches and headlands. (What I call "deep cuntry.") This battery vibrator has brought me to some lovely comes!

Is noise a factor? Some folks share apartments with thin walls and are embarrassed by noisy battery vibrators. The only virtually silent vibrators in existence are the coil-operated electric vibrators, but many of the new battery vibrators are much quieter than they used to be. Check Good Vibrations' website for a noise rating for each vibrator. You can also try vibrating under the covers, because the blankets muffle the noise quite a bit. And if keeping your vibrator a secret is important to you, please note that sometimes an electric vibrator plugged into the same circuit as a TV or radio can interfere with the reception!

My roommate in college had a vibrator. We lived with three guys who laughed every time she said she was tired and would go to bed early...five minutes later the TV would be fuzzy.

Is price a factor? You'll find battery vibrators offer a much greater variety of styles and colors at lower prices than electric vibrators. However, you may go through so many battery vibrators during the life span of one electric vibrator that the electric model could turn out to be the better value in the long run.

Where to Buy Vibrators

You'll find the largest selection of vibrators at adult bookstores and sex boutiques. (By "sex boutiques" we're referring to the more upscale sex stores like Good Vibrations that are popping up more frequently in urban areas.) Purchasing a sex toy is easiest if you can see it in person. You won't get a proper sense of the toy's size, texture, smell, or vibration unless you can pick it up and turn it on. We understand there are many people reluctant to patronize a sex shop, but shopping at department stores can be awkward, too. We suggest asking for the "personal massagers"—you'll most likely get a clerk who feels sorry for your sore muscles. If they're wise to the fact that massagers are used for sexual purposes, it's probably because they have one, in which case they'll give you that secret "welcome to the club" smile.

If you aren't up for shopping at your neighborhood sex shop, or you're too shy to purchase a massager at Macy's, there are other ways to get satisfaction. The most convenient and discreet way to shop for sex toys

---

Vibrator Care and Cleaning

- Don't drop the vibrator onto the floor. This will almost surely end in disaster.
- Remove the batteries when you're not using your toy. This will prevent the vibrator from being accidentally left on and wearing out the motor, and will keep the batteries from leaking and corroding the motor.
- If you've got one of the quiet plug-ins (like a coil vibrator), remember to turn it off, as these will overheat if left on too long.
- If your battery toy is not working, try blowing on the parts to clear out dust. You can also tinker with the wires a bit; sometimes two are crossed and just need to be separated. Make sure the batteries are removed first.
- Check that the batteries are inserted correctly and the base is screwed on tightly.
- Don't immerse the vibrator in water (unless it's specifically billed as waterproof).
- Clean nonporous vibrators with a damp cloth. Use condoms on porous toys or wipe them down with a clean cloth. Refer to the Dildos chapter for cleaning tips specific to different materials.

---

is with companies that have websites or catalogs—check the resource listings for our recommendations. While adult catalogs have been around for years, many people still resist ordering because they don't want the mail carrier (or the kids or the roommate) discovering their penchant for sex toys. Fortunately, the World Wide Web now removes that barrier. You are able to shop at leisure from your own home, without ever receiving a catalog. On top of that, many websites offer far more educational and consumer information than they do in their catalogs, and the proliferation of adult stores online (and that marvelous "search" function) mean you can comparison shop quite easily. For more information on online shopping, check out our World Wide Web chapter.

Finally, in-home pleasure parties—the sex toy equivalent of Tupperware parties—have made something of a comeback since their debut in the eighties. Ask your favorite toy store if they offer this service. Good Vibrations offers pleasure parties in the San Francisco Bay area.

When we receive battery vibrators named the "Hunk Multi-Speed" or the "Vibro Super-Cock" from our adult-industry vendors, we like to rebaptize these toys with more euphonious names before putting them out on our shelves. Over the years, our enthusiasm for catchy captions has landed us into some unexpected hot water.

For example, we thought nothing of listing all our dual-style vibrators under the heading "Double Your Pleasure" in our mail-order catalog—it seemed the obvious motto for vibrators that are designed to provide simultaneous clitoral and vaginal stimulation. We hadn't realized we were trespassing on a trademark until we received a letter from the attorneys for the William Wrigley Jr. Company (the chewing gum people), requesting that we cease and desist employing their copyrighted slogan. While this was an eminently reasonable request, we bristled at the attorney's comments that "Our client cannot allow its trademark to be used in connection with vibrators and the other products you advertise because of the unwholesome associations." Our indignant publicist wrote back, pointing out that vibrators are by no means unwholesome and that "a company that sells a tooth-decay promoting product with television advertisements that promise to 'double your pleasure' while promi-

nently featuring images of comely young twins is not really in a position to criticize anyone for 'unwholesome associations'." We received the soothing response that "scientifically conducted tests indicate that Wrigley's chewing gum is not a tooth-decay promoting product."

After this experience, we probably should have thought twice before naming a sleek, icy blue vibrator the "Popsicle Vibe." The folks at the Good Humor Corporation lived up to their name and were considerably better-humored than the Wrigley's attorney when they wrote to politely inform us that "When you selected this name, you were likely unaware that *Popsicle* is a registered trademark of our company." The pleasure of knowing that our mail-order catalogs are making the rounds in the offices of major corporations more than compensates for the minor inconvenience of devising a new name.

And not all major corporations are sex-negative. In honor of Good Vibrations' fifteenth anniversary, we commissioned chocolates made in the shape of the Hitachi Magic Wand electric vibrator, our perennial best-seller. Not only did the sales executives at Hitachi's corporate headquarters contribute to the cost of casting the chocolate mold, but they ordered five hundred chocolates to distribute at their annual sales conference.

Vibrators and Partners

Vibrators can enhance partner sex play in countless ways—you can vary your lovemaking routine, explore different paths toward orgasm (alone or together), or incorporate vibrators into your foreplay. Keep in mind that this is an area where success depends as much on your communication skills as it does on your positive attitude about sex toys. You might be excited about the introduction of vibrators into your sex life, but your partner may not necessarily be on the same wavelength. A few important things to remember:
- Don't assume you want the same things.
- Talk, listen, and avoid judgment.
- A vibrator can never replace a partner.

- Vibrators bring pleasure. If it brings you pleasure, your partner will probably like it.

Sharing Your Own Toy

It's amazing how much easier it is for us to share our vibrators with friends or roommates than with our partners. It's as if there's a sign posted over the conjugal bed that says "No appliances allowed." Seriously, it's stunning how many people assume their partners won't like vibrators and refuse even to consider broaching the subject. No matter how often we tell you how much fun two people can have with sex toys, unless you can raise the topic, the issue is moot. Here are a few common concerns people have cited for keeping vibrators out of their relationships, along with our suggestions for handling them:

He'll feel like he hasn't been pleasing me all these years. It's possible to be sensitive to a partner's ego without forgoing your own sexual pleasure. You can assure your partner that he has been pleasing you, otherwise you wouldn't have kept coming back for more! Introduce the vibrator as a way to increase pleasure for both of you, illustrating the many ways two people can enjoy it where one cannot. For example, if your vibrator orgasms are more intense, the pressure on his penis will probably be more intense during penetration, allowing him to experience a new sensation. Offer him control of the vibrator so that he can learn how to use it on you and get comfortable handling it himself. Suggest, but don't insist, that he might like using it on himself as well.

She'll think I don't need her anymore. Again, reassure your partner that there are countless ways vibrators fall short as sex partners (they're predictable, they have no sense of humor, and they make lousy kissers, to name a few). Treat your vibrator as an accessory to sex, not the main event. If vibrators are necessary for your orgasm, have her hold it, or encourage your partner to explore the rest of your body's infinite erotic terrain.

He thinks I shouldn't have to rely on something besides him for sex. Everyone employs some type of stimulation—in addition to a partner—during partner sex. For some people it's a certain fantasy, for others it's special clothing or a mood or setting. This stimulation may not always be necessary for you to reach orgasm, but it does enhance your sexual experience. You can try to find out what sorts of stimuli he responds to and then draw a parallel between that and your desire to bring a vibrator into your sex play. If you haven't talked about it before, find out if he masturbates (odds are he does) and suggest that this is an example of his not relying solely on you for sex. If it's orgasms he feels he should be giving you during partner sex, teach him how to hold the vibrator.

> One lover asked me, "Why would you want to use something mechanical?" to which I responded, "Wouldn't you rather machine wash than hand wash? Vibrators are quick, efficient, and get the job done!"

If none of these approaches works and you feel the need to choose between the partner or the toy, you might consider these words from Betty Dodson: "My advice to women just starting a new affair is: When you bring out your vibrator, it separates the jocks from the lovers. If he can't handle the concept that after you fuck you want to come with your vibrator, I'd recommend keeping your vibrator and getting rid of your lover. Men or women who love women don't make an issue over how their partner gets off, just as long as she does." In our ideal world, our lovers would care only about helping us reach new heights of pleasure:

> My most enjoyable toy experience, without a doubt, was the day I bought my then-girlfriend a Hitachi. She had only recently become orgasmic, and only had orgasms while fucking me (not that I minded!). But I had always been fascinated with women's masturbation. So when I gave her the vibe, she got right down to it. Within a couple of minutes, she had a lovely orgasm, her toes curling, thrashing around on the bed. Then laughter and smiles. I had given her the gift of being able to come on her own!

Buying a Toy for Your Partner

Think about why you're buying a vibrator. Do you have some expectation around improving your sex life that your partner might not be aware of? Do you think her orgasms should be different? How will she react? Are you buying him a vibrator because you want to use it yourself? What message will this send?

Talk to each other about your expectations beforehand (as opposed to whipping the toy out in the heat of passion). If your partner is feeling pressured or intimidated, don't push the issue. Try to get at the root of the anxieties, but do not pass judgment. In this example, it appears that the couple spoke about vibrators at some point, which may have contributed to the success of the surprise:

> My lover knew I had never used a vibrator. I was blindfolded and tied up and she had been talking dirty to me. Then all of a sudden, I hear this buzzing and I felt the vibrator on my clit. Then she started fucking me in the ass with her fingers while she kept the vibrator on my clit. The fact that I couldn't see it, only hear it, made it exciting. I found out later that it was the Hitachi Magic Wand. From that day on, it was the only vibrator for me.

Using Your Vibrator with a Partner

Throughout this chapter we've identified a variety of vibrators and pointed out ways you can use them alone or with a partner. Different models offer different kinds of access or stimulation, depending on how you want to get off. Any vibrator can be used to engage in a form of mutual masturbation, where you simply take turns coming in each other's presence. Toys like anal vibes or vibrating nipple clamps can be used to accessorize whatever sex act you're engaged in. But what many couples really want to know is: *How can we incorporate a vibrator into intercourse, or penetrative sex?* Here are a few of the most common ways, but as usual, we encourage you to experiment! Since women so often find it easier to orgasm with a vibrator, the following discussion assumes that at least one partner is a woman.

THE MISSIONARY POSITION: Toys with long arms, like the wand vibrators, can be wedged in between two people in the missionary position. The arm is easy to hold if the woman is on the bottom, and the large head vibrates the clit and the penis or dildo; the vibrations are so strong they can be felt on a penis buried inside the vagina. Pregnant women, people with limited mobility, or those with big tummies prefer vibrators with long arms or heads curved to more easily reach the clit. If there isn't much space between the partners (that is, if the partner on top can't prop himself or herself up very high), there may be only room enough for a smaller battery vibrator like the Pocket Rocket, one of the Natural Contours models, or the Fukuoku finger vibe (see the Trends and Innovations sidebar). Another simple solution is to try one of the smaller, hands-free vibrators, though you may not get as much pressure as you need. Vibrating cock rings can also offer a simultaneous buzz for both partners.

> *The first time I had sex with a friend of mine, he got up and came back with a vibrator. I looked at him with some dubiousness but more lust. He penetrated me, then tucked the vibrator between us and turned it on. Wheeeeeeee. I don't think I can separate orgasms in that experience; I turned into a thrashing little puddle of joy.*

> *I LOVE the Fukuoku. I enjoy clitoral stimulation while being penetrated by my boyfriend. With Fukuoku's help, I get off easily.*

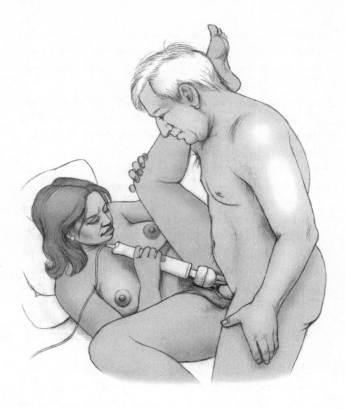

Sharing a wand vibrator

WOMAN-ON-TOP: A woman on top can hold almost any style of vibrator against her clit. In this position she's got all the control, not just of the vibration, but of the thrusting motion as well, so that she can adjust rhythm and speed accordingly. It's a less passive role than the missionary position, and often a total turn-on for the partner on the bottom. The hands-free vibes and cock ring vibes can both work well in this position, since a woman on top has better control of the clit stimulation they provide than if she's on the bottom.

> *The bunny jelly cock ring is both enjoyable and amusing. It's silly, and it works great for face-to-face penetration for a hetero couple or over a strap-on in girl-to-girl play.*

REAR ENTRY: Since rear entry penetration affords direct stimulation of the G-spot, this position can be particularly explosive when combined with clitoral stimulation. A wand vibrator with a big head can be propped up on a pillow so that the woman's clit presses into it with each thrust. A partner's hand, equipped with the Fukuoku finger vibe, can reach around easily and stimulate a partner's clitoris. Hands-free vibes are nice if you require your hands for support—just move the thong-style strap to one side during penetration. Experiment with positioning; you might find that standing beside the bed while your partner kneels on it is more comfortable (and gives you more room for toys) than having you both on the bed.

SIDE BY SIDE: Spoon or side-by-side positions are a little more awkward for vibrator use, yet still good options for those with bigger tummies or limited mobility. In the spoon position, a woman lies on her side with a wand vibrator propped up against her clit, while her partner penetrates her from behind. Alternately, the spooning partner can reach around and hold a smaller vibrator against her clitoris. In a variation on this position, the woman reclines back slightly, opening her legs and placing one over her partner, who can be lying behind her on his or her side or at more of a right angle.

DOUBLE PENETRATION: Plenty of women have fantasized about and finally discovered the thrill of double penetration, thanks to dildo-type vibrators. Your partner's dildo or penis goes in either your vagina or anus, a vibrating dildo (the cylindrical style) goes in the other, and a clit vibrator tops off the adventure. Sometimes it feels like you need extra hands or a helper to coordinate all the activity, but with a little experimentation you might find just the right combination. Dual vibrators like the Rabbit Pearl can give you both vaginal and clitoral vibration at once, though you may need to hold the base to keep it from sliding out. In woman-on-top you can squat on a dildo vibrator, but the drawback is that you're juggling a lot of movement at once. In the missionary position you can more easily spare one hand to hold the toy in place, and in the side-by-side position you can use your legs to keep a firm grip on a vaginally inserted toy while your partner penetrates you anally. If you don't want to worry about the toy falling out, you might try wearing a vibrating plug.

I love having a partner straddling a larger sit-on-top type vibrator while I penetrate her anally. The vibrations go through her to me with a mind-blowing intensity.

Common Questions about Vibrators

Which is the best vibrator? This question can usually be interpreted in two ways. Do you mean "Which is the best vibrator for reaching orgasm?" Only you can be the judge of that. People respond to all different kinds of stimulation, so what works best for one person may be completely irritating to someone else. The only way to find the best vibrator for *you* is to experiment.

The other way to interpret this question is, "Which is the most popular vibrator?" If you want to use popularity as a litmus test for which toys are more likely to please you, that's your prerogative. At Good Vibrations, the Hitachi Magic Wand, the Wahl Coil, the Smoothies, the waterproof vibes, the dual vibrators (like the Rabbit Pearl), the Fukuoku, and the Ultime all have large and faithful fan clubs.

Will I get addicted? There's absolutely no physiological basis for addiction to any form of sexual stimulation. It is true, however, that many of us become habituated to whatever stimulation reliably produces orgasms. Some of us prefer sex in a specific position, sex with a specific fantasy, or sex with a specific partner. It is equally possible to become habituated to sex with a vibrator. There's nothing wrong with it—what's wrong are the people or the voices inside our head saying we "should" have orgasms a certain way and that therefore we "should" wean ourselves from our vibrators. Unfortunately, many sex manuals, experts, and mainstream media perpetuate the addiction myth:

I read a Dr. Ruth manual in my early twenties and became concerned that I would be a slave to the vibrator or water jets.

If you enjoy your vibrator, keep buzzing! If you want to learn other ways of orgasming, here are a few tips for breaking your sexual pattern with the vibrator: Set aside more time to explore alternative sexual activities. Or try the "stop and start" method—bring yourself to the edge of orgasm in your usual way, and then switch to another type of stimulation (you'll find it can be as much fun to go for heightened arousal as instant gratification). Or experiment with different positions, fantasies, and sensations.

Will my genitals get numb? Continuous use of a vibrator will not damage the nerve endings in the clitoris or the penis. You may experience a temporary numbness of your genitals caused by the vibrations, but your sensitivity always returns. You may be concerned that you'll build up a tolerance to the intense stimulation offered by a vibrator and question whether you'll ever be able to masturbate manually again. The answer is yes, you will build up a tolerance, and yes, you can masturbate manually again. Employ some of the suggestions above to break your pattern, and in time your clit or penis will be jumping for your hand like it used to.

What's that mysterious warning about calf pain? Vibrators and massagers sold in the United States are packaged with a label advising against using on unexplained calf pain because there's a risk of shaking loose a blood clot, which could cause serious heart damage or death.

Will I get electrocuted? Not unless you immerse your electric vibrator in the bath, the shower, the Jacuzzi, or any other body of water. Some people have been concerned that bodily fluid in contact with vibrators is dangerous, but to date we've never heard of anyone receiving a shock from even the most copious lubrication or ejaculation.

Can vibrators be dangerous? If you apply common sense (don't leave your vibrator home alone and running when you leave for vacation, don't fall asleep with it on your stomach), there is no cause for concern. We do, however, try to warn people about certain types of vibrators, because of the potential for injury. Electric vibrators that have a heating element can cause minor burns on tender genital tissue. One dildo-type battery vibrator, which moves up and down in a slinky-like movement, has been known to pinch. Some vibrators have a metal rod in the center of the material that can cause damage if it pokes through; check to make sure the material covering the motor is thick and strong and doesn't tear easily.

What about safer sex with a vibrator? If you're using your vibrator alone, you are engaging in safe sex. But you should avoid inserting a vibrator anally and then inserting it vaginally without cleaning it, as this will transmit bacteria that could cause infection. Remedy this by using condoms (or by having more than one sex toy within arm's reach).

If you're using a vibrator with a partner, you should clean the vibrator before sharing it. Many of the plastic attachments can be washed in hot soapy water; dildo-type plastic vibrators can be wiped with a wet cloth. You can avoid the inconvenience of interrupting sex play to bathe your toys if you use condoms—simply strip off the used condom and replace it with a fresh one between uses.

And They All Buzzed Happily Ever After!

Now that we've imparted practically every bit of information in our possession regarding vibrators, it's time for you to go play with them! Our dream is that one day vibrators will become as commonplace and acceptable as any other appliance in your house.

Thanksgiving dinner was at my house last year. My mom looked into my room and saw my vibrator peeking out from under the bed, then she went into my sister's room and saw hers. "You girls," she exclaimed, "aren't you even embarrassed that your guests will see?" I laughed. I don't even notice them anymore. I hope if my guests see my vibrator, they'll just smile and want one, too.

Magnifique! Ultime! Jolie!

Don't worry, we're not about to wax ecstatic over vibrators in French. Rather, these are the names of a new crop of vibrators created by the adult filmmaker Candida Royalle. Her line of toys, called Natural Contours, are so discreet, stylish, and well-designed that they evoke similar superlatives from fans around the world.

Just as she had seen the need for adult films that would place women's sexual gratification front and center—a need she met with her pioneering Femme videos—Candida saw the need for a vibrator that would reflect women's experience of arousal and orgasm. "The clitoris is outside," she explained, "so why were all these toys shaped like phalluses?" Designed to rest on the pubic bone and stimulate the entire vulva, Candida's toys are a welcome alternative to the focused spot stimulation afforded by most other vibrators. "Now that we know the clitoris is not just a little button, but a whole band of erotic tissue, it makes sense to massage and exercise the whole area, which is what my vibrators do."

Upon discovering that the largest of her initial vibrators, the Magnifique, could also be used effectively for G-spot stimulation, Candida went back to the drawing board and debuted what has become her runaway bestseller, the Ultime. The model is curved somewhat like a horseshoe, and one end of it is inserted vaginally for G-spot stimulation, while the other rests comfortably against the clitoris.

After only three years on the market, Natural Contours sales are up to an astonishing 250,000 units per year. If you think the idea of nearly a quarter million women buzzing off is impressive, consider the fact that Candida's vibes are the first openly marketed sex toys ever to cross over to a mainstream market. Traditional retailers have shied away from battery vibrators, not wanting to offer anything with sexual connotations. True, "personal massagers" like the Hitachi have been commercially available in department stores for years, though they are never advertised as anything but muscle massagers, despite the fact that they've been popular sex toys for decades.

Because Candida Royalle's toys are so discreet, attractively packaged, and well-made, they've been picked up by drugstores and women's health catalogs. "The challenge was how to say what these toys do without being too explicit," says Candida. "I came up with the phrase 'stimulate internal and external pleasure points,' but then the health catalogs actually started using words like 'clitoris' and 'G–spot' for the first time. What a breakthrough!"

Candida is anything but surprised at her toys' crossover appeal. "My inspiration is in giving women permission, and helping them really achieve sexual empowerment and fulfillment. I wanted to reach all those women who are afraid to go into adult stores. They deserve access to toys or movies that are great for them."

If you're tempted to try one of Candida's toys, make a night of it and pick up one of her videos as well. Femme videos seek to "give adult movies a woman's voice and explore what women desire and want from sex." Expect more romance, foreplay, safer sex, attractive women *and* men, and, of course, real women's orgasms.

You can visit Candida Royalle's website at www.royalle.com.

"My inspiration is in giving women permission, and helping them really achieve sexual empowerment and fulfillment."

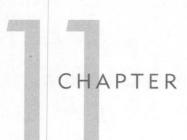

CHAPTER

Penetration

In this chapter, we'll discuss the varieties of penetration you and your partners can enjoy and the ways in which we use our fingers, fists, dildos, and penises to explore each other's bodies.

Vaginal Penetration

There are abundant physiological explanations of why a woman would seek out vaginal penetration. During sexual arousal, the outer vagina becomes congested with blood and the vaginal opening narrows, while the inner two-thirds of the vagina balloons open. The uterus and cervix become elevated, which accentuates the expanding space in the inner vagina. For many women, this ballooning sensation is accompanied by a desire to be filled. And many women find the experience of orgasm enhanced when the vagina contracts around something.

Dildos really improve orgasmic sensation.

I enjoy anything and everything vaginally, from a fist to a little finger. I love the feeling of being filled.

Sexual behavior isn't inspired solely by physiological capacities, however, but by desire, willingness, and trust. We learn to trust our bodies' capacities only after repeated pleasurable experience. If a woman experiences penetration when she's not relaxed, aroused, and lubricated, she certainly runs the risk of feeling pain and coming to associate penetration with pain.

I've noticed the more turned on I am, the more lubricated and open I am, the more I enjoy intercourse.

Penetration usually hurts at first, but lubrication helps. Then it stops hurting after I am aroused more.

"Vaginismus" is the term used to describe one reaction in women who have had traumatic and painful experiences with penetration. The Kinsey Institute has estimated that anywhere from 2 to 9 percent of women experience vaginismus, a psychological response to physical experiences such as rape, childbirth, or painful intercourse. A woman with vaginismus will involuntarily and automatically contract her vaginal muscles whenever penetration is imminent. Treatment for vaginismus has a very high success rate and involves undertaking an exercise program in which the woman practices contracting and relaxing the muscles in her thighs and pelvis, and inserts progressively larger dilators (that is, dildos) in her vagina over the course of several months. The process is one of relearning conscious control over voluntary muscles as well as regaining confidence in the capacity to experience pleasure.

Of course, many women are perfectly happy with a sex life that involves little or no penetration of any kind. After all, one person's erogenous zone is another person's neutral zone, and everyone has different preferences as to which types of stimulation are most arousing. Assuming that all women find vaginal penetration pleasurable makes about as much sense as assuming that all men find anal penetration pleasurable. Furthermore, there's a psychological component to penetration that affects our responses. When you enter your partner's body, you're crossing a boundary emotionally as well as physically. For some people, this merging is profoundly erotic, yet for others it is profoundly invasive. We hope it goes without saying that you should always respect your partner's wishes in this matter.

To be honest, I could do without penetration. If a man just plays with my clit, I'm a happy camper. I don't like sticking things in my vagina.

Fingers

WHY USE YOUR FINGERS? When an early sex therapist polled a group of men and women as to which part of their partners' bodies—fingers, tongues, or genitals—gave them the most sexual pleasure, fingers took top honors. Hands are exceptionally sensitive, skillful instruments. The touch of your hand on your partner's genitals is a form of intimate communication, which creates a fine-tuned range of sensations.

Fingers are definitely the most sensual and loving— also the most responsive.

I like fingers inside me. I like to feel my cunt squeeze them, and I like how warm they are when they're pulled out.

I would have to say that my favorite type of penetration is with fingers. There are so many nooks and crannies fingers can find that a penis just can't hit.

Of course, not every woman will have the same attitude toward digital penetration:

Don't like fingers in my vagina due to childhood sexual molestation experience.

Fingers are hard and dildos are cold. I like a penis.

Personally, I can't even handle putting a tampon in, but I love penetrating my partner. There's nothing like sliding my fingers into a woman's body and heading toward that magical spot.

HOW TO USE YOUR FINGERS: Before you dive in, take the time to remove any rings and bracelets, as these could scratch your partner. It's also a good idea to wear a latex glove. Latex gloves are not only a safer-sex precaution, but in addition they can enhance manual stimulation for both parties involved. We aren't suggesting that you approach your partner clad in thick, vinyl dishwashing gloves. Far from it. Thin latex surgical gloves are available from medical or dental supply houses (and many sex boutiques)—they come in in a rainbow of colors and a wide range of skintight sizes. If you or your partner are allergic to latex, synthetic alternatives are available that are just as thin as latex gloves. Either way, try to find unpowdered gloves, or if you can't, wash the potentially irritating powder off the gloves before use. You'll be able to feel every warm, moist inch of your partner's vagina, but you won't have to contend with the sting of her vaginal fluids, and she won't have to contend with your ragged cuticles, sharp nails, and rough skin.

I like to use gloves because my hands are often irritated by the juices; also, I feel more comfortable probing a lover's vagina with gloves instead of worrying about scratching, even with the shortest of fingernails.

I like fingers very much, but one advantage of penises, by the way, is that they don't have fingernails.

Some folks prefer using finger cots—they are more commonly available in pharmacies and resemble the cut-off fingers of a glove. Finger cots are okay if you really are going to restrict your dabbling to one finger, but given the limited amount of surface area they cover, they aren't the most practical or versatile choice.

So you've got your gloves on, and you're wondering how best to let your fingers do the talking. Only your partner knows for sure. Tastes in finger-fucking vary just as much as tastes in any other sexual activity. Some women prefer to be penetrated with only one or two fingers and others prefer several. The same woman will have varying preferences as to how many fingers she wants inside her, depending on her menstrual cycle and her level of arousal.

I'm crazy about finger stimulation, especially four or five fingers at once.

Occasionally, I like someone's finger inside me, generally when I'm ovulating and very wet. Sometimes after I come, I like someone's finger inside me—it feels very comforting.

Nobody likes being poked at or penetrated before she's turned on, so start by teasing your partner's clitoris, labia, and vaginal opening until her genitals are swollen and warm. She may or may not lubricate heavily—it's always a good idea to add some water-based lubricant. If she's fairly aroused, your partner may slide right onto your finger(s) herself. Or you can start by inserting one finger and attend to her body language to see how to proceed from there.

You can move your fingers straight in and out, or twist them in a corkscrew motion, or tap and press around the vaginal walls. Some women prefer no movement at all, others a gentle stroking, and still others a vigorous thrusting. If your partner enjoys G-spot stimulation, you can crook your fingers up and firmly stroke the front wall of her vagina behind the pubic bone with what's aptly called a "come hither" motion. Some women enjoy massage of the perineal area between the vagina and anus. Some enjoy pressure against the cervix and would welcome deep strokes, while others find it painful to have the cervix jarred. Experiment by stroking and pressing all around

her vagina to find her "hot spots," and ask her to let you know when your touch feels pleasant, neutral, or irritating. Every woman has different responses, so the technique that puts one lover on cloud nine might put another lover to sleep.

Several fingers engaged in very specific ways (up under the bone) is really enjoyable.

A woman's fingers (a woman who knows my G-spot) do lead me to orgasm. But a lot of friction vaginally without G-spot stimulation is more annoying and painful than enjoyable.

Most women find the experience of penetration enhanced when their whole bodies are involved. You can both enjoy several kinds of stimulation at once—try rubbing your bodies together, sucking her nipples, licking her clitoris, fingering her anus, switching on a vibrator, or kissing. And remember, latex gloves make it easy to move between vaginal and anal play. You can simply change your gloves rather than hopping up to wash your hands.

I like a tongue in my ear and on my neck; a hand lightly touching the small of my back; and clitoral and anal stimulation. In fact, in a perfect world, I could have all of that at the same time. Might overload my system, though.

Fingers that stroke my G-spot firmly are great, especially when accompanied by a tongue licking my clit.

I really like to kiss and do things orally while I'm being penetrated. I definitely like the rest of my body touched at the same time.

Vaginal Fisting

WHAT IS IT AND WHY DO IT: "Fisting" is the term used for inserting an entire hand in someone's vagina or anus. Although the word "fisting" sounds vaguely menacing and seems to suggest that the fister slams his or her clenched fist into the fistee's vagina, fisting is a downright tender sexual activity that requires great patience and trust on the part of its practitioners. With your hand planted deep inside your partner's body, you can expect to feel simultaneously humbled and all-powerful. With a hand filling your vagina, you can expect to feel sensations ranging from profound passion to meditative tranquility. For some practitioners, fisting is an almost spiritual experience of union.

I call it "wearing the gauntlet" because fisting sounds so rough and my partner is very slow and solicitous of me when we play like that.

If your first reaction to the idea of fisting is to reject it as violent, painful, and potentially dangerous, you might want to stop and review a few truths about female anatomy. The vagina is made of muscle, and nature has designed it so that it can expand to let a ten-pound baby come through. It is certainly physiologically possible to get a human hand into a vagina without causing damage.

We're not suggesting that every woman try fisting simply because she's physically capable of it. But if you're someone who particularly fancies the sensation of being filled up vaginally, or if you've always enjoyed the subtleties of finger-fucking, you may be curious about what your partner's entire hand might feel like. What follows are some tips for exploring fisting safely. The only women who should never attempt vaginal fisting are male-to-female transsexuals, because a surgically created vagina is far less elastic than a biological vagina. Women who have had total hysterectomies—in which the cervix or the upper part of the vagina has been removed—may experience a loss of vaginal elasticity, which could make fisting painful and unappealing. The same is true for postmenopausal women.

Please do not ever embark on a fisting session if either you or your partner is drunk or in any chemically induced, altered state. Fisting demands attentiveness and concentration on the part of both participants, and you would be foolish to choose this time to dull any of your senses. The first rule of penetration is: If it hurts, you're doing something wrong. Alcohol and drugs can raise your pain threshold to the point where you're unaware you're causing damage until after the fact.

FISTING HOW-TO'S: First things first: Take off all your rings and bracelets and put on a latex glove. For safer sex, you might want to wear a glove on each hand, as you'll be reapplying lube to your fisting hand at regular intervals. A well-lubricated glove not only protects your skin and your partner's vagina, it also transforms

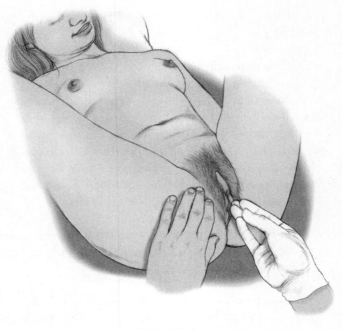

Vaginal fisting

your hand into a sleek and slippery surface. Furthermore, fisting is an activity that demands a slow buildup, and both you and your partner may discover unexpected benefits to instituting some preparatory rituals.

Before being fisted, watching my partner put on the glove and put lubricant all over it, very slowly and methodically, drives me insane.

The fistee will probably want to lie either on her back with her knees bent or face-down propped on her elbows and knees. The fister will want to have both hands free and to be sitting or kneeling in a comfortable position. Take your time coaxing her vagina into a relaxed, receptive state and incorporate plenty of whatever additional stimulation she finds most arousing. Insert one finger at a time until you're up to four. Your palm should be facing her stomach, and your knuckles should be pressing in the direction of her perineum, rather than grinding painfully against her pubic bone. Your partner may find it helpful to coordinate her breathing with your movements: inhaling as you withdraw your fingers and exhaling as you insert your fingers. If she bears down with her vaginal muscles as she exhales, she'll slide further and further onto your fingers. Take regular breaks to relubricate your entire hand and wrist. There are no Olympic medals for speed-fisting, and if you tease her to the point that she's begging for more, so much the better for both of you.

As you're working more and more of your fingers into her vagina, you'll probably find yourself instinctively adopting the hand position referred to as either the "duck" or the "swan." In this crucial fisting position, you tuck your thumb across your palm and narrow all four fingers together in a shape that resembles a beak (hence the bird names). The goal is to make your hand as narrow as possible, to sneak it through the tight ring of muscle around the vaginal opening:

I like being fisted, if they listen to my instructions to make the little duck thing before jamming their whole hand up my cunt.

You may find it helpful to incorporate a twisting motion as you gradually work more and more of your hand into her vagina. If she's sufficiently aroused and your hand is sufficiently lubricated, the moment will arrive when the widest point of your hand across your third knuckles slips inexorably into her vagina. When your hand has pushed past the muscles ringing the vaginal opening, it will naturally fold up into a fist, snugly surrounded by the strong, hot walls of her vagina.

Once inside, there are a variety of ways to move your hand. You can rock it slightly back and forth; circle it slowly; clench and unclench your fist; tap the inner walls of the vagina; or even thrust deep into her vagina. Many women have sensitive cervixes, so unless your partner specifically likes this kind of stimulation, you should refrain from pummeling her cervix.

Fisting—opening and closing my hand while it is inside—is great. Touching her cervix is a charge. Needless to say, I love having it done to me, too.

Vaginally, I enjoy a whole hand or rapid, vigorous hand thrusts.

While your partner's vagina may feel like the center of the universe to you during fisting, that's no reason to neglect the rest of her body:

My partner's best orgasms are when I have one finger up her ass, my whole other hand in her vagina, and my mouth on her clit.

I like to be gently stroked somewhere else (feet, ass, face) while being forcefully penetrated. I also like her to use her tongue to penetrate my mouth in the same hard rhythm as she is fucking me.

Your partner may or may not orgasm during fisting. Some women find the sensations of being fisted so transcendentally intense that orgasm seems irrelevant. Whether or not she comes, you'll eventually find yourself at the point where you need to remove your hand. If she has just orgasmed, her vagina may feel a lot smaller all of a sudden. Don't be alarmed. What went in must come out. Ask her to bear down with her vaginal muscles as you slide your hand slowly out, unfolding it as you go. If her vagina feels suctioned shut, you can break the seal by slipping another finger into her vaginal opening.

Fisting is a powerful experience for both parties involved. Both you and your partner may experience an altered state of consciousness. Allow yourselves plenty of time to come down from your high. Your partner will probably feel conscious of her vagina for several days thereafter. It's conceivable she could spot a little blood, but unless the bleeding is heavy, there's nothing to worry about.

Vaginal Intercourse

We're purposefully allotting neither more nor less space to vaginal intercourse than to any of the other sexual activities and playthings addressed in this book. The myth that intercourse is the be-all and end-all of sexual experience, and that most other activities are "foreplay" to the main event, is one that has something of a stranglehold on our collective libido. In reality, intercourse need only be the "main event" when procreation is the goal (and in today's world of reproductive technology, even this is not always the case). An emphasis on the primacy of penis–vagina intercourse devalues not just the experience of gay and lesbian couples, but also the experience of bisexual and heterosexual couples who have learned that there's more to sex than just sticking the proverbial plug in a socket. The negative results of this single-minded approach to sex are manifold: If the pleasures of "outercourse" were openly acknowledged, surely we'd see a decrease in the rate of teenage pregnancies, the spread of sexually transmitted diseases, and the number of preorgasmic women.

I do think there is this standard (even in the lesbian/bi community) that penetration is the real thing—the ultimate thing—and that if you don't like being fucked you are uptight or boring. We have to get over that. Life is too short to spend trying to conform to other people's standards for pleasure. Claim your own desire!

With this disclaimer off our chests, we hasten to add that intercourse certainly deserves a place in the Sexual Activities Hall of Fame. Intercourse provides full-body contact, mutual stimulation, and an intermingling of flesh that is highly arousing on many levels, both physiological and emotional. The discussion of vaginal intercourse that follows is equally applicable both to opposite-sex and same-sex couples and to penis/vagina intercourse or dildo/vagina intercourse.

EXPECTATIONS: You and your partner should be clear about your respective expectations and assumptions around intercourse. If you're in agreement that intercourse is just one facet of your sexual interaction, you'll probably have fewer concerns about whether it will lead to orgasm. If you do have orgasm as your goal, you'll need to bear in mind that anywhere from 50 to 75 percent of women do not achieve orgasm from penetration alone, as penetration does not provide enough of the clitoral stimulation that most women need to reach orgasm. Do yourselves a favor and don't get stuck on the physiologically unlikely goal of a no-hands orgasm for both partners, for this will only limit your enjoyment of intercourse.

Sometimes it's hard to get penetration and stimulation at the same time. Sometimes it's too awkward (physically or because of my partner's feelings) to do it myself.

I much prefer oral sex over fucking. I do love both, but the fucking part is mostly for my honey so he can come inside me. He's a hard come and does it best inside me.

Another popular intercourse expectation is that of simultaneous orgasm. Marriage manuals of the fifties and sixties touted this as the summit of sexual bliss, thereby establishing a standard that is extremely difficult for most couples to live up to. Arousal patterns vary from person to person and from occasion to occasion. If you're monitoring your partner's level of arousal, you're bound to be a bit distracted from your own. Simultaneous orgasm promotes an ideal of egali-

tarian reciprocity that doesn't have a whole lot to do with the average Joe or Jane's sexual responses. Of course, if you do experience simultaneous orgasm, that's grand. Just don't be surprised if it happens more by sheer accident than by design.

LUBRICATION: A key accompaniment to any type of penetration is lubricant, and intercourse is no exception. Unless your partner has a great deal of natural lubrication, consider adding some from a bottle—this will make intercourse more comfortable for both of you:

We use condoms with extra Astroglide even though I naturally lubricate a lot myself. We apply it periodically as we go, to stay nice and slippery at all times. It makes it feel better and allows us to go on for a long time.

We do occasionally hear from men and women who complain that "too much" lubrication makes it hard for them to get enough friction to reach orgasm. If this is the case, you can try adjusting your angle of penetration so that the penetrator is rubbing against the edge of the vaginal opening, rather than sliding straight in. Or you can wear condoms—latex tends to suck up lubrication and to add friction to the proceedings.

DIFFERENT STROKES: One final consideration to bear in mind is that different individuals have different tastes in terms of their preferred style, angle, and depth of intercourse. You might like long, leisurely strokes or shorter, rhythmic strokes—or you may enjoy combining shallow and then deep strokes in a pattern. You might like to keep your hips close together, grinding against each other, or you could prefer rocking your hips away from each other. If you and your partner have different tastes, you can incorporate both your preferred methods into one intercourse session.

I've always enjoyed unhurried, exploratory, playful penile penetration.

Psychologically, I dig just about any hard and rapid fucking.

The angle of penetration can also affect the level of stimulation you both receive. A man may want to angle his penis against the edge of the vaginal opening to get the maximum stimulation on the sensitive glans and underside of the penis. Or, if he angles his penis high against the top of the vaginal opening, each stroke can tug on the woman's clitoral hood, thereby indirectly stimulating the clitoris. Women may enjoy pressure on one part of the vaginal wall more than another.

I like to have sex in several different positions. I need friction on my cock from different areas to easily reach orgasm.

G-spot stimulation occurred with a partner whose penis was curved to the left a little bit, so I guess he hit the spot!

Women have a wide range of preferences when it comes to the depth of thrusting they're comfortable with. Different positions accommodate deep thrusting better than others, and some women find this quite pleasurable. Others, including women with sensitive cervixes or women who have had hysterectomies, may prefer a shallow thrusting, focusing on the outer third of the vagina. The vaginas of many male-to-female transsexuals are too shallow to accommodate deep thrusting.

I enjoy shallow thrusting with fast movements, especially in the early stages of arousal—I find it actually stimulates me both physically and mentally.

I think a lot of my pleasure in intercourse or penetration comes from stimulation of the cervix, so length is important.

I enjoy penetration with a cock but really have to focus on staying open and relaxed. The only position that works for me is on my back with legs wide open and bent. I can't take too much thrusting.

Depends on where I am in my menstrual cycle. Right before and after my period, deep thrusting can suddenly jar my cervix (ow!). The rest of the time, I like deep penetration, so having my knees up, sometimes over my partner's shoulders, makes me happy. It's all good.

Whenever you are on the receiving end of any kind of penetration, you should always feel you can control the depth of thrusting. You can manage this unobtrusively by wrapping your hand in a donut-shape around the base of your partner's penis or dildo. You'll easily be able to control the depth of each thrust, while keeping the penis pleasurably enveloped with your hand.

POSITIONS: There has probably been more written about intercourse positions than any other topic in the history of sex manuals. Folks have been snapping up illustrated copies of the *Kama Sutra* for the past fifteen centuries, not for the Hindu philosophy of the text, but for the chance to admire images of couples entangled in the "yawning position" or the "lotus-like position." The sixteenth-century Arabic manual *The Perfumed Garden* lists forty different "postures for coition." And no modern guide—including this one!—is considered complete unless it includes numerous illustrations of couples with their limbs entwined. Obviously, position books have a powerful and timeless appeal.

What's behind this obsession? Well, as any ballroom dancer can testify, it takes a little practice to get two bodies moving in time on the dance floor. It stands to reason that it would also take a little practice to get two bodies moving in a way that's mutually arousing, stimulating, and comfortable off the dance floor. Just as no one instinctively knows how to waltz divinely, no one instinctively knows how to perform intercourse divinely. Yet most position books on the market should be taken with a grain of salt. Either they promote one sure-fire patented technique that is guaranteed to please each and every reader, or they present 101 different sexual positions, all of which are minor variations on the same basic themes. Don't be intimidated by either extreme—position books are fun for their erotic visual content, even though the advice they offer is of dubious value. There are really only a handful of basic sexual positions, and you and your partners can have a great time adapting these positions to your unique body sizes, physical capabilities, erogenous preferences—and the whim of the moment.

As you read the following, bear in mind that we address the active partner in all sexual situations in the second person; "you" may be a man or a woman.

Missionary: In the missionary position, the receptive partner lies on her back while you lie on top of her. Legend has it that the missionary position derived its name from Pacific Islanders, who were surprised to observe Christian missionaries having intercourse in a position they themselves never used. It's certainly true that Western missionaries promoted intercourse positions in which women lay below men as being most "natural." Given this historical link to institutionalized male dominance, the missionary position is frequently disdained as being somehow old-fashioned or "oppressive" to women. Yet, even though it limits the receptive partner's movement and, by itself, provides little direct clitoral stimulation, many women find plenty to love about this position.

The much-maligned missionary position actually works great for me! Sometimes it's just nice to be nailed to the bed.

I like to be on my back. I like to feel the weight and skin of another person on my body. So much more of my body gets stimulated that way. When I sit on another, only one small part of me gets stimulated.

Oh God—I'm still a feminist if I like the missionary position, aren't I? I like it because I can still reach my clit that way. I can't come when I'm on top.

There are several enjoyable variations on the missionary position. In a male/female couple, the woman can keep her legs down straight, thereby narrowing her vaginal opening and increasing pleasurable friction on the man's penis. This variation also makes it more likely that her partner's pubic bone will rub against her clitoris. Another alternative is for the woman to spread her legs and bend her knees—this allows for deeper penetration and also makes it easier for her to move her hips. For some women, freedom of movement is crucial to reaching orgasm during intercourse.

This is the way I have an orgasm: my partner on top, my legs on his shoulders or chest, while I grasp his shoulders for leverage with my legs, so I can help pump.

I do orgasm with penis penetration if I can move my body freely.

We like to vary the missionary position—she'll put her knees at my shoulders and I'll wrap my hand around her to hold her ass up nicely. Or I'll get on top of her with one leg between her legs and one leg outside her leg—this allows for a lot of clitoral stimulation from the penis.

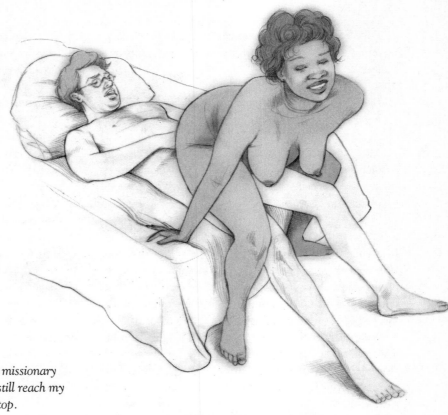

Vaginal intercourse, woman on top

Woman-on-top: Although the name of this position implies opposite-sex intercourse, it's equally delightful whether there's another woman-on-bottom or a man-on-bottom. In this flip of the missionary position, you lie on your back with your partner straddling you; she can be facing your head, facing your feet, or lying down with her back on your chest.

I have very strong orgasms when my legs are bearing my weight, but I don't always want to stand, so I kneel or squat over my partner.

Woman-on-top is excellent for women who would like to control the depth of thrusting, such as those recovering from vaginismus or childbirth or those who have had hysterectomies. It's also a particularly comfortable position for pregnant women or women who are considerably smaller than their partners. The woman-on-top position is versatile and allows easy stimulation of her nipples and clitoris. Many men find that they are more relaxed and experience less intense stimulation when they're on their backs, so they can delay ejaculation more easily in this position.

For me, the best clitoral stimulation comes from being on top. I love to tower over my lovers while sitting on their cocks.

I have very large breasts and like to be on top with my partner licking and sucking them.

Me on top means I get to control the whole thing, including when he comes. I can do it slowly and move in twisty ways that just seem to get me in the right place. Plus, I get to look at him from a neat angle.

Rear entry: Also referred to as "doggie-style," this position places your partner on her stomach or on her elbows and knees while you either stand or kneel behind her. It's very comfortable for women in the later stages of pregnancy, larger women, and those who are smaller than their partners. This position has a lot of fringe benefits—it's great for G-spot stimulation, it allows easy stimulation of the nipples and clitoris, and it's conducive to vibrator play. The woman can lie on her stomach or on pillows with a vibrator pressed against her clitoris.

Rear entry penetration gives me the best internal sensation. I like the debauched feeling of being taken from behind. It's really intense stimulation.

My fave is "doggie" style. I get the most G-spot stimulation, and I can better control how much penetration I get.

My personal favorite is doggie-style. Mostly because I love the feeling of balls flapping against my clit hood piercing. For me, penetration is most stimulating in that position and I get the free clit stimulation as well!

In rear entry, the natural curve of the vagina coincides with the curve of the erect penis or curved dildo, so deep thrusting is more comfortable in this position than most others. And there's no question that it's arousing to hang on to your partner's hips and move her to and fro—rear entry allows both of you a pleasurable freedom of pelvic movement.

I love getting slammed from behind—really having my husband pound into me as hard and fast as he can.

My partner has repetitive stress injury, so he can't support himself on his hands for too long. We like to do it standing up with me bent over the bed and him behind me. It's easy for both of us to push up against each other that way.

Some people find it depersonalizing not to be able to see a partner's face during intercourse, and associate rear entry with sex between animals:

Doggie-style is nice once in a while, but it seems a bit impersonal despite the stimulation opportunity.

I prefer face-to-face positions. I love to kiss, and I love to watch his expression; it's part of the turn-on and makes it more personal.

Rear entry is also commonly associated with anal intercourse—even though it's only one of many possible positions for anal sex. Being the sexually diverse and creative animals that humans are, many people find these two factors erotically inspiring.

I like being penetrated from behind. We often play-act as a gay male couple, so penetration from behind adds to that fantasy.

Side by side: In this position, you and your partner either lie facing each other—with thighs intertwined—or lie facing the same direction in a spoons position. A slight variation puts your partner on her back, draping her legs over your thighs. Side-by-side positions are good for long, leisurely intercourse, as the stimulation they provide is somewhat less direct than that of other positions.

Side by side is a great warm-up—it builds the tension.

We call it the "X" position—my partner and I lie cross-wise, she lifts one leg over my body, and I put her other leg between the two of mine. She's on her back, and I'm on my side, facing her. That one seems to work well if I don't have a particularly stiff erection, and makes it easy for her to masturbate with her hand while we're screwing.

The spoons position allows the receptive partner to control the depth of thrusting, and since it ensures

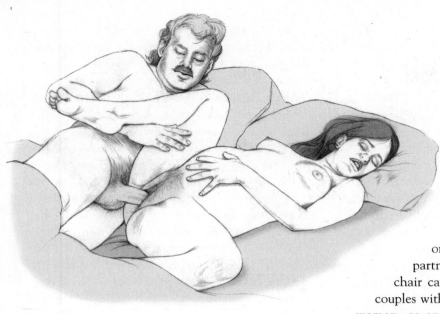

Vaginal intercourse, side by side

I love vaginal or anal from behind, usually while lying on my side. This is useful for times when my hips and legs are painful from the fibromyalgia. I love face to face as well, though I can't be on top for long because my arms don't always hold me up very well. Sitting usually works better for face to face if I'm going to be on top, as it's less stressful on my joints.

You can sit intertwined on a bed or you can sit on a chair, with your partner straddling you. Intercourse on a chair can be a particularly good position for couples with a wide discrepancy in size, pregnant women, or any women who want to control the depth of penetration.

Definitely my favorite position is with my partner sitting "Indian style" with my legs around his waist and our arms wrapped around one another. This not only gives the richest penetration, but it also allows us to touch and have our hands free to roam one another's body. It is a good intimate, as opposed to sexual, position.

My current favorite is a variation of the woman-on-top position—screwing on a chair. The chair position is great, because it's restful, allows full stomach-to-stomach contact, and gives the man the chance to caress the woman's neck, back, shoulder blades, ass, and anus—hmm, delightful!

that neither partner will have to support the other's weight, it's another excellent position for women in the late stages of pregnancy. It's similarly convenient for two people with a wide discrepancy in size or height. Finally, side by side is a good position for older people or those with disabilities that limit stamina or mobility.

My partner is quite fond of the spoon position, and I love it because it gives him access to my neck. I have a bit of a neck fetish and love him to bite my neck while we do it. He likes this position because he can thrust hard and deep like with doggie-style, but he doesn't ram my cervix quite as much.

Once I did something fabulous when we were in the spoons position. I bent over so that I was perpendicular to his body. It was very easy to move and set rhythm freely, and penetration was at a very nice angle.

Sitting: The sitting positions create a relaxed and intimate mood. They allow for lots of full-body contact without intense genital stimulation. Like side-by-side positions, they're good for older people or those with disabilities that limit stamina or mobility.

Standing: Couples who happen to be the same body-type may enjoy intercourse standing up. While standing up is not the most common position for intercourse, you may enjoy variations of this position in which your partner is sitting on a counter, tabletop, or airplane bathroom sink while you stand facing her. Standing positions lend themselves to the fantasy that both of you are so swept away by passion that you have to grab each other no matter where you are—which gives them an undeniable and widespread appeal.

I love to sit on the bathroom counter with my feet up on the counter while my lover moves right up to my pussy. We can watch ourselves in the mirror.

Anal Penetration

There are just as many physiological reasons for both men and women to enjoy anal penetration as there are for women to enjoy vaginal penetration. The anus is rich in nerve endings and participates with our genitals in the engorgement, muscular tension, and contractions of sexual arousal and orgasm. Pressure and fullness in the rectum feels pleasurable to some men and women, just as vaginal fullness feels pleasurable to some women. Anal penetration can stimulate both the perineal area and G-spot in women and the bulb of the penis and prostate gland in men. Many of us find anal stimulation intensely pleasurable.

I enjoy both vaginal and anal penetration. I think my anus is more sensitive than my vagina, and I don't admit this to a lot of people.

You may already have discovered that anal stimulation greatly enhances and intensifies masturbation, oral sex, or intercourse. After all, it's hard to miss that power-packed little bud of erogenous sensitivity located only inches from your genitals. Anal stimulation is an integral part of many folks' sex lives. Some individuals with disabilities that numb sensation in their genitals retain the capacity for pleasurable sensation in the anus. Women who have grown to be uninterested in vaginal penetration, perhaps after childbirth or with the onset of menopause, may prefer exploring anal penetration. Anal penetration offers men the experience of being physically entered, while countless men and women alike describe anal penetration as being a uniquely relaxing and meditative experience.

Despite these physical truths, those of us who enjoy anal play are understandably reluctant to stand up and be counted. From the time we're old enough to start toilet-training, we're taught that the anus is the dirtiest part of our bodies and that it needs to be brought under strict control. The same orifice that was a source of innocent pleasure during infancy becomes a source of shame and confusion in childhood. Many of us learn to hold a lot of tension in our anus, and the resulting health problems such as constipation or hemorrhoids convince us that the anus is, at best, a neutral area and, at worst, a painful one. It's no wonder that many adults are unable to conceive of the anus as an erogenous zone.

As for anal penetration, I've never tried it because it seems kind of awful. Doesn't appeal to me personally though people I know enjoy it.

Although our focus here is on encouraging you to get to know and love your anus, we should note that feelings of shame and transgression can be highly erotic, and that some people doubtless enjoy anal play in part because they feel they're messing around where they shouldn't. If the anal taboo is preventing you from taking pleasure in this sensitive and stimulating portion of your anatomy, we hope the information in these pages will help you overcome your negative associations. But if the anal taboo is enhancing your pleasure, let us be the first to assure you that anal play is naughty, kinky, and downright nasty.

Recent years have seen a slight lifting of the anal taboo: Anyone in the adult entertainment business can testify to a surge of interest in anal pleasure. On the one hand, the AIDS epidemic has spawned general confusion around the relative risk of anal play—popular perception has conflated anal sex and disease-transmission to such an extent that many people incorrectly believe that HIV can be transmitted via anal intercourse even if neither partner is infected with the virus. On the other hand, the mere fact that anal intercourse is now routinely referred to in newspaper articles, public health brochures, and schoolrooms across the nation has brought anal stimulation out of the closet. Once something is normalized as a topic for discussion, it's just a hop, skip, and a jump to normalizing it as an activity.

Inhibitors

FEAR OF FECES: Probably the most common factor that inhibits folks from experimenting with anal play is the fear of encountering feces. To address this appropriately, let's review a little anatomy. The anal canal is less than an inch long and leads into the rectum, which is anywhere from five to nine inches long. The rectum leads, in turn, to the colon, which is where feces accumulate until you're ready to defecate. The rectum is only a passageway, not a storage place, so it's unlikely you'll come across more than a few traces of feces in the course of your explorations. The fact that the rectum's sexual status suffers due to its participation in the digestive process is somewhat arbitrary. After all, the digestive process starts with your mouth, and nobody considers kissing a disgusting activity.

Still skittish? You might want to take a bath together before indulging in anal play, or, better yet, you could pop on a latex glove or condom before making your first foray. Some people feel more confident if they rinse their rectum out with water, using a turkey-baster syringe or an enema. Unless you're preparing for some deep penetration or anal fisting, we wouldn't encourage the use of enemas. Enemas take time and finesse—you have to monitor the temperature of the water you're using, the water pressure, and the height of the enema bag. A simple dip in the tub is sufficient preparation for most anal activities.

FEAR OF DISEASE: The second primary inhibitor to anal experimentation is the fear of disease transmission. Anal sex is so linked in the popular imagination with gay male sex, and gay male sex has unfortunately become so linked with HIV transmission, that many people assume that anal sex in and of itself will cause disease. Neither of these associations is particularly logical. Plenty of gay men never engage in anal intercourse, and plenty of heterosexuals and lesbians *do*. Specific activities don't transmit disease; viruses transmit disease. Unprotected anal intercourse, like unprotected vaginal intercourse, is simply one way in which someone infected with an STD can conceivably transmit it to his partner.

The lining of the rectum is considerably more delicate and richer in blood vessels than the walls of the vagina, so it's easy to scratch or tear the tissue of the rectum, and easy for bodily fluids to pass from the rectum into your bloodstream. You should never insert anything into your anus that does not have a completely smooth surface, and you should never engage in unprotected penis-anus intercourse without putting a condom on the penis, unless you and your partner have both tested negative for STDs. To prevent possible bacterial infections, never switch your attentions from a woman's anus to her vagina without stopping to wash your hands, change your glove, or change your condom.

Forget my behind; that's not a turn-on for me. All I can think of if someone messes with it is, "Quick! Scrub up with soap so you don't give me an infection!"

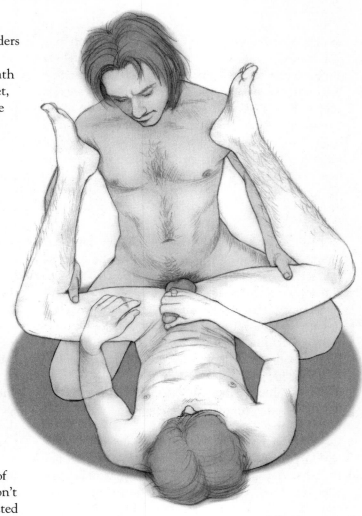

Anal intercourse, missionary position

HOMOPHOBIA: Anal sex is inextricably linked in many people's minds with gay male sex.

I have occasional anxiety about the homosexual act of anal play, but I like the forbidden nature.

I've discovered that I really enjoy anal penetration, but I'm afraid my wife thinks I'm going gay.

This is just one more manifestation of the tyranny of the notion that intercourse is the main event of any sexual encounter. If by definition sex presumes sticking a penis into a vagina, then gays and lesbians are presumed to simulate this one "true" sex act by engaging in anal intercourse or by strapping on dildos to penetrate each other. In fact, sexual orientation is not defined by how you fuck, but who you fuck. There are gay men who never engage in anal intercourse, lesbians who've never seen a dildo, and heterosexual couples who love anal sex. The fact that the taboo against anal sex is partially motivated by homophobia is one more example of how homophobia restricts not only the freedom of gay people, but ultimately the freedom of all sexual people.

Anal Do's

DO RELAX: The anus is ringed by two sphincter muscles, one right on top of the other. The external sphincter is the one you voluntarily control when you allow yourself to defecate. The internal sphincter is involuntary. This muscle will tighten up reflexively if you try to force your way into your anus, resulting in the excruciatingly sharp pain familiar to anyone who has rushed anal penetration. With practice and patience, it's possible to gain some control over this internal sphincter, but it will always serve as the guardian of the gateway, tensing up if you try to insert too much too soon.

Before you try to incorporate anal play into sex with a partner, set aside some time to do some anal exploration yourself. Lubricate both your finger and your anus, and position your finger at the anal opening. Concentrate on your breathing: Inhale and tighten your pelvic muscles, exhale and release those muscles. As you exhale, try bearing down slightly with your muscles, and sweep the tip of your finger into your anus. Leave your finger in place while you continue to inhale and exhale. You should be able to feel your two sphincter muscles contracting and releasing around your fingertip. If you're comfortable with the way your fingertip feels, you may want to insert your finger all the way into your rectum. Try moving your finger in and out or in a circular movement. You'll probably find it pleasant to angle your finger toward the front of your body: toward the perineal sponge and G-spot in women and toward the bulb of the penis and prostate in men. Maintain a relaxed pace. If anything hurts or causes your muscles to tense up, stop moving or stop what you're doing altogether. The point is to enjoy yourself and to learn about what feels good.

DO USE LUBE: The anus and rectum don't produce any lubrication of their own, and you absolutely must use some kind of lubricant anytime you engage in anal penetration. Bear in mind this cautionary understatement:

Trying to put a dildo up my butt when I did not have lube was not a good idea.

Since water-based lubricants dry up more quickly than oils, some folks feel that oil-based lubricants are optimal for anal play. We would still suggest that you avoid the risk of using oils. Instead, shop for thicker varieties of water-based lubricant and use them lavishly. Look for lubes that don't contain nonoxynol-9, as this is a potentially irritating to delicate rectal tissue. As a fundamental precaution, if you've been on the receiving end of an oil-based lubricant, you should refrain from being on the receiving end of penis-anus intercourse for the next few days, as oils could linger in your rectum and destroy the next condom that comes your way.

Unfortunately, some lubricants and lotions containing anesthetic ingredients such as benzocaine are specifically marketed for anal sex. What's wrong with this picture? The last thing you want to do is to numb sensation in your anus, thereby deadening your awareness of what's going on in your body. The network of nerve endings in your anus and outer rectum is your best defense against hurting yourself. As with any kind of penetration, pain is a warning signal that you should stop what you're doing.

DO RESPECT YOUR ANATOMY: The anus and rectum are made of smooth, highly expandable tissue, so it's physiologically possible for your rectum to expand to accommodate an entire hand if you're anesthetized during surgery or if you're a practitioner of anal fisting. As with vaginal penetration, physiological capabilities have little to do with personal preferences. You may be perfectly happy with a pinkie's worth of anal attention, or you may enjoy anal intercourse with a large dildo. If you insert anything longer than nine inches, you'll come to the entrance to your colon. Devotees of deep anal fisting may wish to delve into the colon, but average aficionados of anal penetration are happy to restrict their paddling to the relative shallows of the rectum.

Knowledge of the shape of the rectum is especially relevant to comfortable anal penetration. The outer or lower rectum tilts toward the front of your body for about three inches, at which point it curves back to the spine for another few inches, and then tilts slightly forward again where it meets up with the sigmoid colon. You'll need to keep these curves in mind when you insert a finger, dildo, or penis. You'll want to angle toward the front of your body to follow the initial tilt of the rectum while simultaneously angling gently upward to negotiate the first curve of the rectum. Practice by feeling your way along slowly while experimenting with body positioning—just as no two snowflakes are alike, no two rectums are alike, and you'll need to adjust to your own idiosyncrasies. If you're inserting anything more than four inches long, it should be flexible enough to adapt to the curves of your rectum.

DO USE COMMON SENSE: Anything that goes into your anus should be smooth, seamless, and free of rough, scratchy edges. It's all too easy to damage the delicate tissue lining the rectum. This means you may need to file down the plastic seams on your anal beads.

You should also make sure that there's no way you can lose hold of whatever is going into your anus. That butt plug or battery vibrator you're wielding should have a flared base, so that even if you let go, it won't slip out of reach into your rectum. At a bare minimum, your toy should be over seven inches long so that you can keep your grip on it. If you do happen to let a toy slip into you, it's more than likely that if you wait patiently in a relaxed position, it will come back out the way it went in. Many of us, however, find it hard to be patient and relaxed with a rudderless sex toy on the loose in our bodies, and in certain instances, the toy can get pushed all the way up into the colon, at which point surgical intervention will be necessary to remove it. Save yourself the possible headaches: Choose and use your toys carefully.

DO COMMUNICATE: If you're on the receiving end of anal penetration with a partner, you should feel as much in control as you do during solo play. It's up to you to help your partner negotiate your rectum safely and comfortably. Communicate about what feels good, and let your partner know immediately if you experience any pain. You should be able to stop what you're doing at any time. Anal play can be an extremely intimate encounter with a partner, provided you trust each other sufficiently to relax and enjoy.

Fingers

Probably the most common source of anal stimulation is the finger. The light, sensitive touch of a finger is the ideal way to titillate the anus and coax it into opening up. If you're going to play with your partner's anus, we suggest you put on a latex glove or a finger cot. Not only will this take care of any hygiene concerns you or your partner might have, but you'll also be protecting your partner from your fingernails and any rough skin. Start by applying lube around the anal opening and circle your finger around the soft folds of anal tissue. Take the time to look at your partner's anus: You may be surprised at how sweet and innocent it looks—not like an "asshole" at all. Many people find that gentle stroking of their highly enervated anal opening is all the anal stimulation they desire.

I like the feel of a finger pressing lightly against my asshole.

I adore digital pressure to the outside of my anus.

If your partner becomes sufficiently relaxed, she or he may bear down and slide right onto your finger. Your fingertip should be reaching toward the front of the body, rather than crooking up toward the tailbone. The sphincter muscles may tense up automatically as soon as you enter, so hold your finger still at first until the anus relaxes around it. Then feel free to insert your finger more deeply, exploring the outer rectum. You can circle your finger, tap and stroke the walls of the rectum, or move your finger gently in and out. If your partner is experiencing anal penetration for the first time, she or he may find the sensation a little unsettling. The primary association we all have with pressure in our rectum is that we're about to defecate, so your partner may feel briefly uncomfortable while adjusting to the sensation.

We hope it goes without saying that anal penetration is a great adjunct to other types of stimulation. In fact, many couples regularly incorporate anal fingering into their oral sex or intercourse routine.

During sex, an occasional fingering by my girlfriend while I'm inside her is great.

I enjoy my partner putting a finger in my anus during oral sex. But it makes me come a lot faster. I also like her tongue on and in my anus.

My favorite position is when I'm on my back in a pleasure swing, with my knees to my chest, while my cock is sucked and stroked and a finger is penetrating my butt.

Anal Fisting

Like vaginal fisting, anal fisting is something of an art form, and is spoken of in almost spiritual terms by its practitioners. At first blush, the notion of anal fisting strikes many of us as impossible at best and dangerous at worst.

Fist? Don't people need diapers after that?

The truth is that the rectum is highly expandable, and every human being's rectum is capable of accommodating a hand without sustaining damage. The proportion of human beings who are able to voluntarily relax their anus to this extent is, however, relatively small. People who engage in anal fisting frequently take hours to build up to any one session, and experience it as almost a meditative union of mind and body, involving total relaxation and receptivity. Fisting is an esoteric sexual discipline that has been practiced around the world throughout history.

All the basic rules of anal play—relaxation, lubrication, and communication—apply ten-fold where fisting is concerned. Never go into a fisting session if either you or your partner is drunk or stoned. Drugs can numb your awareness of pain, and pain during anal penetration is always an indication that what you're doing is not right for your body. Given the delicate nature of the rectum, it's especially important to make sure your nails are filed short and smooth and that you're covering them with a latex glove.

Since water-based lubricants dry up more quickly than oils, some people feel that oil-based lubricants are the only way to go when it comes to fisting, arguing that latex gloves are thicker than condoms and are unlikely to break down from contact with oil during the limited time period they're worn. We would still suggest that you avoid the risk of using oils, as noted in the lube section.

Anal fisting is frequently and misleadingly listed as an activity that's high-risk for sexually transmitted diseases. Although it's true that fisting could conceivably cause tears in the rectum, which would be vulnerable to subsequent encounters with infected bodily fluids, fisting is inherently no riskier than any other type of anal penetration. However, the fister should always wear a latex glove to minimize the chance of transmitting infection.

The techniques described in the section on vaginal fisting are applicable to anal fisting. We don't believe, however, that anyone who reads one or two pages on the subject of anal fisting in a general interest book like this one is sufficiently educated to take a crack at this quite sophisticated sexual practice. If you're interested in learning more about fisting, we recommend that you track down an excellent book devoted to the subject, *Trust: The Hand Book.*

Anal Intercourse

An activity that has many fans, anal intercourse has been practiced in all civilizations throughout history.

I've discovered that anal sex stimulates the legs of my clit and makes me come more easily. Anal sex feels more intense and it also feels more intimate than vaginal sex in a way, because it takes more relaxation and trust for it to work.

If you and your partner would like to experiment with anal intercourse, please discuss your intentions ahead of time. As with any anal play, intercourse requires considerable relaxation and good communication, and it's best not to embark on it on the spur of the moment. One bad experience with rushed, forced anal penetration is frequently all it takes to make someone swear off anal sex for life. That dense concentration of anal nerve endings that communicates exquisite pleasure when approached respectfully communicates agonizing pain when handled roughly.

I've only once had anal penetration that was pleasant, because he knew to go slow and use lubrication.

When partners ask if I've had anal sex and it's obvious the answer is yes, they always assume I'll do it with them. Um, sorry guys, no, that involves trust and lube.

The following discussion of anal intercourse applies both to opposite-sex and same-sex couples and to penis-anus intercourse or dildo-anus intercourse.

EXPECTATIONS: Get clear with your partner about your respective expectations. Are you assuming that anal intercourse will be just like vaginal intercourse in terms of preparation, pace, and sensation? Bear in mind that the anus and rectum require a more deliberate and gradual approach than the vagina does. You may not be able to insert your entire penis or dildo, or to thrust as vigorously as you do during vaginal or oral sex. You and your partner should have discussed in advance whether or not it's okay for you to come while inside the rectum. As you approach orgasm, your movements may become a little less controlled, and this could cause your partner to tense up and experience some discomfort. You may find that your anxieties around inflicting pain or the more lengthy process of getting your penis inserted causes your erection to subside. Try not to be too goal-oriented in your approach, and allow yourselves to have fun exploring the range of sensations—let your level of arousal ebb and flow. After all, nobody has got a stopwatch trained on you.

If you're being penetrated, you may have anxieties that you're taking "too long" to relax and feel that you should grit your teeth and bear any painful sensations out of some sense that "the show must go on." Please respect your own responses, and don't buy into the popular misconception that anal sex "has" to hurt. It will be a more pleasurable experience for both of you if you're completely relaxed and receptive. If the physical sensations become too much for you or you feel frightened and out of control, by all means, stop what you're doing.

The pleasure derived from being penetrated results from the internal massaging pressure and fullness in the rectum. Direct prostate stimulation leads many men to orgasm solely from being anally penetrated. Some women, though fewer than men, can also orgasm solely from anal intercourse. If orgasm is your goal, you should certainly incorporate other types of genital stimulation into what you're doing. A vibrator on your clitoris, a dildo in your vagina, a hand around your penis, a nipple clamp tugging your nipple, or a cock ring snapped around your testicles can all contribute to your experience of anal intercourse. Some people feel that anal intercourse produces unique sensations of serenity and intimacy, and it may be that these sensations will be powerful enough to make orgasm seem irrelevant.

Anal intercourse is infrequent, but an exclusive "high."

POSITIONS: Despite the common assumption that anal intercourse almost by definition takes place in a rear-entry position, all the positions used in vaginal intercourse can be adapted to anal intercourse. The most important consideration for any position you choose is that the receptive partner should control how and when penetration takes place. For convenience's sake and to avoid a morass of pronouns, let's assume that Tarzan and Jane are about to try anal intercourse for the first time. Jane has fashioned a beautiful dildo harness out of jungle vines, and Tarzan is eager to enact his fantasy of feeling Jane moving inside him.

Before Jane attempts penetration, she starts by teasing Tarzan's anus with her finger. She applies plenty of lubricant with her fingers, taking the time to really work the lubricant past the anal opening and into the rectum. (Some people find it helpful to co-opt a vaginal cream applicator to insert lube well into the rectum.) Once Tarzan's anus is happy and relaxed and able to comfortably accommodate two of Jane's fingers, Jane positions the tip of her banana-shaped dildo at Tarzan's anal opening and holds it there. Tarzan inhales and exhales a few times, while contracting and relaxing his sphincter muscles. When he feels ready, he bears down onto Jane's banana. Jane moves forward into him ever so slightly, but she holds the dildo still just inside his rectum while his muscles adjust to the sensation. After Tarzan has gotten used to the sensation of fullness, he asks Jane to move her hips slowly back and forth.

Tarzan and Jane quickly become expert in anal intercourse, and try all the following positions. In missionary position, Tarzan lies on his back with his knees pulled to his chest and his feet over Jane's shoulders. This allows for deep penetration, prostate stimulation, and face-to-face contact, though Tarzan doesn't have much freedom of movement and sometimes his legs get cramped.

In rear entry, Tarzan is on his elbows and knees, while Jane penetrates him from behind. Jane likes the fact that this position allows her to do a lot of pelvic thrusting, while Tarzan likes the deep penetration it affords, not to mention that Jane can easily reach around and play with his penis. Sometimes they try a variation where both are standing up with Tarzan bent slightly at the waist and bracing himself against a tree. When Tarzan wants total control of the rate of penetration, Jane lies on her back while he straddles her and sits down on the dildo. This is a convenient position in which to stimulate each other. When neither of them wants to support the weight of the other, they lie side by side in a spoons position. While this does not allow for deep penetration or much thrusting movement, it's a comfortable, intimate position that allows for lots of full-body stimulation.

You may want to try all the same positions as Tarzan and Jane, or you may make up your own variations. Just stick to the golden rule of anal sex, and make sure that the receptive partner has ultimate control over the movement and pace of penetration. Some people get an added erotic thrill by identifying anal intercourse as a power play, in which the receptive partner is the submissive bottom under the control of his or her dominant penetrator. This dynamic can enhance your experience, especially if you are aroused by the taboo of anal sex as a forbidden activity. There are just as many people for whom power play would be distasteful and who prefer to experience anal intercourse as an equal melding together of two bodies.

When being fucked I like to straddle my partner who is lying on his back. I like to have control of how the penis enters me until I've loosened up enough to actually be fucked by him. When fucking I like to be sitting up with my partner sitting in my lap so that we can kiss and play with each other's nipples—so that it seems more equal than dominant/submissive.

Intercourse Enhancers

Additional Stimulation

People's preferences with regard to how much and what kind of additional stimulation they crave during intercourse can range from "less is more" to "more is more."

I don't like a lot of extra stimulation during fucking, preferring to concentrate on the act.

I don't think two people have enough hands to stimulate everything that wants to get stimulated on me!

There is nothing better than vaginal, anal, and clitoral stimulation all at once, especially if I have my nipple clips on at the same time!

We ourselves, as you may have guessed, are of the "more is more" school, and we encourage you to experiment with a wide range of sensations during intercourse. Take advantage of the fact that intercourse is a full-body experience. While you are joined at the hips, your hands and mouths can roam freely over each other's chests, backs, shoulders, butts, and thighs. You may want to focus attention on traditional erogenous zones, or you may find the unexpected arousing.

I love having the hair on my head pulled, especially at the back of my neck.

I really enjoy being scratched on my legs, not too hard, but hard enough. I enjoy having my nipples bitten and my chest rubbed (I sound like a pine cabinet!).

I like it when a man slowly introduces his tongue in my mouth and fucks my mouth with his tongue the exact same way his cock is fucking my cunt. At that point, my mouth comes alive and my imagination soars.

During penetration, I love having my breasts touched at all times. The whole breast, not just the nipple.

Fingers are a bit of a turn-off quite honestly unless they are inserted with a penis, preferably on the perineum side of the vagina. Doing this with two fingers and moving them around while the penis is fully inserted (and holding still) I find very sexy and physically stimulating.

As mentioned above, the majority of women need clitoral stimulation to reach orgasm during intercourse. Who provides the stimulation may depend on what position you're in. In the missionary or woman-on-top positions, it can be easier for a woman to stimulate herself.

I usually only climax with clitoral stimulation, so this for me is a must. I prefer to do it while I enjoy my partner stimulating my nipples. Oh yes, put a tongue in my ear and your teeth across the back of my neck.

Rear entry or spoons are convenient positions if you want to reach around and stimulate your partner's clitoris. Some women find that, once they are sufficiently aroused, the indirect clitoral stimulation from intercourse is enough to bring them to orgasm, and that additional direct clitoral stimulation might numb them out.

Sometimes clitoral stimulation distracts me when I'm getting ready to come while fucking.

I like clitoral stimulation beforehand, but if I get too much I lose sensitivity.

Both men and women can appreciate having their nipples stimulated during intercourse. Face-to-face positions allow you to suck, lick, and bite each other's nipples, while nearly all positions allow for nipple pinching and tweaking. Many people find that the more aroused they are, the more vigorous attention their nipples crave.

Nipple stimulation is practically mandatory to a "hot" experience. I can practically come with a combination of tit biting/licking and lip kissing. The hotter I get, the harder I like my nipples tweaked/pinched. I get annoyed if my partner is gentle with my nipples.

I love breast stimulation even to the point of it hurting—actually, that really gets me hot.

Nipple stimulation gets me "over the top" and into orgasm faster than anything.

I have neurological disabilities. It took me a long time to understand that it's okay to have my nipple pinched while I masturbate—it speeds up my ejaculation time.

I have a nipple piercing, which feels good if it is gently played with.

Anal stimulation is another popular intercourse enhancer for men and women alike. Preferred techniques range from the simple pressure of a finger or thumb stroking the anal opening, to some form of penetration: a finger, several fingers, a dildo, or a plug. Nearly every intercourse position lends itself handily to one or both partners reaching around to play with the other's anus. Men may enjoy feeling a finger stroking the prostate gland during intercourse—to do so, reach about three inches into the rectum, and stroke toward the front of his body.

Some women find double penetration extremely arousing. It provides stimulation of the sensitive perineal area between the vagina and anus, while the sensation of pressure on both sides of the vaginal wall can be quite exciting for both parties involved. Of course, for every woman who finds double penetration double the fun, there's a woman who finds it unpleasantly overwhelming.

My favorite thing is to have a butt plug in while I'm fucking a penis, a finger, or a dildo. That's a great feeling—like you are totally filled.

I enjoy anal stimulation/penetration, but combined with vaginal penetration, it's sometimes distracting.

Many men also appreciate having their testicles played with during intercourse. Try reaching between his legs and forming your fingers into a ring around his scrotum and the base of his penis. Either hold on, applying a gentle pressure, or tug gently on the scrotum. You could also try palming each testicle separately, but bear in mind that a fluttering, light touch may feel more ticklish than sexy.

My favorite stimulation during intercourse is a firm yet gentle grasping of the entire scrotal sac. It conveys a sense of control that overcomes my wife's sexual reticence.

I like to have a woman stroke and squeeze my testicles during sex.

Spatial Arrangements

From the humble pillow to the elaborate pleasure swing, devices that adjust your physical positioning are time-honored intercourse enhancers. If you're penetrating a woman who's lying on her back, try raising her hips by placing pillows beneath them. This elevated posture allows for deeper penetration—also, the angle of penetration will follow the natural curve of the vagina, allowing your pubic bone to rub against her clitoris. Similarly, if you're penetrating a man who's lying on his stomach, he may enjoy having pillows piled beneath his pelvis. Some men (and women) prefer to masturbate by rubbing against a pillow or bolster and can easily employ this useful technique during rear-entry intercourse.

You can also enhance your positioning by having one person sitting or lying down, while the other person stands. For instance, your partner can lie on his or her back at the side of the bed, while you stand on the floor or kneel against the side of the bed. This allows your partner the leverage to raise and lower his or her legs and hips for different angles of penetration, while it provides a delightful weightless feeling. Alternatives include intercourse with the receptive partner perched on a table or counter. Different heights will obviously work better for different-sized people.

For the ultimate weightless sensation, try a swing or sling. Hanging chairs have been in existence since ancient times, testament to the timeless appeal of being suspended in midair. Your partner can sit in the swing, being rocked to-and-fro onto your penis or dildo, or your partner can straddle you while you lie in the swing. Many people find that being cradled in a swing creates a relaxed, receptive state that greatly enhances and facilitates deep penetration, G-spot stimulation, or fisting. Swings are enjoyed by pregnant women and large people, who may particularly appreciate a temporary release from gravity. They're also a boon to folks who suffer from debilitating back pains or other disabilities that limit stamina and mobility.

Whether you're using a simple hammock or a genuine sex swing complete with adjustable straps and stirrups for the legs, installation is a far simpler undertaking than you might think. All you need are two or three eyebolts and some lengths of chain, both of which are easily purchased at any hardware store. Make sure to screw the eyebolts into ceiling beams, rather than into plaster, and use the lengths of chain to adjust the height of the swing to your specifications. Voilà. Not only will you be the envy of all your friends, but you'll never have trouble getting a housesitter when you want to go on vacation!

Vibrators

The same toys that provide delightful stimulation during solo sex are ready and waiting to serve you and your loved ones during partner sex. One of the most common reasons a male/female or female/female couple gives for buying a vibrator is that they'd like to increase clitoral stimulation during intercourse. Penetrating a partner provides direct stimulation to

the most sensitive part of a man's penis—his glans—and therefore the vast majority of men reach orgasm from intercourse alone. The majority of women, however, require additional attention to the clitoris to reach orgasm during intercourse. This is where a vibrator can be of invaluable assistance.

Any and every style of vibrator can be incorporated into intercourse. It's easy to tuck a battery vibrator or vibrating egg between two bodies, and it's even possible for a woman to take a no-hands approach and wear a vibrator between her legs in a leather pouch or harness. You may be worried that introducing a Hitachi Magic Wand into your intercourse routine will be the equivalent of slipping between the sheets with a Mack truck, but it ain't so. Even the larger plug-in vibrators rest unobtrusively against a woman's clitoris when you're in woman-on-top, rear-entry, or side-by-side positions. Some people also find it comfortable to slip a wand vibrator between their pelvises while in missionary position. Coil vibrators are a less convenient shape to position between two bodies, but you may find that a long G-Spotter attachment on a coil vibrator provides the perfect way to reach the clitoris while holding the vibrator off to the side of your bodies.

As even the most attentive lover can become distracted by his or her own pleasure during intercourse, your best bet would be for the receptive partner to hold the vibrator and control its intensity, pressure, and positioning. You may want to experiment with placing a vibrating cock ring at the base of your penis or dildo, though since this moves on and off your partner's clitoris in time with your thrusts, the cock ring won't provide reliable, consistent clitoral stimulation. Yet it will provide consistent stimulation to the penis, which some men like (and some men find overwhelming).

Men whose partners are using a vibrator during intercourse are often pleasantly surprised at how good the indirect vibrations transmitted through their partner's body feel on their own genitals. A man being penetrated may enjoy holding a vibrator against his penis in all the ways described above.

French Ticklers

These are devices that look like a cross between a condom and a Creepy Crawler. They fit like a cap over the head of a penis or dildo, and they're covered with rubber nubs and fronds. The idea behind French ticklers is that the sensation of the little tickling fronds going in and out of a woman's vaginal opening will somehow be unutterably pleasing to her. Presumably, French ticklers sprang from the same great minds who brought us textured condoms. While we certainly believe there are some women who might derive pleasure from the sensation of rubber nubs or ribbed condoms whispering in and out of their vaginas, the whole notion has about as much in common with the average woman's experience as does the story of the princess and the pea.

French ticklers and a few other stimulus-styled condoms didn't work with women and annoyed me.

About ribbed condoms: Thanks for making me feel like I have no nerve endings. I couldn't tell the difference. Can anyone?

On the bright side, whether or not they float your boat, French ticklers are often good for a laugh:

In my late twenties, I was visiting a friend in England and we were traveling around the countryside in a VW van, visiting various tourist attractions and pubs. One night as we got ready to turn in, he went to take a leak and came back from the restroom sporting a bright red French tickler. All I could think was, "It looks just like a little rubber rooster!" Unfortunately, I let that comment slip out, and we both dissolved in laughter that made sex impossible.

One variation on the French tickler has some pleasure potential. This is a rubber ring with a knob protruding off one side. The ring is designed to fit around the base of a penis or dildo, with the knob positioned upward, so that it will rub against the woman's clitoris during intercourse. Not every woman will be able to get the knob positioned comfortably or to get consistent, sufficiently intense stimulation from it, but at least this device reflects a rudimentary knowledge of female anatomy. We suspect the primary function of these doohickeys—for lack of a technical name, called "clit rugs"—is as a communication tool for initiating the subject of clitoral stimulation during intercourse.

My favorite sex toy is something we call "the rubber thing." It came in the mail with a box of condoms.

I refuse to call it a "French tickler," since it looks like it came from a factory in New Jersey. Some may call it a "cock ring." It has an added appendage for strategic female stimulation during the act of union. But whatever you call 'em, they're great!

Cock Rings

These are rings designed to fit around the base of the penis and the scrotum, restricting blood flow out of the penis. The resulting pressure can be very pleasurable and can heighten sensation in the penis and testicles. Since cock rings act to constrict the veins that would allow blood to drain out of an erection, some men find that wearing cock rings prolongs their erection or even makes their erection firmer, a side effect that can enhance intercourse for both parties involved.

My most enjoyable sex toy was a cock ring. It was interesting and added about two hours until my orgasm, and when I came—Wow, Bam, Pow, Shazam....

I like when he uses a cock ring and fucks me with his enlarged and super-hard cock.

I enjoy the feel and look a cock ring provides. When I get aroused without the cock ring, my balls pull way up into my body and almost disappear. With the ring around my scrotum, they stay out. It looks great without being painful or uncomfortable.

Of course, this sensation of pressure that some men find arousing may be downright antierotic to others.

Our most disappointing sex toy was a cock ring. My partner said it hurt too much for him to enjoy anything else.

If you wear a cock ring that is too tight or if you wear it for too long, you'll cut off your circulation and you may experience bruising. In most cases, the damage from burst blood vessels is minor and only temporary, but why risk it? Stick to wearing easily removable cock rings and don't wear them for more than twenty minutes at a time. Try not to fall asleep with your cock ring on. Some men do enjoy wearing cock rings for hours at a stretch, but you should only do this after you've gained enough experience to have a realistic sense of your own limits.

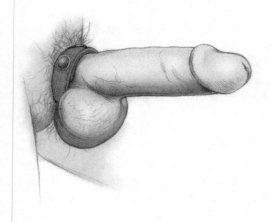

Cock ring

Cock rings come in three varieties: metal, latex, or leather. The only way to don the solid metal or latex variety is to put them on before you're erect. You'll need to drop one testicle at a time through the ring and then tuck your flaccid penis down through the ring. Metal cock rings should really only be used by men who have considerable experience with these toys. After all, once you've got the darn thing on, and it's constricting the flow of blood out of your erection, orgasm will be the only pleasant way to make your erection subside. If your metal cock ring begins to feel painfully tight, and you want to remove it, you have two options. One option is to apply ice or cold water to your penis, which should shrink that erection down to size. An even less appealing option would be to go to the emergency room and have the ring clipped off. Latex cock rings are slightly less problematic, as you can cut these off as necessary in the privacy of your own home without resorting to power tools.

My boyfriend and I decided that it would be fun to try a cock ring, so he bought one to take on holiday with us last year. He thought the quick-release styles looked like torture instruments, so he bought a metal one, reckoning it would be a safer bet!!! How wrong he was. One night, after a couple of drinks, we decided to try it out. I took a while to get the thing on, as he kept getting hard during the process, but once it was in place it looked pretty good, and so I got on top and started to work my magic. After a few minutes I jumped off to try something different and noticed that his balls had gone a funny shade of blue. I started to panic and had images of having to phone for several

Cypriot firemen to appear at the door with bolt cutters to free my boyfriend's cock. After running around the room laughing, I tried cooling him off a bit with some ice but this didn't do much. When he finally went limp, I whisked off the ring and we breathed a sigh of relief— no need for the bolt cutters! Since then, we have warned many of our friends never to experiment with a metal cock ring!

When all's said and done, you're better off with the leather strap variety. These fasten with either snaps or Velcro, and the moment you begin to experience any discomfort you can unfasten them and release the pressure. Furthermore, leather cock-and-ball toys are available in a delightful array of styles: Some have straps that separate each testicle; some have straps that stretch the testicles downwards; some are fitted with D-rings, so that you can attach a leash to them; and some are decoratively studded. Leather cock-and-ball toys provide not only sexual but also aesthetic stimulation to the wearer and his partner.

Kegels

Don't forget that one of the easiest, most effective ways to enhance any type of penetration is to keep your pelvic muscles well toned. Kegel exercises can provide a delightful way to "warm up" before intercourse, because they increase blood flow to the genitals and heighten awareness of genital sensation. A toned muscle is a flexible muscle, and you're likely to experience a great deal more pleasure with strong pelvic muscles than without. Your partner can also enjoy feeling you rhythmically contract and relax your pelvic muscles during intercourse.

Safer Sex

Please don't ever engage in either vaginal or anal intercourse without following some basic safer-sex guidelines. Penis-vagina and penis-anus intercourse are activities that transmit viruses and bacteria with alarming efficiency. The friction of intercourse can easily create minute breaks in the tissue of the vagina, rectum, or penis, through which bodily fluids can pass. We encourage you to refer to the Safer Sex chapter for a detailed discussion of safer sex techniques and risk management.

Intercourse without Penetration

One of the reasons people frequently give for enjoying intercourse is that it allows them simultaneous genital stimulation and full-body contact. We didn't want to leave the topic of intercourse without pointing out that it's possible to reap these simultaneous benefits independent of penetration. Penetration by a penis is fraught with so many consequences, from pregnancy to disease transmission, that it's a shame the variety of full-body "intercourse" techniques aren't more widely discussed and encouraged. Dry humping is dismissed as an archaic adolescent activity simply because it doesn't involve sticking one body part into another. Yet few things feel better than rubbing two bodies against each other, and as anyone who's ever humped a lover's thigh until she or he saw stars knows, there's nothing "dry" about dry humping.

I love to rub against both men and women. I can easily have an orgasm by persistently rubbing against anything hard, like legs.

Dry humping can be a big turn-on, especially when my boyfriend has an erection, and I can feel it through his clothes.

Certain terms for dry humping have come to be associated exclusively with lesbian sex: *frottage* (from the French *frotter*, to rub) and *tribadism* (from the Greek *tribein*, to rub). Both describe the activity of rubbing your clitoris against any part of your partner's body that gets you off, such as her pubic bone, thigh, hip, elbow, or knee. One of the great things about dry humping is its ease and versatility. You can be naked or clothed; rolling around the floor in the privacy of your own home or climbing onto each other in the back seat of a parked car; locked in a full embrace or poised on one another's knees.

I really enjoy tribadism with women—I lie on my back, wrap my legs around them, and rock—thrilling.

My girlfriend jokingly tells me it's not her I love but her leg. When we're naked, I love to close my eyes and straddle one of her delicious thighs, rubbing my cunt slowly and firmly up and down.

Given the full expanse of your partner's body as your playground, you may be surprised to discover how creative you both can be.

I love riding my lover's back. When he's too tired or worn out for sex and I'm raring to go, my lover rolls over to offer me his tailbone. It works very well. I straddle his lower back so that my clit is against the hardness of his tailbone right above the beginning of his bum. I usually lean forward with my hands on his shoulders. I ride just like I would if his cock were inside me. It's plenty of stimulation for my clit and when I do the downward stroke the bump of his tailbone almost feels like the very tip of a penis on the verge of entering me. A highly enjoyable and easy way for me to cum. Also, tired or not, my lover loves the noises I make when I'm getting off so this is a favorite activity of his as well.

Once I was about to take my girlfriend's boots off, and I got inspired to rub my cunt on the toe of her boot. She just lay back in a chair watching me, while I gave her a "shoeshine" she'll never forget.

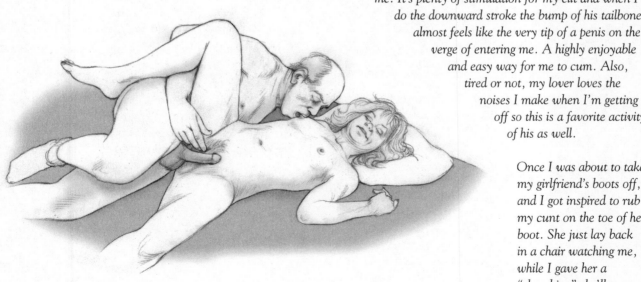

Intercourse without penetration

Another variation on dry humping especially for men is *interfemoral* or *intercrural intercourse*. These are the terms for rubbing your penis between your partner's thighs and getting off from the friction this creates. Some classical scholars speculate that this was actually the primary type of intercourse indulged in between Athenian male citizens and the young boys they initiated into adulthood. So much for the popular notion that all those classical Greeks were obsessed with anal intercourse! Variations include rubbing your penis against your partner's perineum, between the cheeks of his or her butt, or in his or her armpit. Tit-fucking— rubbing your penis in between your partner's breasts— is yet another variation on this theme.

There's a lot of pleasure awaiting you if you let your imagination lead you beyond the confines of traditional sex.

Once, after some time apart, my boyfriend and I made love simply with his hand stuffed inside me and me making love to his cock with my hand wet with my juices, lying as if we were having intercourse, and it was wonderful—like taking apart the elements of traditional fucking and intensifying them.

Dildos

A dildo is any object designed (or recruited) for vaginal or anal insertion. Dildos don't vibrate, though many battery vibrators are dildo-shaped. They don't even move unless you put them into motion. Dildos have been around in one form or another, in one culture after another, since the beginning of civilization. In fact, according to *The Prehistory of Sex,* dildos *predate* civilization—three-dimensional "phallic batons," including a gorgeous sculpture that clearly resembles a double dildo, have been found in Upper Paleolithic art created more than thirty thousand years ago.

Dildos are represented in Greek vase paintings of the fifth and fourth centuries B.C. and were worn by actors in classical Greek stage comedies. Throughout the Hellenistic Age, the coastal city of Miletus in Asia Minor was well known as the manufacturing and export center for dildos made of leather or wood. In a Greek dialogue from the third century B.C., one woman complains to another that all their acquaintances are borrowing her beautiful new scarlet leather dildo before she's had the chance to try it herself. The *Kama Sutra* refers to dildos made from wood, tubular stalks, or reeds tied to the waist, while a nineteenth-century Chinese painting depicts a woman acrobatically entertaining herself with a dildo strapped to her shoe.

Dildos may be sex toys with a long and honorable history, yet in this day and age they just can't get no respect. Kids use the word as a pejorative; sex toy shoppers hesitate over how "unnatural" it seems to play with what seems a disembodied phallus; and many bristle at the implication that they would crave a "penis substitute." The bottom line is, dildos make people nervous. Yet it's well worth overcoming your dildo-induced anxiety.

Why Would I Use a Dildo?

The truth is that it's natural for the vagina to balloon during sexual excitement, leading many women to crave the pressure and fullness of penetration. It's natural for those of us who appreciate anal stimulation to enjoy feeling the anus contracting around a dildo. Isn't it a bit arbitrary to insist that anything that goes into the vagina or anus should be attached to a human body? After all, we work out on Stairmasters and whip up romantic dinners à deux in our Cuisinarts with no concern that we're indulging in "unnatural" pleasures. Instead, consider the theory that the word "dildo" derives from the Italian word *diletto*, or *delight*—for dildos are unquestionably among the most delightful sex toys around.

Sometimes a Cigar Is Just a Cigar

The notion that a dildo is a substitute for nature's fine creation, the penis, implies that dildos are second-rate stand-in's for "the real thing." This second-best status has given dildos a bad rap. Women who have fought to overturn the notion that intercourse alone defines a sexual experience sometimes throw out the baby of pleasurable penetration with the bath water of preconception. For years, it was assumed that lesbians played exclusively with dildos in a simulation of heterosexual intercourse—after all, what else is there for two women to do in bed? In a classic example of cutting off your nose to spite your face, many lesbians responded to the stereotype by condemning dildos as tools of the patriarchy. After all, if a dildo is supposed to be a replacement for a penis, the desire to wear a dildo could be seen as a form of penis envy. Similarly, men who are led to believe that dildos are "fake penises" may react by taking an adversarial stance toward the very toy that could bring them so much pleasure in bed.

Let's set the record straight: A dildo is not a penis substitute any more than riding a bike is a substitute for taking a stroll. A dildo is an object that allows you to penetrate yourself or your partner in a marvelous variety of ways. Dildos are a logical, dare we say natural, response to the fact that while many of us enjoy having our vaginas or anuses filled, no two of us have exactly the same preferences in terms of the length, width, and shape of the object filling us. Why should your experiences with penetration be defined by the dimensions of your current partners' penises or fingers? Few of us limit our dining experiences to eating only whatever is in the refrigerator at home. Think of dildos as the take-out food of the sexual realm; they

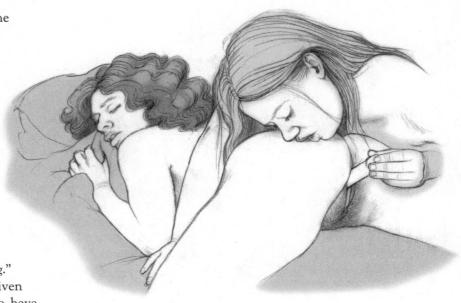

Playing with a dildo

offer novelty, spice up your routine, and teach you about the range of your appetites.

Variety

Not only are no two vaginas alike, but no one vagina is alike all the time. At different times in her life, at different times during the menstrual cycle, and in different intercourse positions, a woman's vagina will accommodate different-sized objects. A wardrobe of variously sized, shaped, and colored dildos is just as crucial to the well-equipped penetration maven as a wardrobe of clothes for all seasons.

In some positions, the contractions of my cunt are too strong for my partner, so we'll use the dildo.

Dildos are good when you can't get enough.

My most enjoyable time with a sex toy was when my boyfriend took pictures of me using my Jelly cock. It's about eight inches long, and he wanted to get pics of it all the way out, half way in, and all the way in to show how much cock I could take. For some reason that amazed him. I was turned on, simply because he was.

Safety

The primary distinction between sex with a penis and sex with a dildo is that sex with a penis requires a certain amount of negotiation with your partner, whereas sex with a dildo puts you squarely in the driver's seat. You and you alone are in charge of your experience with a dildo, which can take some getting used to. Many of us unconsciously rely on our partners to set the pace of a sexual encounter. Even those of us who regularly masturbate with vibrators may be inclined to abandon ourselves to the vibrations rather than to direct the flow of sensations. Dildos are the ultimate self-assertion tool—it's up to you to manipulate them for your own pleasure. And they're great self-awareness tools, allowing you to experiment with penetration without the performance anxiety of having a partner present.

Once I left my dildo in the bedside table at a women's writing retreat. I'm told it now has a place of honor on the Self-Help bookshelf!

Women who are nervous about penetration, or those suffering from vaginismus, can gain confidence through playing with dildos. Postmenopausal women may want to use dildos to keep their vaginas toned for intercourse. Male-to-female transsexuals are required to exercise with dildos (referred to by the medical establishment as "dilators") to keep their surgically created vaginas from contracting shut. Both men and women who want to experiment with anal penetration often find solo play with dildos a great way to learn their own preferences and limits. Furthermore, dildos are the ultimate safe-sex fuck-buddy. As long as you keep your dildo clean and condom-clad, it will never infect you or your loved ones with any virus or bacteria.

Fantasy

Best of all, dildos can provide the key to unlock many an inspiring fantasy. Whether you're playing alone or with a partner, dildos offer an easy, safe, fun way to enact scenes from your erotic imagination.

I especially enjoy using a dildo while getting fucked or sucking my partner —partly for the ménage à trois fantasy—partly because it's a turn-on for my partner.

My favorite method of masturbating is riding a dildo with a vibrator. I guess it reminds me of riding a horse!

Dildo Do's

Do Relax

The key to comfortable penetration of any kind is to relax. Your vagina and anus are surrounded by pelvic muscles, and if these muscles are tense or contracted, you won't find penetration a pleasant experience. A lot of us carry tension in our genitals without even being aware of it. Before you settle in to play with a dildo, bring some attention to bear on your genitals. Do Kegel exercises to get the blood flowing throughout your pelvis. Put the tip of the dildo at the entrance to your vagina, inhale and contract your vaginal muscles, then exhale and bear down with your vaginal muscles. As you bear down, slip the dildo inside your vagina. If you feel your muscles tensing, deliberately contract and relax them around the dildo.

You may find you enjoy squeezing and releasing a dildo, as this enhances awareness of sensation in your vagina. Try combining muscular contractions with moving the dildo: For instance, tighten your pelvic muscles as you slowly slip the dildo out of the vagina, then relax your muscles and let the dildo sink back inside. Whatever you choose to do, keep breathing and don't force any more of the dildo into your vagina than you can comfortably accommodate. The same considerations apply to anal play with a dildo. Remember, you're the one in control of the experience.

Do Use Lube

Dildos are dry. They don't self-lubricate the way genitals do. Furthermore, dildos frequently have a slightly gummy, porous texture that absorbs moisture. Please always use lubricant with dildos. We don't care how much lubrication you produce on your own—two slippery surfaces slide together much more comfortably than one slippery and one dry surface. Apply lube to the dildo and to your vagina or anus. Nobody likes dildo burn, and there's no reason to experience it. The dildo that struck you as impossibly large when you took it for a dry run could well seem the perfect fit once you lube it up.

Do Keep Your Dildos Clean

Dildos come in all types of material. Some dildos are completely smooth and nonporous; others have tacky surfaces and are quite porous. You could transmit infection if bacteria and viruses linger in the pockmarks of your porous dildo. At the very least, wash your dildo with mild soap after each use. Rinse it thoroughly and let it dry completely before putting it away. Viruses and bacteria won't live on a dry surface.

You can save yourself time and trouble by using condoms with your dildos. Even if you use your dildo exclusively in your own vagina, you can benefit from using condoms; they'll prevent you from reinfecting yourself with a yeast infection and can add years to the life of a cheap rubber dildo. Change the condom every time you swap a dildo with a partner or every time you move the dildo from your anus to vagina. After all, no dildo will ever complain of being forced to wear "a raincoat in the shower."

Do Use Common Sense

Babies will put just about anything into their mouths, and adults have been known to put just about anything into their vaginas and anuses.

> I've been penetrated by a pickle, a long-neck beer bottle, and a big stick ice cream.

Although we applaud this kind of enterprise and ingenuity, we implore you to use common sense and not to put anything fragile, anything sharp, or anything with rough, jagged edges into your body. If you're using a plastic hairbrush handle, make sure that the plastic seams are filed down. Don't use anything wooden that could splinter or anything glass that could shatter, and don't insert an open bottle neck-first—the resulting suction could make it very difficult and dangerous to remove.

Certain dildos produced by the adult industry contain wire rods that allow the dildo to be bent or cranked into all kinds of interesting configurations. In the case of more cheaply made toys, the metal can tear through the soft rubber of the dildo all too easily. In a worst-case scenario, the wire could poke through the dildo and perforate your vaginal or anal walls. Look for toys with plentiful, thick casings, and don't be afraid to pull and prod it with your hands to ensure that the rod isn't going to come through. There are other options for those of us who find the idea of an adjustable dildo appealing. Certain jelly rubber and cyberskin dildos contain flexible plastic spines segmented into plastic "vertebrae." These dildos can be bent into a variety of different angles without fear of the plastic spines tearing through the surface as uncovered metal wires might.

Styles

Whereas vibrators can be found camouflaged as "massagers" in department or discount stores, the natural habitat of the dildo is and always will be the sex shop. When Good Vibrations first opened in 1977, the only type of dildo commercially available was the great-big-Caucasian-penis look-alike. As more and more sex-positive entrepreneurs moved into manufacturing, dildo design diversified, and there are now more styles and sizes than you can shake a stick at. Even the mainstream industry is making an effort to produce dildos in a greater variety of skin tones, as well as in playful colors and materials.

As discussed in the Vibrators chapter, many battery vibrators are dildo-shaped and can be used for penetration both before and after their motors give up the ghost. This chapter focuses on dildos: nonvibrating toys designed purely and simply for penetration.

Adult-Industry Dildos

Mainstream commercial dildos, marketed as "novelties," are made of either vinyl or synthetic rubbers molded into flexible, more or less representational penis shapes. Here's a quick tour of what you can expect to find on the shelves of your local adult store.

VINYL AND RUBBER: Dildos made of vinyl or rubber are generally produced in either the unique peachy-orange tint that the adult industry has designated Caucasian skin color (think "flesh"-colored Band-aid) or in a flat black color. While this black color doesn't remotely resemble any human being's skin color, it does go nicely with all your evening wear. Some styles are set on a handle for greater maneuverability; some flare at the base, allowing you to wear them in a dildo harness; and some feature rubber nubs at the base, ostensibly as clitoral stimulators for women. All tend to be inexpensive.

Vinyl dildos are lightweight (either they're hollow or they have a foam core) and less porous than rubber, making them easier to keep clean. Rubber dildos are heavy, porous, and difficult to keep clean. Grime works its way into the air bubbles under the surface and is impossible to scrub out. Furthermore, scrubbing will only produce unappetizing little rubber pills all over the surface of your dildo. If you own a rubber dildo, your best bet is to use condoms with it at all

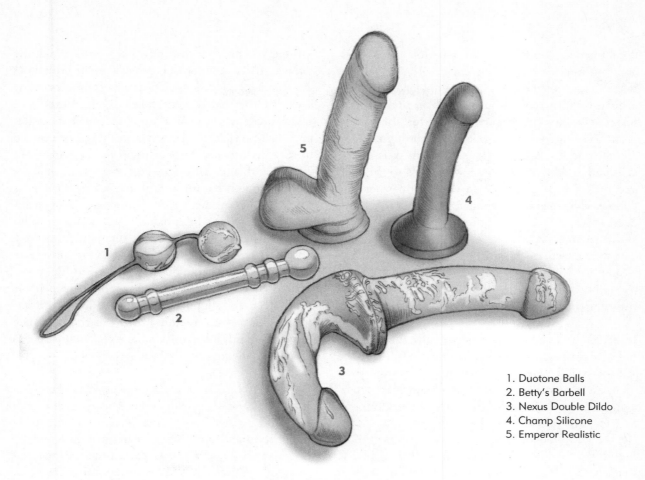

1. Duotone Balls
2. Betty's Barbell
3. Nexus Double Dildo
4. Champ Silicone
5. Emperor Realistic

Various styles of dildos

times. On the bright side, rubber dildos are quite flexible, and they will soften up with time, handling, and heat to become even more flexible.

REALISTICS: Realistic dildos are supposedly molded from live models to, as one manufacturer puts it, "capture every vein, bulge, and crease of a real erect cock." This marketing ploy has resulted in dildos that are cast from the genitals of famous male porn stars (and there are similar lines of rubber vaginas cast from the genitals of female porn stars). Most realistics are available in Caucasian skin tones, some in black skin tones, and all are sized from big to bigger—few are less than two inches in diameter or eight inches in length. Uncircumcised realistics come complete with sculpted foreskins—we've yet to find a model with a retractable foreskin.

The larger realistics are so long and heavy they frequently sag under their own weight, giving the

impression that your porn star pals don't have their hearts in their work. What keeps these drooping dildos from falling off Good Vibrations' display shelves are their suction cup bases. The removable suction cups adhere to any nonporous surface, such as glass or bathroom tile, for easy mounting.

While realistics have a unique aesthetic niche, they're not cheap, they're hard to keep clean, and they're too bulky to be very comfortable when worn in most harnesses.

PROSTHETIC PENIS ATTACHMENTS: These are hollow vinyl shafts, usually attached to an elastic strap. The idea behind what we call PPAs is that some men may have trouble sustaining erections, may want to continue penetrating their partner after they themselves have reached orgasm, or may want to penetrate their partner with a longer, thicker "penis" than the one nature gave them. A man can slip a PPA over his flaccid penis, snap the elastic strap around his waist, and continue to have intercourse with his partner. Sometimes women express interest in buying a PPA as a budget alternative to buying a dildo and harness. Without some kind of stuffing, however, the PPA is prone to being squeezed out of shape. Furthermore, an elastic strap is a highly inefficient means of fastening any kind of dildo to your body—it's hard to thrust in and out of your partner with conviction when the dildo is wobbling and snapping against your torso with every move.

In general, PPAs strike us as inefficient sex toys. They also seem to be uncomfortable for both the wearer and his partner—at the very least, you'd want to slather the inside and the outside of the vinyl sheath with lubricant.

JELLY RUBBER: In the nineties jelly rubber burst onto the scene and spawned a minirevolution in the sex toy industry, releasing manufacturers from their focus on "realistic" styles and skin tones and encouraging the development of truly playful-looking toys. While jelly rubber probably contains some latex (jelly toys degrade when exposed to oils), its primary ingredient is PVC. Polyvinyl chloride is a plastic that's used in everything from fetish fashion to floor tiles to children's toys. Adult jelly toys are soft and pliable and have sleek, smooth surfaces. They're available in luminous jewel tones and bright neon colors; some models have a festive carbonated appearance from air bubbles floating beneath the surface.

> I love your Jelly Boy dildo! (There's a "plug" for you—no pun intended.) Good size, texture, pliability/hardness ratio, and I love that pink Day-Glo color!

Jelly rubber is a popular material for dildos, plugs, and vibrators because it's inexpensive, supple and pretty. However, it is porous and difficult to keep clean. Some people complain that it smells too much like petrochemicals, and its elastic texture is not to everyone's taste:

> I bought a gummy double-headed dildo…not only does it feel weird in the hand, but it feels totally weird anywhere else you put it as well. The girlfriend and I were both pretty cracked up about "fucking Gumby."

One recent study has raised concerns about the safety of PVC. A group of chemicals called phthalates are commonly added to PVC products as a softening agent—yet phthalates tend to leach out of the PVC. Unfortunately, phthalates are environmental pollutants and possible carcinogens that have been linked to liver, kidney, and testicular damage in humans. In 2001, health authorities in several European countries recommended banning children's toys, such as teething rings, made of PVC. Although a subsequent German study found that adult toys contain a significantly higher phthalate content than children's toys, no one has yet proposed a ban on PVC sex toys. Are jelly dildos really hazardous to your health? It's impossible to say. After all, adults don't spend as many hours sucking on (or slipping in) a jelly dildo as infants spend sucking on a teething ring. But the phthalate debate certainly offers one more excellent reason to keep your jelly toys covered with a condom.

CYBERSKIN: An amazing product, cyberskin is so named because it really does feel eerily similar to real flesh and because—or so the story goes—it's made using an injection-molding machine designed by NASA engineers. We're talking space-age material here, folks. Cyberskin is to the turn of the millennium what jelly rubber was to the previous decade—it has quickly become a must-have ingredient in vibrators, dildos, and sleeves. The folks who trademarked this material are fiercely proprietary regarding the details of their formula; our best guess is that cyberskin is some form of thermal plastic, possibly blended with jelly rubber.

Cyberskin is unique both for its resiliency—you can yank away on it, and it will always return to its original shape—and for its life-like density. When you heft a cyberskin dildo in your hand, it feels like yielding, velvet-soft skin surrounding a core of erectile tissue. It also warms quickly to body temperature.

The downside of cyberskin is that it is just about the most porous sex toy material around and is notoriously hard to keep clean (we recommend using condoms with any cyberskin toy). And, it doesn't mix well with other materials—direct contact with everything from silicone-based lubricants to oils to other rubber toys has been known to "melt" the surface of cyberskin toys. It's also on the pricier side. Despite these caveats, cyberskin's amazingly realistic properties have won it a legion of fans.

Silicone Dildos

The dildo revolution got its start in the early eighties when Gosnell Duncan, a holistic health practitioner in Brooklyn, began experimenting with molding silicone into prosthetic devices that would be more pleasurable and comfortable to use than what was then available in the disability community. As word about these unique products spread to the owners of women's bookstores and sex boutiques, demand increased, and an industry was born.

Silicone—the same substance used in surgical implants—is an expensive and delicate raw material, which must be kept sterile and dust-free. Manufacturers continually tinker with their formulas to make their silicone products both resilient and strong, and they must monitor the degree of moisture in the air for successful casting. Silicone manufacturing is a labor-intensive process—each toy must be hand-poured into handmade molds. Consequently, the demand for silicone dildos far outweighs the supply. So far, the prohibitive cost of silicone as a raw material and the difficulty of mechanizing production has kept adult-novelty manufacturers out of the field. (Although novelty companies label certain toys as being made of "silicone," these don't feel anything like the genuine article.) Instead, silicone manufacturing is the exclusive province of cottage industries, whose owners have put imagination and empathy into their work, are responsive to their consumers, and take personal pleasure in the products they create. There are probably fewer than a dozen silicone sex toy manufacturers around the world.

So what's so great about silicone dildos? Texture, for one thing. Silicone is delightfully firm yet flexible, neither too floppy nor too hard. Yes, if Goldilocks and Baby Bear were to select one dildo to take into their sweet tiny bed, it would doubtless be made of silicone. Furthermore, silicone has a smooth, nonporous, velvety surface that is enticing and easy to clean. It retains heat and warms quickly to body temperature. Hygiene fiends are always pleased to hear that you can safely boil silicone products for up to three minutes, while the efficiency-minded can pop silicone dildos into the top rack of their dishwashers.

Best of all, silicone manufacturers have created a wide variety of colors, sizes, and styles. You'll find silicone toys in richly hued jewel tones, marbled swirls, pastels, even glitter. They're available finger-slim to fist-wide in both representational and abstract styles.

Because of the high costs and low volume of production, silicone dildos aren't cheap, but they're certainly heirloom quality toys.

Silicone also conducts vibration exceptionally well. A couple of silicone models are available with hollowed-out shafts, so that you can insert vibrating eggs inside them for an extra treat. And some companies have begun to produce silicone vibrators plus vibrator attachments.

While silicone is highly resilient and can be yanked, tugged, and mauled with no ill effects, if you break the surface of the silicone in any way, your dildo will rip right through with distressing ease. So watch out for teeth and nails. Silicone-based lubricants may ruin the surface of a silicone toy—stick to water-based lubes. If you follow these precautions, your silicone dildo can provide you with literally decades of pleasure.

Latex Dildos

Real latex dildos are made of the natural rubber from rubber trees, and they're produced only in Europe. As a result, they're hard to find in this country. They're available only in black (just like your tires) and generally consist of a latex sheath enrobing a foam-filled core. One real show-stopper you may encounter in a sex boutique is an inflatable latex dildo, which can be pumped up from about one-and-a-half to three inches in diameter. We've also seen a latex whip consisting of a dildo-shaped handle attached to numerous long latex strips. Now if you can crack this whip while the handle is inside you, we'll know you've been doing your Kegels.

Latex is nonporous, so these dildos are easy to keep clean. But latex deteriorates if exposed to heat or light, and oil will transform it into a tacky, gummy mess.

Acrylic Dildos

Dildos made of acrylic are elegant enough to display on any art-lover's coffee table or altar. With colors ranging from clear to translucent rose, blue, or lavender, these shapely sculptures allow you to satisfy your glass-slipper fantasies without risking an accident. Acrylic dildos are smooth, nonporous, and safe for insertion, but they are completely unyielding. They provide a firm pressure that some folks find ideal for G-spot or prostate stimulation and that others find unappealing. Whichever side of the fence you fall on, make sure to use plenty of lubricant when you experiment.

"Barbells"

The Kegelcisor is a stainless steel rod that resembles a barbell. Marketed as a PC muscle toner, the Kegelcisor is packaged with instructions for doing Kegels and sold as a health care product. Nobody needs a resistive device in her vagina to do Kegels correctly—however, many women find that this cool, heavy, space-age toy makes an appealing dildo. Sex educator Betty Dodson, who told us the following anecdote, has been a longtime advocate of these self-awareness toys and has produced her own model called "Betty's Barbell."

> My first vaginal barbell was taken away from me by an airport security guard, who claimed I couldn't get on the plane with this potential weapon in my purse. Of course, they lost the barbell before returning it to me, so I wrote a letter to the airline officials asking just how many times one of their airplanes had been hijacked by an elderly woman brandishing a sex toy. Eventually, they reimbursed me for my "item."

Ben Wa Balls

While they aren't exactly dildos, we're including ben wa balls in this category because they are insertable toys. Many women and men have heard exaggerated claims about the pleasure potential of these marble-sized balls. Even if ben wa balls really were decent sex toys, they'd have a hard time living up to their hype. According to legend, the women of ancient Japan used to insert two hollow ivory balls filled with mercury into their vaginas, then sit back and enjoy the sensation as the balls rolled around inside them. This legend has some lapses in logic: Mercury is a highly toxic substance, and the vagina is not a gaping cave that anything is likely to "roll around" in.

Probably, ben wa balls were small ivory spheres inserted during intercourse to enhance sensation. The modern-day incarnation consists of two gold-plated ball bearings about three-quarters of an inch in diameter.

Some women enjoy ben wa balls for their fantasy value or use them to tune into subtle sensations in the vagina. You probably won't feel any more sexual sensation from ben wa balls than you would from a tampon, though we have heard from women bus drivers and motorcycle riders who say they enjoy wearing ben wa balls on the road, as their vehicle's vibration sets the balls in motion. Some women find that ben wa balls provide stimulation during intercourse, even though they don't move around much. Bear in mind that you shouldn't use ben wa balls anally, as they could easily slip into your colon and out of your reach. We'll discuss anal beads in the chapter on anal toys.

> Over time I've purchased many toys and all have been fun and exciting EXCEPT ben wa balls. Last Halloween I put them in while I took my child trick or treating—I figured I should have fun too. They immediately popped out and rolled around in my underwear the entire night. I was scared that one would pop out and roll down the street. Since then, I keep them on my night stand in hopes that I will come up with a good use.

Duotone balls are a variation on ben wa balls that have more potential: Each metal ball bearing is encased in a hollow sphere about one-and-one-half inches in diameter, and the spheres are leashed together with a nylon cord. Since the heavy ball bearings roll around inside their casing when you rock your hips or tug on the string, they create a sensation of movement that can be stimulating. You might want to position duotone balls half-in/half-out of your vaginal opening for maximum effect. You can find duotones made of jelly rubber, plastic, or silicone; strands with up to four balls; and duotones that vibrate.

> I think duotone balls are especially fun to wear in public for secret surprise stimulation. They were a great pick-me-up when I was on crutches (swinging hips).

> Duotone balls are interesting—I like having them tugged while I'm being masturbated or anally fucked. I was once vaginally fucked while I had the balls in and we both couldn't believe there was room! That was a powerful encounter.

With a little ingenuity, you can devise your own variations on this theme:

> I also enjoy this fake pearl necklace that I wash (of course), wad up, and shove inside my vagina. Then I pull the pearls gently and slowly out and up, so they hit my lips and my clit.

Some women adopt a "bigger is better" approach and insert Chinese healing balls instead of ben wa balls. Slightly larger than a golf ball, healing balls are made of weighted metal that produces a lovely tone, like a distant wind chime. These two balls are designed to be rotated in your palm, thereby stimulating acupressure points and improving the circulation of vital energy through your body. Perhaps you'll find acupressure points inside your vagina that you never knew you had!

Vegetables

We once received a testy note from a customer who was tired of our unremitting praise of silicone dildos—she wrote to let us know that in her opinion "a microwaved zucchini" was infinitely superior to any dildo on the market. You too may be among those who are happiest with a cornucopia of nature's dildos. If you do play with produce, make sure to avoid potentially irritating pesticides—either peel your vegetable or slip a condom on it. If you don't own a microwave, you might want to blanch your chosen vegetable in some boiling water to render it warm and flexible.

> I thought using a carrot for penetration might be nice. It was cold!

In a classic example of art meeting postmodern life, you can find silicone dildos shaped like corn and zucchini, for those folks who want the relationship with their dildos to last past dinnertime.

Buying a Dildo

You may find yourself a little overwhelmed by the sheer number of options available to the dildo-buyer, but you can quickly narrow the field by considering the following variables:

Aesthetics

Would you like a dildo that resembles a penis or one that doesn't? The choice is yours. We've rarely come across a customer who doesn't have a distinct aesthetic preference, and there's no predicting tastes in the matter. The blushing baby-dyke just back from

---

Dildo Shopping Checklist

Some things to consider before buying a dildo:

✓ *Aesthetics:* Would you prefer a dildo that resembles a penis or one that is nonrepresentational?

✓ *Color:* If you'd prefer a dildo in skin tones, select a vinyl, cyberskin, or rubber realistic. If you'd prefer a dildo in decorator colors, select a jelly rubber or silicone model.

✓ *Expense:* If you're experimenting to determine your preferences, you may gravitate toward an inexpensive vinyl or jelly rubber model. If you know what you like and you're making a long-term investment, treat yourself to a silicone model.

✓ *Material:* If you want a flexible dildo, try models made of rubber, jelly rubber, or cyberskin. If you want a dildo that's resilient and easy to clean, get silicone. If you enjoy firm stimulation of the G-spot, try models made of acrylic, metal, or firmer silicone.

✓ *Size/width:* Confirm the diameter that's right for you before you buy!

✓ *Length:* If you or your partner plan to wear the dildo in a harness, select one that's at least six inches long.

✓ *Function:* If you or your partner plan to wear the dildo in a harness, make sure to select one with a flared base.

✓ *Shape:* Contoured or smooth, the choice is yours.

---

the Michigan Womyn's Music Festival may well demand a realistic dildo complete with scrotum and testicles, while the biker dude who just rode in on his Harley may be purchasing a Dolphin dildo for his old lady.

Even though that dildo is destined to go where the sun don't shine, color will probably influence your selection process. Folks who are disappointed by the limited palette of realistic dildos are frequently relieved to find silicone dildos in purple or jelly rubber dildos in green. Others look for a realistic dildo that most closely approximates their own skin color.

Intentions

Different sizes and styles of dildos suit different circumstances. Many people find that they enjoy a thicker dildo when they're playing alone and can control the pace and timing of penetration. If your partner is manipulating the dildo, you'll probably want it to be slimmer than one you'd masturbate with. If you plan to insert it to the hilt, select a shorter model, but if you want to manipulate the dildo, or if your partner plans to wear it in a harness, you'd be better off with one that's at least six inches long. Several of the adult novelty dildos on the market have the shaft set on a handle like a nightstick for easy control. Or you can get creative with a double dildo.

I like to use a long double dildo, putting one end in my cunt and stroking the other end, pretending it's my cock.

Size

While it's true that the average person can accommodate many different sizes of dildos, it's also true that most of us have a decided preference for one size or another.

I like small penises, or better yet, dildos. With very small penises, I orgasm easily. The dildo shouldn't be more than five-and-a-half inches long and one-and-a-quarter inches in diameter, and penises should be even smaller.

I love the feeling of being filled up, so big dildos, lots of fingers, and a fist make me real happy. When they say that size is not important—well, it is for me.

Stores such as Good Vibrations stock a wide range of sizes, and first-time dildo buyers are frequently intimidated by the abundance of alternatives. Male customers seek reassurance that some of the models are "awfully big, aren't they?" while women wonder which model is "average." Frequently, shoppers ask salesclerks, "Which size should I get?" as though dildo dimensions were as easily identifiable as glove or shoe sizes. The truth is, there's simply no way anybody else can select dildo sizes for you. Here are some things to consider in making your own decision:

Obviously, the diameter of the dildo you're selecting is more important than its length, as you can control how deeply you insert the dildo, but there's no way to adjust for an uncomfortable width. Are you currently enjoying penetration from someone's fingers or penis, a candle, a hairbrush handle, a cucumber? You may want to select a dildo that approximates the measurements of an object you already know and love, or you may want to seize this golden opportunity to size up or down. Perhaps you've always fantasized about trying out a two-inch-thick dildo, or maybe you'd like a dildo slimmer than your partner's penis.

If you're a woman who has recently undergone genital or abdominal surgery, if you've never experienced penetration, or if it has been a long time since you did, you should take the time to measure your vagina before purchasing a dildo. Don't be afraid to think small. Medical dilators sold to postoperative male-to-female transsexuals start at about one-third of an inch in diameter and go up from there, while dilators sold to women with vaginismus start at just under an inch in diameter. Some women take advantage of the fact that butt plugs are often available in slimmer sizes than dildos.

I use butt plugs in the vagina—dildos are too big.

One easy (and affordable) way to take your measurements is with vegetables. Head for the nearest produce stand and select some carrots, zucchinis, and cucumbers. Wash them well, dress them in condoms, and try them on for size. When you've found a vegetable that suits your taste, cut it in half and measure its diameter (remember, diameter is the distance across, not around a circle). The same considerations apply if you're selecting a dildo for anal penetration. Take the time to research your preferences before you make your purchase—you'll be glad you did.

My most disappointing sex toy experience was the purchase of a too-large dildo when I first dared to buy one. I was all excited—got it home, practically tore off the wrapper, and hopped into bed with it only to find that its width was an irritant, even with lube. I felt embarrassed that size didn't equal pleasure for me and kept trying to use it for a while. Eventually I braved the trip to the sex toy store again and got other sizes!

Most dildos run between one and two inches in diameter. While people who enjoy vaginal or anal fisting may want dildos greater than two inches in diameter, the average Joe or Jane is generally content with this range.

Shape

Dildos vary greatly, not only in length and girth, but in their shape as well. Some are textured with "veins," some are rippled, some have a head larger than their shaft, and some of the more creative silicone styles undulate in unexpected ways—imagine slipping first the arms, then the head, then the breasts of a "diving-woman" dildo into your vagina. This is another instance where previous experience with penetration can help you make your selection. Do you particularly enjoy the sensation when your vaginal opening expands and then contracts around something? If so, you may find yourself intrigued by a rippled dildo. If you enjoy vaginal fisting, you may be drawn to a dildo with a large head and slimmer shaft. Or you may be someone who has never understood what all the fuss about "textures" and "ribbing" is about, and you'll be perfectly happy with a simple, smooth model.

Playing with Dildos

You can use a variety of methods to incorporate dildos into your sex life. We recommend that you experiment by yourself first, so that you can get a sense of what sizes, styles, and strokes you enjoy before springing a dildo on your partner. You may find you want to insert the dildo and simply rest with it inside yourself; you may want to tantalize yourself with gradual insertion; or you may want to pump away vigorously.

> I like to put my dildo up my butt and just lie there motionless.

> Initially I like to hold the "head" of the dildo just at the opening of my vagina, usually with some lubricant. My orgasm may occur at this point, or one inch inside, or all the way in.

In any case, have respect for your anatomy. Cover the dildo with lube, position it to correspond with the angle of your vaginal or anal canal, and insert it gently. If you're playing with a curved dildo, angle the curved tip toward the front wall of your vagina, rather than down toward your perineum. The firm pressure of a dildo can be popular with women who enjoy G-spot stimulation. Be particularly cautious when inserting a dildo anally, and don't jab it into the walls of your rectum.

Dildo Care and Cleaning

To avoid wilting your dildo, store it in a cool dry place away from bright light or heat. Acrylic dildos are the exception—feel free to display these on your sunniest coffee table. Wash dildos after each use, and let them dry completely before putting them away. Viruses and bacteria won't live on a dry surface.

- *Vinyl, hard plastic, and latex:* Less porous than rubber, so condoms aren't essential. Wash with mild soap and water, rinse well, and air dry. Oils will ruin the surface of latex toys.
- *Rubber (including jelly rubber):* These porous toys are hard to clean, so we recommend using condoms. Wash with mild soap and water, rinse well, and air dry. Oils will ruin the surface of jelly rubber toys.
- *Cyberskin:* Made of a mystery blend of thermal plastic and rubber, cyberskin is highly porous and soils easily—condoms are the single best way to keep it clean. Wash with mild soap and water, rinse well, and pat dry with a clean cloth. You can help prolong your toy's life span by dusting it with cornstarch before storing it away (don't use talcum powder, which some studies have linked to cervical cancer). Oils, silicone-based lubricants, and direct contact with other rubber toys have all been known to melt the surface of cyberskin toys.
- *Silicone:* Completely nonporous and easy to clean. You can sterilize silicone by boiling it for up to three minutes; popping it in the top rack of your dishwasher; or simply washing with mild soap and water, rinsing well, and air drying. Silicone-based lubricants may ruin the surface of a silicone toy—stick to water-based lubes.
- *Acrylic:* Completely nonporous and easy to clean. Wash with mild soap and water, rinse well, and dry with a clean cloth.

The first time you and a partner play with dildos together, take turns manipulating the dildo by hand and show each other what angles, strokes, and speeds feel good. If you're penetrating your partner with a dildo, be especially attentive to his or her body language as well as any expressions of discomfort. When you have a finger, fist, or penis inside somebody, the direct skin contact makes it easy to follow the shape of the vagina or anus and to respond immediately to any resistance or tension. You can't expect the same immediacy when wielding a dildo, and you need to pay close attention to your partner's reactions. With time and practice, the dildo may come to feel like an extension of your own body.

I love using dildos on a female partner by hand, not a strap-on, to really adjust to her pleasure.

I've used dildos with male and female partners, because they enjoy them, but it's sometimes awkward (handling, that is) because dildos aren't as "natural" as fingers.

If you crave a no-hands experience, dildos may seem kind of frustrating. They're certainly not going to move unless you take them firmly in hand, and if you let go of them they're apt to shoot right out of your vagina when your PC muscle contracts. But if you're willing to experiment, you should be able to come up with some options for hands-free fun. For instance, try slipping your dildo into a harness and strapping the harness around the seat of a chair or a pillow so that the dildo is ready for you to mount. Of course, some great ideas are simply ahead of their time:

I've always wished there was a sex toy built like a Thigh-Master (the exercise device that looks like a butterfly, which you put between your thighs and squeeze) with an angled arm that was attached to a dildo and went inside when you squeezed your legs together. Hee-hee, a thigh workout and an orgasm! Score!

Teaming Up Dildos and Vibrators

If you like the way a vibrator feels, and you like the way a dildo feels, you've probably already figured out that playing with both at once is an extremely pleasant experience. We mentioned some of the ways you can combine vibrators and dildos in our Vibrators chapter, but we'll review them briefly here.

Many battery vibrators are phallic in shape, reflecting their designers' blissful disregard for the fundamentals of both anatomy and sexual response. The clitoris, the vaginal opening, and the anal opening contain nerve endings that can respond to vibration. The rectum and the inner two-thirds of the vagina contain fewer nerve endings, which tend to be more responsive to pressure than to vibration. Therefore, if you insert a battery vibrator that has vibration concentrated in the head, you're not really going to feel the vibrations where they're likely to do you the most good. We suspect that many women who say they've been disappointed by vibrators have tried shoving phallic battery vibrators in and out of their vaginas, to little effect.

Really, the best way to enjoy penetration and vibration is to use two toys at once. Yes, specialized technology provides the best results every time. Select a dildo whose size and shape appeal to you, and hold your vibrator against the base of the dildo—the vibrations will ripple throughout your entire genital area. Many coil-operated vibrators are packaged with a funnel-shaped attachment that, when placed against the round base of a dildo, creates a suction transforming the dildo into a powerfully vibrating toy. Battery vibrators can also be pleasantly combined with dildos: Some folks tuck a vibrating egg against the clitoris while playing with a dildo, and some attach a vibrating cock ring right onto the dildo.

My favorite method of masturbating is using a lubed-up dildo that one hand is pushing in and out, while the other hand is either rubbing my clitoris or using a vibrator on my clitoris. If using a vibrator, I'll also hold the vibrator against the dildo and up against my anus. Yeow!

I particularly enjoy double penetration. My favorite is to lie absolutely still, with a dildo and anal plug inserted, and a vibrator on my clit. All my attention is focused on the sensations from the vibe, and the orgasms start strong and just keep building.

Soft rubber dildos tend to absorb vibration, but silicone is a divinely effective transmitter of vibration. Certain silicone dildos are especially designed to be teamed up with vibrators—their hollowed-out shafts accommodate vibrating bullets.

You may be thinking, "It all sounds so complicated!" The truth is, it's actually far easier to enact sex toy combinations than it is to describe them. The great thing about sex toys is not only the sensations they provide, but also the sense of unlimited possibilities they inspire. We've learned a lot over the years from our creative customers, some of whom have graduated from buying sex toys to designing and manufacturing them for others. All it takes is a sense of humor and a spirit of adventure to whip up some unique sex toy recipes of your own.

Double Dildos

These consist of a shaft anywhere from twelve to eighteen inches in length with a "head" at each end. In theory, you mount one end of the dildo (either vaginally or anally), your partner mounts the other end, and you both ride the same dildo like a seesaw to mutual orgasm. The reality of a double dildo experience does not always live up to the ideal. As always, if you expect the dildo to take on a life of its own, you'll be disappointed. One or the other of you will need to hold the middle of the double dildo and get a push-me/pull-you motion going.

While the vast majority of double dildos are one size throughout, which can be problematic for couples with different size preferences, a few styles have different diameters at each end. Vixen Creations' Nexus is a silicone double dildo with separately molded ends; it's also the only double currently available that fits easily into a harness. And Good Vibrations sells the brilliantly simple "Coupler," a neoprene pad perforated with three holes—you can slip any two dildos with bases through the holes and fasten them together.

Although they have an undeniable fantasy value, you may find double dildos just aren't all they're cracked up to be.

Double dildos haven't worked as well as I've always hoped. They're fun sometimes, but generally take too much effort and coordination for me to be able to really let go. This has been true for me with both men and women.

Unless you and your partner are roughly the same body size, it may be hard to coordinate riding the same toy. By far the most reliable position is one in which both of you lie on your sides facing opposite directions with your legs scissored together. If you're trying to

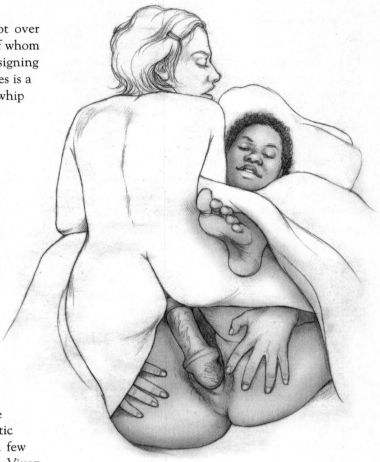

Sharing a double dildo

use a double dildo for anal-anal insertion or vaginal-anal insertion, you may need to crouch doggie-style facing away from each other. People are frequently disappointed that a toy that promises simultaneity and intimacy actually puts them at arm's length from a partner.

Double dongs are disappointing. Can't get one to work right—always flops out or pulls you too far from your partner.

If you'd like to experiment with double dildos, your best bet would be to keep your expectations low and to approach the experience as a novel type of acrobatic foreplay. If you're disappointed with the results of your experimentation, you can always keep that double dildo around as an extra-long single dildo. If you're thrilled with the results, more power to you!

Dildo Harnesses

Harnesses are made to fit around your hips and hold a dildo in place against your pubic bone, enabling you to penetrate your partner while your hands roam free. At Good Vibrations we sell dildo and harness combos to couples of all sexual orientations and field plenty of requests from folks who are looking for X-rated videos featuring dildo and harness scenes. If our customer base is at all representative, dildos are being routinely strapped on all across this great land of ours. Women are wearing them with women; women are wearing them with men; men are wearing them with women; and men are wearing them with men.

Strapping on a dildo is the ultimate genderbender. A woman who pops on a phallus can expect to feel everything from ridiculous to sublimely powerful. After all, when a woman looks down and sees the archetypal symbol of male privilege bobbing between her thighs, the experience can subvert all preconceptions of who she is and what her role is during sex.

The first time I strapped on, my partner was way more experienced than me, so that was a bit intimidating. I asked her which of her plethora of dildos she wanted me to use, and she picked this large, bright turquoise one with lots of bumps and ripples. I remember strapping on and standing there, buck naked with this large turquoise thing dangling between my legs, and I felt absolutely ridiculous. I think I laughed for about five minutes straight. But the sex was fabulous, and I've never looked back!

Similarly, a man who straps on a dildo is accepting the radical idea that his penis isn't necessarily center stage in every sexual scene, while a man who is anally penetrated by a dildo-wearing partner must embrace his own receptive, submissive side. Dildo-wearing presupposes a willingness to explore a range of emotions, fantasies, and roles.

My male lover enjoys getting fucked by me wearing a harness and dildo. As a woman, this experience has been extremely empowering for me. It changes the way you view sex—suddenly the "shoe is on the other foot," so to speak.

While strap-ons are most commonly associated with lesbian sex, probably half of all harness sales are to heterosexual couples who plan to explore male anal

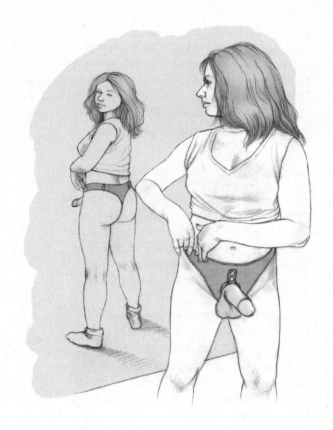

Single-strap harness

penetration. Since its release, *Bend Over Boyfriend*—an educational porn video loaded with hot scenes of "the gals givin' it to the guys"—has been a runaway bestseller with Good Vibrations' customers.

Heterosexual and gay men also strap on dildos—to penetrate their partners if they can't sustain an erection, to enjoy a method of penetration that is completely risk free, to penetrate their partners while having their penises stroked, or to double-penetrate a female partner both vaginally and anally. What people of all sexualities enjoy about dildo harnesses is the variety, adventure, and drama they add to a sexual encounter.

Most of all, I love to fuck my partner with a strap-on. I love to make him suck my realistic cock and then slowly and lovingly fuck him and talk dirty to him till he screams with pleasure and comes explosively.

Being in front of a full-length mirror, watching my lover's expressions and reactions while I take her from behind with a strap-on, now that's a real turn-on.

HARNESS STYLES: Dildo harnesses have waist and leg straps that radiate out from a central ring or a flap of material with an opening cut in it. You slip the dildo through the ring or the opening in the flap—the base of the dildo rests against your body and is secured when you tighten the harness straps. Any dildo you strap on must have a flared base or it will fall out of the harness.

When you're wearing a dildo in a harness, the dildo rests against your pubic bone, higher up on your body than a penis is or would be. This positioning gives the wearer more control over the movement of the dildo. A harness with some sort of central flap of material generally supports a dildo better than one that consists solely of a ring attached to straps.

The majority of harnesses found in adult bookstores are cheaply made with vinyl or stiff leather bodies and elastic waist straps. Unfortunately, elastic is not an ideal material to use in securing a relatively heavy object to your body. It sags, stretches out of shape, and snaps back and forth, making it difficult to control the dildo.

Better quality harnesses are made of leather, latex, or fabric and have waist straps that fasten securely with D-rings or buckles. Harnesses come in two basic styles: those that have one center strap running between the legs and those with two leg straps, one running around each thigh. Devotees of the single-strap style like the simplicity of the fit and find the thong effect of the center strap either unobtrusive or pleasurable. Devotees of the two-strap style prefer strapping a harness around the thighs, thereby leaving their own genitals unimpeded. Men can comfortably wear the single-strap style only if they're using the ring of the harness as a cock ring—that is, with the ring worn around the base of their penis and scrotum—rather than wearing a dildo in the harness. For strapping on a dildo, men should use a two-strap harness and position the dildo above their own genitals.

Of course, plenty of people jerry-rig their own harnesses using men's briefs or button-fly jeans. But you're guaranteed a more secure fit and more skin-to-skin contact when you seek out "the right tool for the job." If you find briefs more aesthetically appealing or more comfortable for packing (wearing dildos beneath your clothes), a growing number of boxer- and brief-style harnesses are on the market.

Finally, we should note that not all dildo harnesses fit around the hips. Some are designed to strap over

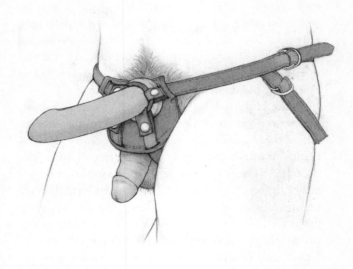

Two-strap harness

the head, positioning a dildo either over the wearer's mouth or chin—which gives a new twist to going down on your partner. The Thigh Harness, which is sold under several different names, fastens a dildo onto the wearer's thigh, offering a whole new dimension to bouncing your loved one on your knee. This model opens up a range of new positions for enjoying penetration, and two partners can each strap on a Thigh Harness to penetrate each other, an alternative to double dildos that allows full-body contact.

BUYING A HARNESS: Price, size, and style will influence your choice of dildo harness. If you're experimenting with harnesses for the first time, you might want one of the less-expensive fabric models. If you know what you like and you're convinced that you have many happy years of strapping ahead of you, you'll probably want to invest in a long-lasting leather model. Adjustable waist straps allow a custom fit—harnesses that fasten with buckles tend to provide a tighter fit and more stability than those that fasten with D-rings. Ideally you'll have a chance to try on the harness before you buy, as style is a personal preference.

Select a harness with an opening or ring that fits snugly, but not too tightly, around your dildo. Preferably the ring in your harness should be made of flexible latex, rather than unyielding metal. While some people prefer the aesthetics of metal, it can be rough on more delicate silicone dildos. Most leather harnesses have a ring around the harness opening as reinforcement—soft leather stretches, and nobody appreciates having the harness opening stretch to the point that the dildo falls right through.

Some harness rings snap on and off, allowing you to exchange rings of various diameters to accommodate a range of dildo sizes. If you favor realistic dildos complete with balls, you should look for a harness like Stormy Leather's popular Terra Firma model. The leg and waist straps of this two-strap harness snap directly around the center ring, holding the dildo firmly against the wearer's body. The ring is positioned in front of the harness flap, so that you don't have to stuff a bulky rubber scrotum beneath the harness flap where it would chafe your skin.

One ingenious sex toy accessory, the Slip Not, is designed to address the problem of what to do when the dildo you want to wear has a very small base and falls through the hole in your harness. It's a donut-shaped foam pad with a tiny hole in its center; simply slide it all the way down to the base of your dildo so that it rests between the dildo base and the harness opening, and it will act like a safety belt for tiny dildos.

Don't forget to keep your harness as clean as you would any other item of intimate apparel. Hand wash with mild soap and water, and let it dry thoroughly before putting it away. You should be careful not to dry leather harnesses in front of direct heat, unless you fancy a cracked, saddle-worn look and feel.

TIPS AND TECHNIQUES: Wearing a dildo in a harness demands a fair amount of coordination, imagination, and attentiveness. When you strap on a dildo for the first time, you may unconsciously expect it to be transmuted into a sentient part of your body, and you may be disappointed at how much energy is required to control it.

Using a strap-on dildo with a lesbian lover was disappointing—because I couldn't feel what was happening with her.

Don't despair—with a little practice and a lot of feedback from your partner you'll quickly gain command of the situation. Ideally, the dildo you wear in a harness will have a slight curve to it, so that it will match the natural curve of your partner's vagina or anus. It's easier to control a firm dildo than a soft, floppy one. Needless to say, you should take care to apply lubricant both to the dildo and to your partner's vagina or anus. Most harness users find that it's best to wear a fairly long dildo, given that the harness itself will take up about half an inch of the dildo's length. Furthermore, if you want to get into a stroking rhythm, it's best to use a dildo long enough that it won't ever pull entirely out of your partner.

With my partner using a long dildo, I can lie on my front, be fucked from behind, and masturbate all at once. The best thing about her wearing a dildo is that her hands are free and she's able to be more on top of me. Plus, she can reach my nipples or clit from behind.

Reinserting a dildo can interrupt the flow of things, as dildos don't have the self-lubricating properties of penises. Remember, you won't be conscious of the dildo you're wearing in the same way you would be conscious of a part of your own body—you'll feel pretty silly if you find yourself pumping energetically away in midair, leaving your partner high and dry.

Of course, some couples prefer the close body contact of inserting a dildo to the hilt and rocking their pelvises together without thrusting in and out—short dildos are perfect for this method of penetration.

All the positions that apply to penis-vagina or penis-anus intercourse are suitable for intercourse with a dildo. A man wearing a dildo in a harness should position the dildo above his genitals—he may even find that strapping on a dildo opens up some intriguing possibilities for double penetration. In the missionary position, he can simultaneously penetrate his female partner in the vagina with his strapped-on dildo and in the anus with his penis; in the rear-entry position, vice versa.

ENHANCERS: Harness-wearers frequently want to know how they can stimulate themselves while penetrating their partners. There are a surprising number of options. Those who crave vaginal penetration can purchase a double harness, which features a second hole positioned over the wearer's vagina accessible to a partner's fingers or dildo. (Note that double harnesses are designed for use with two separate dildos, not with a double dildo.)

A cuff allows you to turn your single harness into a double harness. The cuff is a rectangle of fabric or leather with a hole in the center and snaps or Velcro on each end—simply slip a dildo or plug through the hole in the cuff, insert the dildo or plug into your body, and fasten the cuff in place around the center strap of the harness. Cuffs work best with single-strap harnesses, but some folks are also willing to adjust the leg straps of a two-strap harness to wear a cuff between their legs. Since a cuff will hold the entire length of the dildo or plug inside you, you should make sure to select a comfortably short model.

Small battery vibrators offer the best way for harness-wearers to get clitoral stimulation. Vibrating silicone dildos transmit vibrations beautifully to both the harness-wearer and her partner. Some women obtain clitoral stimulation by tucking a vibrating cock ring around the base of the dildo between flesh and harness, while others substitute a vibrating-egg vibrator.

Dildos and Genderplay

While dildos are so much more than "penis substitutes," we don't want to ignore their fantasy potential. Plenty of women enjoy "packing"—that is, wearing dildos beneath their clothes for sexual role-playing—or to be ready for action when they head out for a night on the town. Female-to-male transsexuals and women in drag pack to simulate the bulge of a penis.

The first thing to know about packing is that the dildo that makes a great sex toy in a harness is not necessarily a great choice to stuff into your boxer shorts. Just as a man finds it uncomfortable to walk around with a full erection, a woman finds it uncomfortable to walk around with a stiff dildo straining beneath the buttons of her 501s. If you're transgendered and seeking the most realistic appearance, you'll want a dildo that is too floppy to actually penetrate anyone with—there are convincing packing dildos made out of cyberskin or silicone.

If you're packing with the intention of using your dildo with a partner, you'll want a firmer dildo, but ideally one that is flexible enough to bend without breaking. If your dildo is fairly long and firm, you might want to wear it snapped onto the leg strap of your harness with a harness cuff. This way, you avoid having the base of the dildo jammed awkwardly into your pubic bone. It's easy enough to move the dildo into place when the time comes to use it.

Dildos also make great toys for any woman who's ever had her erotic imagination sparked by fellatio, with its blend of seduction, submission, vulnerability, and dominance.

My favorite method of masturbation is simply lying on my back with my legs spread far apart rubbing my clit while I fantasize that someone, anyone, is sucking my "dick."

Role-playing with a dildo can be a safe yet arousing way to enact fantasies of fellatio, whether you're watching your girlfriend suck your "cock" or you're pretending to be your husband's gay lover. You and your partner can select the dildo that best resembles the penis of your imagination. And you can truthfully swear that you'll never come in his or her mouth.

Marilyn Bishara

"Vixen dildos are hands down the cream of the silicone crop, combining unbeatable aesthetic appeal and endurance."

Marilyn Bishara doesn't fit anybody's stereotype of a dildo designer. A reserved woman with a mane of silver hair, she never leaves home without a couple of dogs in tow. Her biggest loves are her motorboat, numerous pets, teenage niece—and last but not least, her company: Marilyn is the founder and proprietor of Vixen Creations, the world's premium manufacturer of silicone toys.

Marilyn was inspired to launch a dildo business in 1992 while working as a computer programmer for Good Vibrations. During the hours she spent in the mail order room, she overheard a steady stream of complaints that the supply of silicone products was hopelessly insufficient to meet the demand. When Marilyn proposed that Good Vibrations go into silicone manufacturing, staff voted down the idea, so she decided to do it herself. She knew from her previous job at an outdoor gear manufacturer that production was no great mystery, and she had the curiosity, good humor, ambition, and enterprising spirit required to weather the start-up process.

Silicone is a temperamental material, and it took time to devise the Vixen formula, which is a perfect balance between firm and yielding. Marilyn plugged away at R&D in her own apartment after she got home from work, washing dildos in the kitchen sink, and trimming excess silicone on her bed. She jokes that buyers of her early prototypes weren't thrilled about the cat hairs that occasionally made their way inside the packaging.

But her efforts paid off—Vixen dildos are hands down the cream of the silicone crop, combining unbeatable aesthetic appeal and endurance. They have a silky-smooth finish, come in richly hued colors, and are just about indestructible. Although production has moved out of Marilyn's kitchen, her dildos are still made with pride in the USA—if you always look for the union label, look for the Vixen logo as well. Marilyn's motto is "happy employees make good dildos," so she offers her staff good wages, liberal benefits, and free lunch every day. In return, they devote care and creativity to the time-consuming process of hand molding each and every toy.

Marilyn and her staff put a premium on customer satisfaction. Vixen offers a lifetime guarantee on all its toys, and many of its most innovative products have been designed in response to customer feedback. Best-sellers include the Nexus double dildo; the Mistress, a slender, gracefully curved realistic style; and the Gee Whiz, the first insertable silicone attachment designed to fit onto wand vibrators.

To learn for yourself why Vixen products are "worth every inch," look for them in sex boutiques and online at www.vixencreations.com.

CHAPTER 13

Anal Toys

Like dildos, which have been in existence since time immemorial, anal toys have a long and distinguished history. One European doctor of the Victorian age instructed his male clients to insert wooden eggs rectally—his theory was that the pressure against the prostate gland would help route semen back to the bladder, preventing wasteful ejaculation of precious sperm. We have to assume that those gentlemen who went about their daily duties with a wooden egg up their rectum were enjoying themselves as much as our survey respondent who remarked:

Butt plugs under clothing can put a different twist on your day.

The anus is an erogenous zone for men and women alike, and as children nearly all of us engage in some sort of anal exploration.

From a very early age (6 or 8), I enjoyed inserting objects into my anus but did not actually masturbate until I was 12 or so.

As we grow into adolescence and adulthood, we encounter numerous societal taboos around anal play, ranging from the extreme (indulging in anal pleasure is dirty and perverted) to the subtle (indulging in anal pleasure is immature and potentially risky). Yet the truth is that anal play need be no more dirty or risky than kissing. If you follow a few commonsense precautions, playing with anal toys is completely safe as well as fun. Based on enthusiastic feedback from our survey respondents, we're confident that anal play is sweeping the nation.

Once as my wife reached orgasm, she wound up shooting her butt plug into the nightstand lampshade. The shade suffered a small dent, which my wife thought was humongous. She insisted upon rotating the shade so no one would see the dent—as if they would have known where it came from!

Once More with Feeling

To recap what you've read in previous chapters: Please do take the time to relax your sphincter muscles before inserting anything into your anus, as relaxation is a prerequisite to enjoyable anal play. Do use plenty of lubricant. Make sure that any toy you insert anally is completely smooth and nonabrasive, has a flared base so that it won't slip out of reach into your rectum, and (if longer than four inches) is flexible enough to align with the curves in your rectum. Finally, don't transfer your toy from anus to vagina without either washing the toy or covering it with a new condom. The simplest, most convenient approach is to wear a condom on your anal toy every time you play.

Butt Plugs

Essentially, butt plugs are dildos designed especially for anal use. They are flared at the base so that they won't wiggle out of reach, and many have a diamond shape that tapers to a narrow neck. This diamond shape allows you to "wear" a plug inside your rectum. Once you sneak the widest point of the plug past your sphincter muscles, your anal sphincter will clasp around the narrow neck, holding the body of the plug snugly inside you.

Variations on the diamond plug are generally rippled—some are pyramid-shaped like Christmas trees, with three increasingly larger ripples ranging from the tip to the base of the plug: As you get progressively more aroused and receptive, you can make your way from one ripple to the next. Some have corkscrew-like ridges down the length of the shaft; others have an undulating shape resembling beads strung close together. The rationale for these rippled shapes is that many people enjoy the sensation of the anus repeatedly contracting and releasing around each bump and ridge. Other people find this much anal activity more distracting than pleasurable, and prefer to slip a plug in place and leave it there.

I have a vibrating anal plug of which I am quite fond. I don't much care for a penis in my ass, as they tend to want to stroke in and out, and I prefer just to be filled.

Some plugs are set on a handle, which provides a convenient way to approach what one adult mail-order catalog has coyly termed "the backdoor of Eros' temple." These nightstick-styled plugs have a rippling shaft, a diamond-shaped shaft, or a slim shaft ending in a fat round tip.

Plugs are available in the same range of materials as dildos (see the Dildos chapter for details). Vinyl is inexpensive and easy to clean, but not as flexible as other materials. Jelly rubber, rubber, and cyberskin are quite flexible but hard to keep clean. Silicone combines the best of both worlds—it's flexible and completely nonporous.

Some leather specialty stores or fetish boutiques stock metal plugs and eggs. Metal plugs are cool and heavy, providing a unique sensation. But they're not for novices. Since they're exceptionally weighty and hard, you have to be careful how you move when they're inside you to avoid banging them against your spine or tailbone. These metal toys are completely solid except for a narrow hole running down their center—within the S/M community, folks sometimes attach electrodes to these plugs to transmit electricity. Unless you're very experienced with anal play, you shouldn't insert any toy that doesn't have a base or isn't on a string, so we don't recommend your playing with egg-shaped toys.

Anal Beads

These consist of a series of plastic, rubber, or silicone beads strung on a nylon cord. The beads range anywhere from marble-sized to softball-sized (needless to say, the latter are only for those with considerable experience in anal play). Anal beads are popular with folks who like to feel the anus opening and closing around each new bead. You may be surprised how visually entertaining it is to feed the beads into your partner's anus and pop them back out again. Some people like to pull the beads swiftly out of the rectum while they're coming, as a way of intensifying the orgasmic contractions. Others find this sensation too intense at the moment of orgasm and prefer to remove the beads before or after orgasm.

I've been anally penetrated with fingers, dildo, vibrating plug, and beads, all with enjoyment, but not at the moment of orgasm! A finger in my butt when I orgasm is okay, but the others draw my focus too much and I don't seem to be able to have as exquisite a sensation. But they all get me very excited!

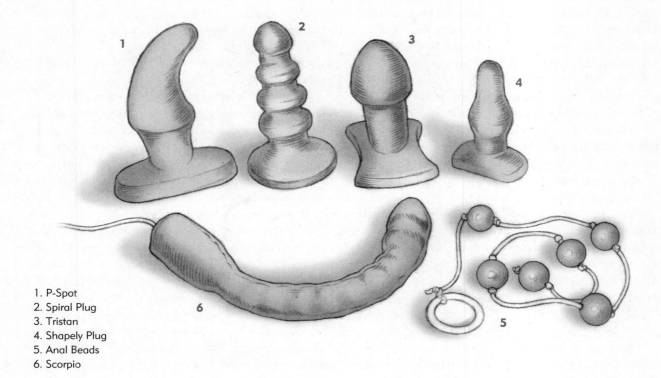

1. P-Spot
2. Spiral Plug
3. Tristan
4. Shapely Plug
5. Anal Beads
6. Scorpio

Various styles of anal toys

Because adult novelties are cheaply made, it's a good idea to do a little safety overhauling on your anal beads before playing with them. Plastic beads frequently have nasty, sharp seams, which might scratch your rectal tissue. But this is nothing that a once-over with a nail file won't solve. Softer rubber or jelly rubber beads can be porous, so if you want to use them more than once, put a condom over them. You can knot the open end of the condom around the last bead.

Vibrators

Vibration provides a fabulous way to enhance anal stimulation and penetration. After all, vibration can titillate the myriad nerve endings of your anus just as it does those of your clitoris or penis. A vibrating butt plug can relax your anal sphincter, distracting you from any involuntary tension or resistance you might otherwise feel. Or you can use a vibrator externally in conjunction with anal penetration.

My favorite method of masturbating is sitting on a silicone dildo, with a vibrator over my cock. I'm filled and exploding all at the same time! It leaves me with a pleasant, dirty, spent glow. The anal sensations the next day or two cause erotic daydreaming.

Battery Vibrators

Many of the plugs described above are available with battery packs, so that you can insert your plug and set it abuzz. Some anal toys feature a flexible plastic spine inside a long, slim tail—you can bend the spine to the angle that best suits your own tail. A variation on this theme is a slim probe that simultaneously vibrates and rotates. And some silicone plugs have hollowed-out shafts that accommodate a battery vibe.

People often use cylindrical battery vibrators for anal play. Some men find that G-spot vibrators, which are curved at their tip, make good prostate stimulators (one more way in which the prostate and

G-spot are analogous). Feel free to use battery vibrators for anal play, provided your vibrator is at least seven inches long and you can always keep hold of it—don't use a toy that lacks a flared base if you think you might lose your grip on it in the heat of the moment. If the vibrator itself seems too large to insert, you can adapt it for anal use with any one of a number of flexible vinyl sleeves. These sleeves fit over the top of a cylindrical battery vibrator and feature the nubs, fronds, and fringes so beloved by adult novelty manufacturers. The most practical styles are the simplest. By the time vibrations get down to the tip of a sleeve, they're considerably diluted.

We don't recommend using egg-shaped battery vibrators for anal play. Granted, the egg is attached to a cord, but if you start yanking on the cord to dislodge the egg from your rectum, it could come loose. Play it safe, and stick with toys that either have a flared base or are long enough to hold onto.

My lover and I were having sex while "wearing" twin egg vibrators. When we were spent, he removed his but I couldn't let go of mine...after a bit of tugging it popped out of my anus with a very clear "pop" sound. We still laugh about it.

Electric Vibrators

For a powerful and penetrating massage, electric vibrators can't be beat. If you're holding an electric vibrator against your clitoris or penis, the vibrations will probably be diffused throughout your genital region and indirectly stimulate your anus.

The insertable attachments sold for use with wand vibrators work well for anal insertion. The curved G-Spotter attachment may be the best shape for anal use. Some men find this attachment just the ticket for tickling the prostate, while others find it a bit too short to hit the spot. The only coil vibrator attachment that should be used anally is the Twig, as even if this should slip off the vibrator shaft, it won't slip into your rectum.

Of course, these vibrator attachments come in a fairly limited range of sizes and shapes. Overall, your best bet for combining anal penetration and vibration is to select a butt plug that pleases you and simply hold your vibrator against the base of the plug. As with the vagina, the nerve endings that are responsive to vibration cluster at the opening and outer third of the rectum, so using a vibrator externally should give you all the stimulation you desire. The funnel-shaped attachment packaged with most coil vibrators is ideal to press against the round base of dildos or plugs—it creates a suction that transforms the two toys into one.

Plug Shopping Checklist

Some things to consider before buying your plug:

- ✓ *Expense:* If you're experimenting to determine your preferences, you may gravitate toward an inexpensive vinyl or jelly rubber model. If you know what you like and you're making a long-term investment, treat yourself to a silicone model.
- ✓ *Material:* We recommend using condoms regardless of the style of plug you select, but be aware that jelly rubber or rubber models are porous and will be harder to keep clean than plastic, vinyl, or silicone.
- ✓ *Size:* Confirm the diameter that's right for you before you buy—using finger-width measurements is probably the easiest way to gauge your preference.
- ✓ *Length:* If you plan to insert your plug and leave it in place, select one that's no more than four inches long. If you want to stroke in and out of your rectum, select a longer probe or slim dildo.
- ✓ *Shape:* If you enjoy the sensation of your anus expanding and contracting, you might want to buy anal beads or a rippled plug. If you prefer penetration without movement, you might want to buy a diamond-shaped model that you can wear in place. If you or your partner want to stroke in and out of your rectum with the plug, select a slim, curved dildo, rather than a diamond-shaped plug.
- ✓ *Safety:* Your anal toy should have a flared base. Make sure that the surface of your toy is completely smooth and nonabrasive, and be prepared to file down plastic seams on some new toys before you play with them.

Buying an Anal Toy

Take the time to identify your personal preferences before you go out and buy an anal toy. Do you like the sensation of having a finger or two inserted in your anus? Then you might want to purchase a plug. Do you like moving a finger in and out of your rectum, or do you prefer holding it still? If you enjoy movement, you might want to buy anal beads, a slim rippled plug, or a dildo. If you prefer no movement, you might be happiest with a diamond-shaped plug.

As with buying a dildo, the most important aspect of selecting an anal toy is deciding what size to get. Plugs range in diameter from pinky-slim to fist-wide, so you won't lack for options. Do your homework, and base your selection on fact rather than fantasy. We still have fond memories of the two female flight attendants who spent their time in front of the anal toy shelf boasting to each other, "My boyfriend's so macho, he only wants the biggest one!" Those of us who are less macho probably have more in common with the survey respondent who wrote:

I bought a two-inch butt plug vibrator and savored the idea of using it only to find that it was too big!! And the vibration of the tiny bit that went in was so titillating.

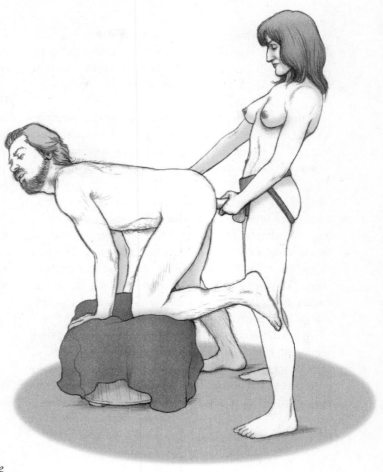

Anal intercourse with dildo harness

Playing with Anal Toys

When inserting any plug, angle it up toward the front of your body. You'll find it helpful to twist the plug slightly to get the widest part through your anal opening. When removing any plug, slowly jiggle it out of your rectum—a gentle twisting motion is also helpful here to ease the body of the plug past your sphincter.

You may enjoy wearing butt plugs during masturbation, oral sex, or vaginal penetration. The pressure and sense of fullness that plugs provide can be highly pleasurable, particularly in combination with other types of stimulation.

Sometimes while masturbating I use a small plug for prostate stimulation.

My wife enjoys inserting a plug while we are proceeding toward orgasm.

Some people like to wear butt plugs under their clothing throughout the day. Anyone who's ever worked in a sex shop has encountered customers who immediately take their new purchase off to the bathroom to pop it in place. Keep this possibility in mind next time an intimidating highway patrolman pulls you over—perhaps he's sitting on something that throbs even harder than his motorcycle.

Why would someone want to wear a plug out and about? For the thrill of a sexual secret, as an act of obedience to a dominant partner, or in order to relax the sphincter muscles in preparation for anal intercourse.

I enjoy inserting dildos into my boyfriend's anus. I also insert butt plugs to relax him in preparation for a dildo.

If you do want to wear a butt plug inside yourself, during either masturbation or partner sex, you can use a cuff fastened around the center strap of a dildo harness. Or, you could take a more prosaic, low-tech approach:

I like wearing my leather cock ring wrapped around the base of my cock and balls, with my butt plug adhesive-taped in my bottom. I wear them while shopping, doing errands, and housework.

Customers buying a dildo harness for anal intercourse frequently make the mistake of selecting a diamond-shaped plug to go with their harness. Why is this a mistake? Well, standard butt plugs are designed to be left in place, not thrust into and out of your anus. You'd find it pretty uncomfortable to have the widest part of a plug yanked through your anal opening with each stroke of your partner's hips.

Instead, select a dildo, rather than a plug, that seems the right diameter to the receptive partner. Use as your gauge the number of fingers the receiver can comfortably accommodate. You'll probably find it helpful to select a dildo that curves up from the base, rather than one that is set perpendicular to the base, as this will align more naturally with the curve of the rectum. And remember that a dildo worn in a harness should be a little longer than a dildo used by hand, so that it will never slip entirely out of your partner's body. Extra length also comes in handy when negotiating any body size discrepancies.

If you have half as much fun playing with anal toys as we've had selling them, you're destined for a good time. It's a pleasure to challenge our society's irrational anal taboo, to spread the word that anal play is safe and stimulating, and to celebrate the sheer entertainment value of the subject matter. As more and more people around the country are discovering, anal toys are sex accessories that can be both fun and funny:

Once when we were staying in a hotel room, we left an anal plug in the sheets and went to breakfast. To our surprise, when we came back, the room had been made up. The plug had been washed and placed on the pillow surrounded by chocolate mints. My wife was embarrassed beyond words and I'm still laughing.

W riter, editor, performer, and entrepreneur—Tristan Taormino epitomizes a new generation of sex educators. Barely into her thirties, she is America's most visible, enthusiastic, and persuasive advocate for the simple pleasures of anal sex.

Tristan began her writing career as publisher of her own pansexual erotic 'zine, *Pucker Up*, moving on to edit the nineties incarnation of the classic lesbian magazine *On Our Backs*. This led to a gig editing lesbian erotica anthologies for Cleis Press, and ultimately to her reign over an anal sex empire: When the folks at Cleis called and asked if she'd be willing to write a book on anal sex for women, Tristan didn't hesitate. As she explains, "I was beginning to really love anal sex, to have a lot of anal sex, maybe what I perceived as more than the average amount—whatever that is. And I thought, I *cannot* be the only one. Well, why isn't anyone talking about it?"

Tristan's resulting book, *The Ultimate Guide to Anal Sex for Women*, has inspired an adult video series and, needless to say, butt plug endorsements (she designed Vixen Creations' Tristan plug). When asked what her favorite sex toy is, however, she gives an answer that resonates with sex educators everywhere: "I feel so strongly that there should be a bottle of lube on every bedside table in America—I'm trying to achieve that. I cannot tell you how much I proselytize about lube."

Tristan writes extensively about sexuality in venues ranging from the *Village Voice* to *Taboo* magazine and also leads workshops around the country—having honed her speaking style as a saleswoman at New York's Toys in Babeland. Sincerely dedicated to improving sexual literacy, she visits college campuses, lecturing to the young men and women whose experiences of abstinence-only high school sex ed have left them in dire need of some straight talk about anatomy and sexual response.

These lectures have inspired Tristan's number-one wish for America's sexual evolution: "We need to change the way we educate teenagers, because all this adult sex education wouldn't be necessary if teens got accurate information." She's an articulate advocate of honest communication about sex and the value of "sex with the lights on"—the signature message she preaches nationwide being "You are the key to your own pleasure."

When asked about her own role models, Tristan credits Joani Blank for paving the way to making careers such as hers possible: "She was ahead of her time. Stores like Good Vibrations are radical places that actually change people's lives." She also admires Betty Dodson's "Let's get in there and look at everything with the lights on approach," and points out that "When I give sex workshops, they are consciousness-raising groups repackaged in a new form for a new historical moment. The idea that we can teach ourselves and each other about our bodies, that we don't need to crack open a textbook or look to the medical establishment, that we have the knowledge and can spread it around ourselves—that's one legacy of the women's movement that is intrinsic to how I teach people about sex."

Visit Tristan Taormino online at www.puckerup.com.

PROFILES *in* PLEASURE:

Tristan Taormino

"I feel so strongly that there should be a bottle of lube on every bedside table in America—I'm trying to achieve that. I cannot tell you how much I proselytize about lube."

CHAPTER 14

Fantasies

I like to fantasize when I'm walking around, in public places preferably. That way I can use my mind and imagination to get myself so worked up that I almost come without touching myself. And when I finally get myself alone, it's guaranteed phenomenal masturbation.

You've no doubt heard that the brain is our largest sex organ, but it may never have occurred to you that it's also an incredibly versatile sex toy. Without the brain responding to stimuli and sending messages to the rest of the body, we'd have about as much sexual feeling as pieces of furniture. But it's the brain's capacity to house a vast reservoir of erotic imagery—known as fantasies—that makes it a powerful sex toy, since fantasies can be endlessly tapped for sexual pleasure.

Sexual fantasies, simply put, are mental pictures that trigger arousal. Their content, importance, and purpose vary greatly from person to person. Some folks summon them when they want to be sexual, others find they have little control over how and when their fantasies emerge, while still others don't fantasize at all.

Fantasizing, like masturbating, is an act of self-love as well as an assertion of sexual confidence and independence. You are responsible for turning yourself on; you don't have to wait for someone else to do it.

A fantasy can be anything from flashing on an act or an image…

Making love on a sailboat in the middle of the ocean under the hot sun with a breeze blowing.

…to a well-scripted sexual encounter:

I am a (very naughty) queen in the 1600s or so. I'm sitting on my throne wearing one of those old-fashioned multilayer slips. It's a huge throne and I have one leg up on the arm of the throne and my slip pulled up while I play with my clit. My court looks on entranced. I'm so turned on that my juices are forming a large puddle on my leather throne. My juices are even dripping off the throne onto the floor. My guards bring in a prisoner from the dungeon who has been screaming at them that he is dying of thirst. They bring the prisoner to me for punishment. When the prisoner (who is very sexy) sees my juices running off the chair, he breaks free from the guards and runs up to me. He drops to his knees and buries his face in my cunt and begins lapping up my juices straight out of me. I'm moaning and screaming while he licks my clit. He laps at me like a cat drinking from a big bowl of milk. He just keeps licking at me like this over and over till I cum. (My lover and I acted out this fantasy. After I'd cum, my lover climbed up to me and said, "Thank you for letting me drink you." Wow. I don't think anyone's ever said something that has made me feel as sexy and desirable as that statement. Grrr!!)

Or fantasies can take a much less literal form:

I don't have sexual fantasies as others do. I don't have situational fantasies, or made-up people in them. I mainly focus on sensations: I try to re-create the feeling of someone's hand on my skin, lips against my breast—not "imagery," just sensation.

Whether it's explicit or vague, short or long, kinky or common, if it gets you hot, it's a fantasy. As a way to illustrate the variety of fantasies, in terms of both content and the way they are expressed, we have transcribed some of our survey respondents' fantasies in this section. Perhaps you will discover new fantasies of your own as a result!

Popular Themes

Despite the fact that no two people's fantasy lives are the same, some popular themes emerge.

Sex with Someone Other Than Your Partner

A favorite fantasy is of being forced to have sex with someone that is not my husband for the purpose of giving this man a child. He is blond and very good looking. I am told to fondle my breasts in a manner consistent to expressing breast milk while he is having sex with me.

A strange man walks into the room wearing dirty blue coveralls and black combat boots. The coveralls are hanging on his waist and under them he's wearing an oil-stained white T-shirt that shows the curves of his arms and chest. He leans on the door jamb smoking a cigarette. He drops the cigarette on the floor and walks over and takes me.

I'd love fifteen minutes with my community studies professor. I'd get her on her desk in her office, or

against the wall. Unbutton the top two buttons of her shirt, suck her earlobe, and run my tongue down her neck, across her right clavicle, over her shoulder, and then untuck her shirt, pull it off, off with the bra, bite gently the outside of her tit, touch the back of her knee, run my spread fingers hard up the inside of her thigh, squeeze her cunt, and then she'd beg me to come home with her.

Voyeurism and Exhibitionism

I enjoy thinking about having sex with an unknown man with a very large and beautiful penis in a rather public forum (not in front of people but with the chance of being seen). He pursues me and then after I make him jack off for awhile we fuck hard and fast wherever we are. I also enjoy making him talk about what he is thinking about (mainly fucking me) and not letting him touch himself until he cannot stand it. Sometimes there are other men who jack off while we are fucking.

Being watched in a clear glass room in a very crowded lesbian night club while my lover and I are having very aggressive sex. We can't see or hear the women watching us, but know they're all getting wet and turned on by what they see.

My latest fantasy is taking a shower with my husband watching. Slowly shampooing my hair, rinsing, then with a sponge working the soap down my whole body, showing him all the areas of me, bending over, washing my feet, and then using the shower head to rinse off the soap. It ends with him towel drying me all over.

Forced Encounters

My favorite fantasy centers on forcing a powerful man to an unwilling orgasm. I don't necessarily need to be the one doing the action, but I want to see him struggle against feeling pleasure, fight his bonds, writhe in hatred and shame against his tormentor, and finally succumb to a force greater than his own. Sometimes the storyline changes a little, and it's a male movie star acting out a titillating sex scene with a desirable costar (male or female). Their significant others are on the set watching, and the man doesn't want to get turned on, but he does, and can't hide his huge erection. His costar realizes the struggle the man is having, and does everything possible to drive the man crazy with lust.

I am a student currently trying to find my first job (this part is true). I finally find a job, but the boss will not hire me until I become his sex slave. Then he has the idea that I should become one for the office. Whenever they want, anyone can grab me and do whatever they want to me right then and there. Men grab me from behind and we fuck standing up. They call me into their offices when they need a little stress relief and we fuck for a while. Sometimes, they even like for me to give them head while they talk to their wives on the phone. I'm the office slut and I love it!

I'm alone on a beach—caught up in watching the sunset. Suddenly there's a man behind me. He says he won't hurt me if I cooperate. He slits several access holes in my jeans so no one passing can tell what's going on. He proceeds to stimulate me with his hands in front while gently and persistently entering me anally from behind. I pretend that I hate it but become so aroused I climax several times before he even thinks about coming. Though this is a rape fantasy, he's really very considerate and gentle, and I feel no threat.

My current fantasy is being given up by my stepmother to be an indentured servant to a wealthy family and being seduced into wet nursing for their kids, then being broken into a bondage and fucking toy for the parents, their other servants, the guard dog, etc.

Sex with Someone of Another Sexual Orientation

I am watching a movie at home with my best (girl) friend. I suggest putting a new movie in the DVD player. She agrees and we start watching a sexual film. She is turned on, but not wanting to show it. I scoot over and lay my head in her lap. As she is intently watching the movie (and not watching me), I start moving her skirt upward. I slowly move my head further into her lap and lick her thighs. She sighs and lays her head back to enjoy. I proceed to give her the best orgasm that she has ever received. We move into the bedroom, kissing all the while, and have wonderful hot sex on my extra-long king-sized bed.

I fantasize that I'm a boy who thought he was straight until he somehow stumbles into a sexual encounter with another boy.

In my fantasy I'm turned on by another woman. It's very romantic, spontaneous, and erotic—the excitement so strong that the veins in my arms feel like they will burst, sweaty palms, rapid pulse, and my pussy so wet it is dripping. When this happens I want my male partner to be there just to watch. I want him to see me kiss a woman for the first time. To see my face as I slide my tongue in and out of her mouth. Kissing her breast, arms, fingers, stomach, and thighs. And then the pure joy of eating my first pussy. The whole picture totally excites me.

I'm in a hotel's health club locker room, shaving. Two gorgeous men come out of the sauna naked except for towels wrapped around their waists. They're talking about meeting "the girls" in the lobby to do something touristy. One disappears to the lockers to dress. The other unwraps his towel and stands naked at the sink next to me.

Sex with the Stars

I imagine Britney Spears giving me oral sex while Justin Timberlake gives her oral sex.

Joaquin Phoenix walks into my bedroom in boxers and nothing else. I am lying in bed asleep. He wakes me up with stolen erotic caresses, until before I have even totally awoken I am already shaking with orgasm. I wake up slowly in his arms, give him a kiss on the scar on his lip, then straddle him and we have very intense, sweaty sex until we both can't move.

A lot of celebrities show up in my dream life. Recently I dreamed I was on a dock waiting for some friends to come pick me up in a boat. I realized at some point that Lisa Bonet and Lenny Kravitz were standing behind me. Somebody's hand slipped into my bikini top and started playing with my breast. I really didn't want to turn around to see who was doing this to me, because I realized I just didn't care. I let whoever it was stroke me till I couldn't take it anymore, then I finally turned around and saw it was Lisa (while Lenny was wanking away beside her). I pulled her into my lap, and started finger fucking her till she screamed through her climax. Then I bent over so that Lenny could do me, but I really wanted him to hurry so I wouldn't get caught by my friends!

I fantasize about mild S/M with five women and one of them must be Cher.

Although (or perhaps because) I am a lesbian, I have really hot fantasies about dominating famous men I find attractive. I've always been caught up in rock 'n' roll idolatry, and one of my favorite scenarios is to dress up in a slutty little groupie outfit—you know, spandex and heels—only packing a vibrating dildo underneath. I gain access backstage and meet my idol. I approach him from behind as he's pouring champagne and press up against his ass, knowing he can feel my bulge. He turns and looks at me somewhat bewildered but before he can speak I push him down on the floor and place a stiletto to his chest and maneuver it expertly to pop the buttons on his shirt. I take off my shirt, revealing a cut-out leather bra, then slip off my skirt and expose my nice cock to him. "I named this dildo after you because it brings me such pleasure. Now I'm going to use it on you so you can experience the ecstasy of being fucked by your own prick." His jaw drops, and I seize the moment to insert my cock into his mouth. Next I fuck him in the ass with my dildo, stopping periodically to sip champagne.

Here's a good fantasy involving my favorite two characters from Love and Rockets comics. Hopey (the more dykey of the two) is between my legs using her mouth, fingers, and tongue on me, while Maggie holds my arms down above my head. Maggie talks to me about what Hopey's doing with a soothing, sexy voice and occasionally Hopey gives Maggie some orders. One of the most important details in my fantasies is what everyone's wearing. Bustiers, schoolgirl-type skirts, Doc Martens drive me wild.

Sex in Nature

My partner and I go on one of these upscale holidays somewhere where there is a remote, uninhabited island that features an optional extra excursion for a couple. They take you there by speedboat with a picnic basket and leave you on this gorgeous sand beach for the day. There are palm trees to shade you. No one says so but it's obvious that you're there so that you can make love as and when you want with no risk of disturbance. The fantasy has a real-life basis, for my husband and I have actually done something similar to this. But the fantasy version has some extra features. One version is that it's

all a clever con trick by a rich voyeur who is watching, and perhaps filming, from a well-disguised hideaway in the trees. Another is that you think you're alone but there is another couple on the island who come and join you on the beach just as you're getting into action. Or maybe the crew of the boat just come back after half an hour.

My girlfriend takes me out in the woods; slowly and teasingly removes my clothes; bends me over a boulder; teases me until I cry out for her to take me; then takes me vaginally with a dildo until I come several times; then takes me anally.

Double (or more) Penetration

I'm being fucked by three guys at once—one vaginally, one anally, and one orally. They all come in my various orifices and then switch positions until they've all sampled every one of my holes.

My current favorite fantasy (perhaps arising from my failed "double penetration" experience with a dildo) is a ménage à trois with my husband's close friend, J. J is very tall and handsome, fun to hang with, and there's been some hint that he was/is bisexual. In my fantasy, J comes to visit and we all somehow end up in bed. There's the usual foreplay, and then my husband fucks me while J fucks him. In my fantasy, the look of pleasure on my husband's face is one of cosmic bliss. I should mention here that my husband is terminally hetero and this will never happen. I think. They both make love to me, with J's (impossibly huge) cock in my cunt and my husband's (more easily accommodated) cock in my ass.

Me and three men. I'm straddling the first and he's on his back and I'm fucking him. The second guy is behind me in my ass, the third guy is lying across the guy lying down, but in front of me, and he's licking my pussy.

Gang Bangs

I'm dressed to the nines in stiletto heels, garter belt, stockings, clingy dress, plenty of cleavage. I go into a kind of rough dyke bar. Sitting at the bar, I feel eyes on me, and I know they belong to the pack of butches and FTMs in leather and denim I noticed when I came in. I sip my drink and feel my pussy get wet under their stares. I get up and go into the bathroom. I'm standing in front of the mirror, breathing deeply to collect myself, when they walk in behind me. They come in one after the other and line up facing the mirror. They watch me watch them, and all of them are strong, solid, hard. The first one approaches me, placing a hand on my throat and pressing a hard bulge into my ass. "You knew what you were asking for when you came in here dressed like that, didn't you?" "Yes." "You want it, don't you?" "Oh, yes." And suddenly, they are all there, and everything is happening: I am triple penetrated; I am spanked; my nipples are bitten; I am whipped; I am passed around, and combinations thereof until I come hard on my hand or my Hitachi.

I am hitchhiking and a van stops that has four guys in it. I can only see the driver (the others are behind a curtain behind the front seats). The guys are grooving on my big tits and when the driver picks me up, he's friendly and nonthreatening. He offers me a drink but says I have to go into the back to get it out of the cooler. I move the curtain, head into the back, and am grabbed by the three guys. They gag me, rip off my clothes, and tie me down. The driver is the leader of the group and he turns down a deserted road and parks. He gets into the back and gets first chance at me. He plays with my tits, tit fucks me, plays with my pussy, then he starts to fuck me. The other guys then move in toward me, playing with my tits, wrapping my hands around their cocks, and all the while they are talking about me— you know, "What big tits this pussy has…. This hole is so tight…. This pussy loves to get fucked…." When I am about to come in real life, the guys start shooting off on me and rubbing it around. (In real life, I hate that!)

Group Sex

One of my current favorite fantasies is to dress up as a girl and with some girlfriends of mine attend a slumber party where we do each other's makeup and such. That turns sexual and I pleasure all of them with my mouth and hands and penis and feet and they teach me how to be the best lover and we enjoy sharing sex toys and each other and develop a long-lasting bond.

My fantasy is that as I sit here thinking and filling out this survey, my wife would be upstairs with some 27-year-old woman and I'd hear the faint buzz of vibrators, laughing, and then moaning. And that eventually it'd get quiet for a while and then they'd call me to come upstairs and join them.

I would love to be the main object of desire for an orgy. I am on top of some sort of altar, but I can't see, because I am wearing a mask over my eyes. I can tell it is dark, though. There are many robed bodies surrounding me. I can tell because I feel the robes being moved, to gain better access to my body. I feel many tongues and hands, vaginas in my face, and penises in my mouth. I also feel penises slide in and out of me, and when I grab at them, I am held down with soft restraints.

This involves sex in a foursome—me and my husband and another couple who are close friends. Although the foursome sex is a fantasy, the situation is based on a real-life event before we were married when we shared a hotel room that had two double beds with these friends. In the middle of the night I woke up beside my husband who was fast asleep and I saw the other couple on their bed making love. Apart from a "live" sex show in Holland and films, it's the only time I've seen anyone else having sex. They were naked and she was on top of her boyfriend. They obviously thought we were safely asleep and I could tell they were trying to be quiet. The room was quite light because the early morning sun was filtering through the curtains. I could see that the woman was masturbating as well as moving herself up and down on her boyfriend. I continued to watch through half-closed eyes for I didn't want them to see that I was awake, of course, though they weren't looking in my direction. Eventually she gasped a bit and stifled a cry and I took it that she had come. Shortly after this she lifted herself off the guy and I could see that he was still erect. Then they repositioned and did it doggie-style with him kneeling up on the bed behind her raised bottom. To my surprise (even shock), he withdrew just before coming and his sperm spurted out onto the bed. All of this really happened and I just went back to sleep some time after they had finished. They never knew I had seen them. But in my fantasy I usually ask them, at some stage while I'm watching, if we can join in, and I wake my partner. My favorite version of what ensues involves the other guy fucking me while I fellate my husband who in turn gives cunnilingus to the other woman. She and I have mind-blowing multiple orgasms while the guys manage to last an extraordinary length of time. It usually ends with earth-moving simultaneous orgasms for all four of us.

S/M, Bondage, and Discipline

My wife in a hot red vinyl corset with matching hotpants, arms tied above her head, legs held open with a spreader bar, blindfolded and teased her until her thighs are moist. Remote control egg for the teasing.

A favorite fantasy is having my car pulled over by a cop. The cop asks me to step out of the car and frisks me. I'm wearing a thin summer dress and no underwear. His frisking gets rough and we end up having sex on the hood of my car with traffic going by.

It's usually variations on my lover asking to "see if I can take it" or some sort of over-the-top size or penetration experience. Sometimes he's directing another man to "get me ready" or "hold her legs" or "stick this into her—she needs it."

I would like to own my own men who speak only when spoken to, live to serve and pleasure me, and wear nothing. They will bathe me, brush my hair, and always keep their asses handy.

A woman controls me and binds me on a couple of chairs or a bed. Then she spreads my mouth open with a ring-gag. She penetrates my anus with a strap-on dildo (and uses plenty of lubricant). After that she invites some people, both male and female, who use me for their sexual purposes. They have fun, and so do I.

Taboo Sex (Animals, Kids, Etc.)

I imagine I'm a little girl and have an older brother (who, in my fantasy, is my fiancé) and we are playing hide and seek and accidentally see our parents having sex. We decide to try what we saw them doing. It's so innocent…and makes me cum really fast.

I currently spend time (with my lover) surfing bestiality websites. My (our) fantasies revolve around the idea of adding a dog to our lifestyle. It is not that we ever would even consider doing this, but it is exciting to fantasize about. We talk about it while lying in bed, and it always leads to wild animalistic sex.

I fantasize about a latex-free party for my very closest friends. Ejaculate is really forbidden fruit these days… just once I want a night when my lovers and I can go bare without worrying about pregnancy or disease.

My favorite fantasy is being a young teen who is lost, and having an older man find me, and eventually having him place my hand on his crotch through his pants to feel his raging hard-on. After a bit of coaxing, he has me unzip his pants and pet his little friend. It feels so silky smooth, like velvet. I keep petting it until he begs me to stop. At this point, he lifts my skirt up, and plays with my clit through the cotton. I gasp, and he continues until my panties get wet. He then tells me that it looks like I've had an accident, and I'd better take them off so I don't get in trouble when I go home. After I do he keeps playing, and then slowly and gently inserts a finger a bit and uses the flat of his hand to massage my clit. While doing this he asks me to pet his little friend again, and we pet each other for a while in the front seat of his old car. All of a sudden, I tell him that I think I feel like I have to pee, but he tells me that that is not what I have to do. He says that I just have to let happen what is going to happen. At this point he is breathing funny, and I ask if he is okay, he says he is having the same feeling that I am having, like having to pee. I ask him if he wants me to stop, but he grunts "No," and asks if he can put his friend in my pee-pee hole. I think for a moment, and finally agree. He takes his hand off me, and grabs a blanket from the back seat and leads me out to the soft tall grass and lays the blanket down for me. He explains that it may hurt for a bit, but then it will feel much better after he "Parks his car." He places his friend at my opening that is dripping wet, and gently pushes his friend in a bit at a time. He is right, it hurts for a bit, but then after he gets in all the way and starts to go in and out it really feels wonderful. I tell him I'm having that feeling again when he starts to breathe and go in me faster and faster. He says to go with it, and I think for sure I'm gonna pee all over him, but then, all of a sudden, my insides are pumping and I'm screaming at the top of my lungs! Not too long after that he yells "Oh God, oh fuck, oh fuck, I'm coming!" and he goes really fast, then almost stops. He kisses me and thanks me. A minute later he rolls off me, and we just lie there. About a half hour later I ask if we could do it again, we do, and it is much better. I ask him what his name is, and he says to call him Mr. Parker. He asks if he could meet me again to park his car, and I tell him he is welcome in my garage anytime!

Miscellaneous Fun Fantasies

My partner and I wake up one morning and usually we start the day with having sex and then we get ready for work. On this particular day, I am rushing to get to work and am about to leave the bed without our normal sex first. She stops me and asks me where I'm going and I tell her I have to get to work for a meeting. She convinces me to at least perform oral sex on her until she achieves one orgasm and then she will let me go. Well, one orgasm turns into four as the first three really "didn't count." She then flips me over and sits on my face to force me to pleasure her, orally. She knows I really need to go to work, but is unusually horny and decides to keep me home for the day. So, she picks up the cordless phone, while still on my face, and calls my office and tells my boss that I will not be in today because I'm sick. She then hangs up the phone and says, "There, now I've got you here to myself all day long so you can f**k me!" We then spend the rest of the day and night having sex like animals.

I love to fantasize about my wife lying on her bed, watching a porn video. As she lies there, she starts to get excited and begins rubbing her breasts. She loves to pull and twist her nipples. Then she slowly starts to rub her pussy with her hand, playing with her lips. She spreads her legs as far as she can. Then with her left hand she spreads her lips open. Then she takes her right hand and draws her index finger over the opening, and it's all slick and wet. Then she finds the clit, which isn't difficult because it's got a pebble in it, and begins to rub on it. This time she uses her middle finger and starts rubbing, beginning gently, then a little harder and faster. Her head is back, her hips are working up and down, and then when she can't catch her breath she starts cumming.

It starts with me having a lot of money. I check into a large hotel suite and call an escort service. I have them send over five to ten girls and tell them that I want them for one full week. When the girls show up, I tell them that I want them to take off all their clothes and remain that way for the entire week. They are not to leave the room. Food will come from room service. While they are with me, they are to be my sexual slaves, doing anything and everything I want, whenever I want it. I would have them do things with me and with each other. I would have one girl in my lap at all times. Even if I cannot possibly come one more time, at least one girl will be either in my lap or in my arms or cuddled up next to

me. We would all sleep together in the big bed. The girls would bathe me from time to time and I would watch and maybe help as they bathed each other.

Enjoying Your Fantasies

I fantasize about my lover (usually) when I masturbate—he kind of creeps into my fantasy like smoke. My hand is rubbing my clit real fast and frantic while I'm thinking how much I totally want him. Before I know it I'm panting and coming and oh, oh....

Most people use fantasies to increase their sexual arousal, whether they're enjoying (or anticipating) sex with themselves or a partner. (More than 70 percent of male and female respondents to a Kinsey survey reported fantasizing during sex with a partner.) Anyone, however, can enjoy a sexual fantasy without expecting to engage in sex. Consider it a recreational activity, like walking in the park or talking on the phone—it's something we do to improve our mood, or relieve boredom or stress.

Sexual fantasies calm me down and stop me from obsessing and worrying.

We asked our survey respondents to share their favorite times and places to fantasize, and these answers topped many lists: during masturbation, during partner sex, during class, before falling asleep, after waking up, when taking a shower, in the car, on the bus, on an airplane, on the subway, while riding a bike, on the phone, at the office, at home, at the library, instead of doing homework, during meetings and lectures, walking down the street, on the beach, in the financial district. These responses deserve special mention:

My fantasies most often occur during masturbation, but every so often they come out of the blue; for example—sitting on a bus, a man's crotch directly in front of my face. I begin to fantasize about taking out his penis and performing fellatio.

I like to fantasize before going to sleep because it increases the chances of better dreams.

Any time or place where I have more than two minutes without anything to do or read.

My favorite time to fantasize is when it is most inconvenient to do so. For instance, when I am with a customer at work, while I am driving, while I am on hold on the phone.

Some people have one reliable fantasy that they call upon when the mood hits. Others maintain a ready supply of favorites, while still others make up new fantasies as they go. When asked about her favorite fantasy, one woman replied:

I don't have a favorite. It varies from fucking whoever my favorite fellow student is, to strangers, dogs, bunches of people, multiple genders, groupies, old people, young people, boys, drag queens, famous people, someone I passed at the grocery store, in public, private, inside, outside, me as male, me as a different female, transsexual, etc.

Fantasies are a powerful aphrodisiac because they offer people a chance to enjoy sexual activities they might not normally experience—or necessarily ever want to. Just as many of us engage in nonsexual fantasizing (daydreaming), like entertaining thoughts of winning a gold medal, living in an exotic foreign land, or being rich and famous, so too can we enjoy the thrill of some chance sexual encounter brought to us courtesy of our imaginations. For most of us, the knowledge that we won't engage in these activities in our real lives only adds to the erotic charge of our fantasies.

Most of my fantasies include situations I have no real desire to fulfill in person. Which is a real relief because when I menstruate I find my fantasies become more violent. I find keeping them my secret is what is most exciting.

We also use fantasies to explore different parts of our personalities. Take the example of the serious, to-be-feared commanding officer who enjoys fantasies of submission and humiliation, or the supermom den-mother who fantasizes about being a professional stripper at the local nightclub. You can try on a new gender, sexual preference, or sexual technique. Experiment with their erotic appeal to learn something new about yourself.

My fantasies are often about being straight, which I'm not! One is of being a secretary, and my boss says he'll pay me extra if I fuck him, so we fuck on top of an executive desk in a high-rise with lots of windows.

I've noticed that in my fantasies I like to be taken advantage of by men in positions of power. It's a real turn-on, especially when I imagine a cop making me fuck him in exchange for not getting a ticket.

Fantasies can also function as a rehearsal for a scenario you would actually like to act out. Perhaps you met someone recently—you could mentally role-play a variety of scenarios about how to intimately approach that person. Maybe you're considering trying out some new toy or technique with your partner, and you want to envision a variety of ways to approach the subject and meet with success. These fantasies can sometimes be as much of a turn-on as the real thing, or even more so. Many couples have found that sharing fantasies is a good way to find out what a partner likes. Of course, if keeping your fantasies private is necessary for them to be effective, you may want to think twice about this!

You may find that your fantasies stay pretty consistent, or they may change dramatically throughout your lifetime. Events in your real life can have a profound impact on your fantasy life:

When I first learned to orgasm, my fantasy life exploded. Before that, I could only vaguely imagine climax, so my fantasies petered out somewhere during penetration. Now I get to have these earth-shattering orgasms!

After the abuse, my fantasies were masochistic. I deliberately played with domination fantasy to empower myself, and it worked. Now my fantasies change all the time. Sometimes a fantasy can "wear out" by being overused!

Because of marital problems, my fantasies seem to arise from frustration rather than fulfillment.

A lot of people discover that their range of fantasies expands as they broaden their sexual experiences.

Since being exposed (via online exploration with my lover) to a greater variety of sexuality (specifically, D/S, vibrators, blindfolds, Literotica stories, spanking, etc.), my fantasies now are much broader, kinkier, as it were. I still retain a very strong emotional connection to my partner in sexual fantasies, but we do more, and more varied, things.

When I was young I only ever dreamed about getting laid as much as possible, with no interest past that. As I have aged, the touching and feeling and holding has become more important.

Acting Out Fantasies

Your fantasies don't have to remain entirely in your head. Transform some of them into reality via a few of the games described below. They can revitalize routine sex and settings. All this requires is a sense of adventure and a willingness to experiment.

Role-Playing

You can play with personalities, themes, or relationships by placing yourself in imaginary situations and letting a new sexual dynamic emerge. If you've fantasized about a life of movie stardom, it's not too difficult to don some sunglasses, adopt a haughty attitude, and cast yourself as the toast of Hollywood. Your partner can be whomever you desire—an adoring fan, the lead in your newest movie, or the casting director.

These folks like to play with a specific theme that excites both of them:

Our favorite fantasies are more or less variations on a theme, a semi-S/M scenario.

My partner portrays a large, heavy gay male in some dominant, fairly dangerous position—we've played with the Star Wars empire, Nazi Germany, the record industry, a Satanic cult, the Victorian era, and we're currently using characters from a Godfather-type Mafia. I'm a woman, but I usually portray a femme-ish gay male in a bottom-type position—a slave, or a loved submissive boy. We do a lot of verbal domination and occasional verbal humiliation.

This couple leaves the fantasy, and the type of sex, up to chance:

All our game requires is some dice and a willing attitude. First we swap fantasies, describing what we'd

like done to us or what we want to do. Then we roll the dice and the high number wins. The loser must perform the desired act, doing everything in her or his power to make the fantasy real. Sometimes it's as simple as giving head. Other times the fantasy can take days and involve a significant amount of work. We do have one rule though: The loser is allowed to say no.

Some common roles people like to play with are:
- Schoolgirl/boy and headmistress/master
- Rich widow and delivery person
- Commanding officer and enlisted soldier
- Truck driver and hitchhiker
- Secretary and boss
- Star and groupie
- Priest/nun and parishioner

Choreographing the sexual encounter can be almost as much fun as engaging in it; the anticipation can be a heady aphrodisiac. Shop for props and costumes or try drafting a script for yourself. If you're intrigued by role-playing and just need a few more ideas, read a book of fantasies, grab some erotic fiction, or watch an erotic movie. You might find characters, settings, or activities you'd like to imitate. There are also game books as well as card and board games that offer some imaginative suggestions.

Talking Dirty

Ever considered bringing someone to a higher state of arousal through your impressive, obscene verbal skills? Unaccustomed as most of us are to hearing and using sexually explicit language, using it with your partner can lend an intense charge to a sexual encounter. And it lends itself well to different locales—you can unexpectedly set someone's pulse racing in a public place or during the middle of the workday (one individual likes to leave nasty messages on his girlfriend's voice mail). Countless respondents to our survey mentioned explicit language as something that turns them on during sex.

I get off on talking dirty and reading erotic literature while we fondle and fuck. I do like crossing the line of propriety.

Using words like cunt, cock, fuck, pussy and others is exciting to me and my partner.

Most folks are intrigued by the idea of explicit sex talk, but don't know how to begin. Start with writing your own list of dirty words. If you need a little help developing a sexual vocabulary, track down a book like *The Dictionary of Sexual Slang* or *The Fine Art of Erotic Talk*. Read a variety of erotic material, from the explicit to the euphemistic. Watch an X-rated movie, paying special attention to the dialogue you find arousing. Take a look at which words hold a special sexual charge for you. Similarly, read and watch erotica with a partner to discover which words are a turn-on for him or her. You may find that you each respond better to one type of language over another. For example, "I crave the feel of your sweet lips on my ripe, juicy peach" might stir your lust more than "Suck on my pussy until I explode" or vice versa. You may find you respond particularly well to certain words or phrases, or just to certain styles.

Dirty talk right up close to my ear is the ultimate. Especially P words, like "pound your pecker" or "pump my pussy, you pud." The air-expunging P-sound is like a Smart Missile running right smack into an erogenous zone, a G-spot inside my brain somewhere.

I enjoy talking dirty as long as it doesn't get explicit—I like it to be very suggestive and mysterious.

If you're suffering from a bit of performance anxiety or are fearful you won't be taken seriously, practice. Talk to yourself in the mirror or while puttering around the house—just make sure no one's home! Practice using your hot words while you're masturbating. If you usually moan, try substituting words as you get excited or voicing the fantasy you're having. Phone sex can be a good place to start; if you're calling a service, you may be emboldened by the anonymity, and we'll talk more about this in the next section.

If you're struggling with your script or subject matter, relax. You don't have to memorize the text of a pornographic best-seller, you've got plenty of material inside your brain. Describe a past sexual encounter or a favorite sexy scene from a movie. If you're with your partner, try relaying the sexual activity you're engaging in at the moment.

My favorite fantasy is my husband, taking my clothes off—very hurriedly—and going down on me. And while he is doing so, he keeps telling me how good I smell, how great I taste, and how hard he is just doing that. And how he can't take it anymore and how he has to be inside me. Knowing that I am turning my partner on is very arousing for me.

Give your partner a verbal list of the many ways you like to be made love to, or elaborate on what you'd like to do to her or him. Fantasies and erotic dreams lend themselves well to storytelling; you can have your partner ask you specific questions to draw out the details. Or make a game out of it by taking turns making up parts of the story.

Keep in mind that your language doesn't have to be explicit to be erotic—role-playing can present you with new options for communicating sexually to a partner. You may find that just hearing your partner speak to you in the commanding voice of a drill sergeant is enough to turn you on.

There's no wrong way to talk dirty! If your partner doesn't enjoy the activity as much as you do, perhaps you don't share the same turn-on around certain stories, words, or themes. You may talk yourself into a frenzy of desire when the subject is dominance, whereas your partner's preference might be for sex with a science-fiction twist. Take turns indulging each other, and you should both be happy. If you like sex talk but it leaves your partner cold, you might ask yourself how important it is to you. Your partner may not want to participate in the dialogue, in which case you could simply get off from your own storytelling.

We play a game called "stay." My lover comes home from work and I greet her at the door in an aggressive manner…kissing her and pressing her to the door. After a bit of heavy kissing, undressing, and grinding, I tell her that she has to do exactly what I say. I move away, get a chair, and set it ten feet away and start removing my clothes, telling her how my skin feels… how hot I'm getting. From time to time I go to her and kiss and caress her, telling her to keep her hands to herself and "stay." I then get out my favorite vibrator and use it to get off, still reminding her to "stay." After my orgasm, I go to her with a dildo strapped on and fuck her up against the wall.

Phone Sex

Although phone-sex lines have been around for years, since the onset of AIDS, phone sex—paid and unpaid—has increased in popularity because it's a completely safe and discreet way to get off. Anyone can understand the appeal of phone sex; just think about the last time you spoke to someone whose voice you found surprisingly sexy. Imagine yourself in a receptive, aroused state while that caller switches from extolling the virtues of a new long-distance service to describing the contours of her or his fine physique!

This popular activity often involves masturbating while engaging in sexually explicit conversations over the phone. Most people think of 900 numbers or paid phone calls to anonymous operators when you mention the term "phone sex," but certainly any two (or more) people can engage in their own version of phone sex.

Masturbating on the phone with my girlfriend is always the hottest turn on for me. I know that she can picture in her mind every touch I am describing to her and I imagine her hands are really touching me. One time I called her and we had been just talking for two hours and teasing and leading up as I masturbated and just seconds before my orgasm I thrashed and hit the button on the phone and hung up on her...so I left her with "blue balls"!!! I called right back and we had to do it all over again.

I masturbated over the telephone with a man I met in a chatroom once. He kept me on the phone for four hours, telling me where to touch, how soft or hard, having me use a dildo, able to gauge from my voice where I was, keeping me on the edge forever. When I finally came it blew my mind.

My first experience of lesbian sex was on the phone with my best girlfriend when we were 15. We were too chicken to actually do anything to each other for a while so we told each other what we wanted to do over the phone.

Cell phones enable you to get pretty creative about where and when you place that provocative call. Think about calling him at the office the next time you're sunbathing nude. Or dial her car phone when you know she'll be stuck in rush-hour traffic and let her know what's really on your mind. Nasty messages on answering machines and voice mail can be another fun game—just make sure you dial the right number!

The phone-sex industry offers several different options for the libidinous caller who's willing to pay for the call:

- You can dial a sexually explicit recorded message.
- You can speak live to one operator who will share nasty thoughts and fantasies tailored to your specifications.
- You can hook up with a party line—one or several other callers who get each other off as a group. For a hilarious and hot transcription of the phone conversation between a man and a woman who hook up via a party line, pick up a copy of Nicholson Baker's novel *Vox.*

Engaging in phone sex can be a great way to learn how to talk dirty—after all, they say immersion is the best way to learn a foreign language. It also enables you to explore some of the fantasies or qualities you find particularly arousing. Southern accents may leave you cold while British accents turn out to be just the thing to raise your temperature. Many folks find that the anonymity of the exchange allows them to be more daring when it comes to vocalizing their desires.

Phone sex is wonderful for connecting my penis and my prostate to my mind. I feel safe talking dirty when I'm not face to face with someone. It's an intensified form of shared imaginations; the negotiations are very different, and they keep shifting with words instead of actions.

To me, phone sex is the ultimate in intimacy. Having to be verbal, explicit, and direct is a potent erotic combination because I'm normally a shy person.

Commercial phone-sex companies cater to every conceivable sexual proclivity. You can sample everything from "the voyeuristic journey of female bodybuilder fantasies" to "cross-dressers waiting to meet you." The FCC does regulate what words and subjects can be discussed over the phone lines, so don't expect to explore fantasies of bestiality, incest, or sex with clergy members with professional phone-sex operators. Phone-sex advertisements can be found in many sex magazines, tabloids, gay newspapers, and directories. Make sure to read the rate information in the ad, as charges can vary drastically between companies.

- *Get in the mood.* Before you make the call, spend a little time relaxing with a glass of wine or some favorite music and fantasize about what you want to talk about. You may want to wear some sexy clothing, or nothing at all.
- *Get comfortable.* Set yourself up in your favorite chair or stretch out on the bed. Find a position that will allow you to hold the phone and play with yourself at the same time. Speaker phones free up both hands, while cell phones allow for maximum mobility around the house (or garden or pool or office)!
- *Be prepared.* Have some lube nearby and some tissues or a sex towel. If you plan on using sex toys, put them within easy reach and make sure they're all plugged in.
- To get your money's worth out of commercial phone sex, be prepared to initiate the sex talk, otherwise you may waste time while the operator tries to figure out what you want. Remember, the longer you're on the line the more money the company makes, so they're in no hurry to get you off (pardon the pun).

Pagers

Once an annoying little beeper used primarily by on-call doctors, the pager is now a sophisticated, affordable device that blends the erotic possibilities of a vibrator, computer, and phone. Everyone from expectant parents to security guards enjoys the instant communication offered by the pager, though not everyone has discovered that pagers can be used for erotic expression and arousal. Invest in a pager with a digital readout and the caller can leave short, steamy messages for the recipient. Combine this with a vibrating model, and your sweetheart will receive your sexy sentiment along with a titillating buzz!

I wanted to eat in the restaurant at Nordstrom's but there was a wait, so they gave me a pager to carry around while I shopped. I put the pager in my breast pocket and when it buzzed I shrieked! I certainly gave the salesclerks a good laugh; they must see that little sex toy work its magic all the time.

Computer Sex

Plenty of fantasy material awaits you on the Web. You'll find sexy stories, fantasies, and images to inspire your erotic imagination. Bookmark pages you want to share with a partner, engage in some online chat together, go surfing together for sexy pictures, or find a naughty game to play. For more on these erotic offerings, see the World Wide Web chapter.

Exhibitionism and Voyeurism

Most people associate exhibitionism with the flasher who gets off by showing his genitals to a shocked stranger, and this activity is illegal. Many of us, however, possess exhibitionist tendencies that we can act on safely with consenting partners. Some people like the thrill of having sex in semipublic places because the chance of getting caught increases their arousal.

On a road trip once, I stayed in a nice hotel where it was possible to get into the pool after hours. The indoor and outdoor pools were connected and you could go from one to the other by just ducking your head under the partition. I got myself aroused by taking off my trunks and swimming nude in this forbidden public place. I stayed near my trunks, knowing that if anyone approached, the water would hide my nudity long enough for me to get into them by the time somebody got close. I started daring myself to venture further and further away. When I couldn't take it any longer, I masturbated under the water.

Once I was in the passenger seat of a car driven by a lover, and he commanded me to masturbate. It took a while to get past the worry of truck drivers looking in, but eventually I got into it.

Some enjoy performing acts of exhibitionism for their lovers' eyes only, because it turns one or both of them on.

I fantasize that I am hiding while watching him stroke himself off.

I like being watched when I masturbate, which works out well since my husband says he gets turned on by watching me.

If there's an exhibitionist in you but you're not sure how to let her or him out, go to a strip club, rent an instructional strip video, check out stripping scenes in erotic videos or on websites, and then practice some of the moves you see. Observe people around you and notice what turns you on so that you can appropriate any of the things you see for your own exhibitionist behavior. You may find that certain clothes, an attitude, even a hair style catch your attention. Experiment with wearing tight, sheer, or revealing clothing. Masturbating somewhere besides your bed can make you feel more exposed or daring. Ask your partner if you can masturbate in front of him or her, or start walking around the house naked. For encouraging guidance on unleashing your sexy inner self, read Carol Queen's engaging book *Exhibitionism for the Shy*.

Voyeurism is the flip side of exhibitionism—voyeurs are folks who enjoy watching others have sex. Voyeurism can be fun when you indulge in it with willing partners. Watching your partner strip or masturbate, peeking through the keyhole as she or he bathes, making X-rated home videos together—these are ways to express your voyeuristic side. Alone, you can enjoy voyeurism by going to strip shows, looking at pornographic materials, and overhearing the neighbors having sex!

I enjoy lingerie (wearing it, being admired in it, taking it off, or doing it with it on). I also enjoy looking at pictures of my lover and me having sex.

Once I watched my best friend make love and it was totally beautiful!

Love voyeurism! When I was in NYC, I could watch hetero sex across the courtyard and homosexual activity across and one floor up. Made me very hot.

Cross-Dressing

If you find yourself partial to the costumes involved in role-playing, or if you're simply fond of your girlfriend's or boyfriend's clothing, dress up! Many of us get an erotic charge out of putting on and wearing the opposite sex's clothing; it's a harmless way to indulge our fantasies. Even though it's often associated with drag queens, cross-dressing is more common among straight men. And there are plenty of women who have "passed" as men over the ages, as well as modern-day "drag kings" with fully developed male personas. We'd like to expand the definition of cross-dressing to include anyone who gets a sexual charge from dressing up in clothing not typically associated with his or her particular sexual identity. For example:

I'm a butch girl who occasionally loves to dress up in sexy lingerie.

Sex Toys

We were tickled to see how many people include sex toys in their descriptions of favorite fantasies. In some instances, they are one of many props that enhance a scene.

I fantasize about being in a ménage à trois with two other bisexuals and a room full of toys, ties, and swings.

I want to have a group of five or six women kissing, sucking, fucking, and touching me all over after I have done the same for each of them. I want to be last so that I am as hot as I can get. We use dildos, feathers, crops, restraints, blindfolds, wax, and oils.

In other fantasies, sex toys play the starring role.

I have this one super fantasy that involves me and my girlfriends simultaneously getting off every night with vibrators in our dormitory at a Catholic girls' school.

I fantasize about fucking a guy with a strap-on while I jack him off.

At Good Vibrations, we like to remind people of the enormous fantasy potential of their purchases. A woman strapping on a dildo and harness suddenly finds herself with a "penis" *and* a new perspective.

Although I am a femme lesbian, I always seem to fantasize that I have a dick.

Cock rings are another example of sex toys with fantasy appeal. Adorning that penis with a lovely collar not only perks it up, it can tease out those stud fantasies as well.

I enjoy the look and feel a cock ring gives. It's ornamental in a way that makes me feel a bit daring and more confident.

Our entire store is often the setting for people's fantasies; some even confess during their visit that they're acting out a fantasy! Some have been sent on a specific mission to visit the shop with warnings not to return empty-handed; at other times folks just visit because the sight of all those dildos, harnesses, and vibrators gives their erotic imaginations a boost.

We go to Good Vibrations if we want to get really, really hot!

Group Sex

FRIENDS AND INTIMATES: Sex with more than one person at a time is a popular, hot fantasy. In a survey of *Men's Confidential* readers, 84 percent of the predominantly heterosexual male respondents said they fantasize about masturbating in front of or with other men. Although more people have an interest in threesomes and foursomes with friends than act this out, several customers shared experiences of multiple mouths and hands exploring their bodies.

The hottest foursome I had involved butch/femme play, dildos, blow jobs, lingerie, and latex. We made a lot of noise and broke my friend's bed.

I like masturbating with other guys—it's quick and just about sex—which is not usually the case when I'm with women.

I like to experiment with threesomes. Usually it has been two women and one man, although I would like three women.

I would like group sex if it were with good friends.

When it comes to sex, the more the merrier! I've managed several times with two women and a man, and am still looking to try two women.

If this sounds like fun, why not throw a party? You could be the first person on your block to do so, and it sure beats sitting around waiting for someone else to do it! Plan it as you would any party—send out invitations (ask for an RSVP) and prepare delicious finger food. You may want to let your guests know in advance what your party rules will be (examples include safer sex, consensual activity, polite behavior). Arrange your home or apartment to ensure that there are comfortable areas to play in, and furnish them with sheets, pillows, and cushions. Cue up an X-rated video or put on some sexy music to help get things started. Make plenty of party favors available to your guests: condoms, gloves and dams, lubricant, vibrators, dildos, massage oil, whipped cream, soft mitts, paddles, and anything else you think will inspire your playmates. You're all set to earn your reputation as the hottest host or hostess in town!

JACK-AND-JILL-OFF PARTIES AND SEX CLUBS: Group-sex parties have become increasingly popular in the age of AIDS. Some (but definitely not all) are governed by strictly enforced rules regarding consensual behavior and no-risk activities. These parties usually feature courteous guests, safer sex accouterments, and toys, and they provide a secure, playful environment for those who want to voyeurize, exhibit, role-play, fantasize, masturbate, or simply experiment.

I love to watch sex between people at sex parties, especially two men having sex together.

Folks interested in exploring group sex, but who are frustrated by the logistics of organizing their own parties, could investigate this alternative. You can usually only find these parties in certain major cities, and attendance is often by invitation only, so getting hooked up with one requires some work.

Larger versions of these parties are sometimes held in clubs and are a bit easier to find. Look for announcements in local sex newspapers or magazines. Although sex clubs are subject to regulations (usually from the local health department) that seek to prevent the spread of STDs, not all clubs follow them, so you won't always find safer sex practiced. Try to find out in advance whether the club adheres to safer sex guidelines—and avoid the ones that don't.

Parties and clubs cater to a gay, lesbian, straight, mixed, or S/M clientele; inquire in advance if you don't know your hosts' particular slant.

Games

If you've ever played strip poker or "spin the bottle" or adapted an ordinary board game for sexual purposes, you've discovered the erotic potential of game-playing. Adult board games, card games, and word games abound and run the gamut from those intended to improve erotic expression to those that script out sexual scenarios. One of Good Vibrations' most popular impulse buys is a pair of Dirty Dice. One die lists a variety of actions—lick, suck, kiss, and the like—and the other lists body parts—lips, below the waist, and so on. Both players win with every shake of the dice!

Games often introduce an element of chance into sex play; the unpredictable outcome of the encounter can be particularly exciting. It's also liberating to simply agree to play by someone else's rules. With many games, not only are you relieved of any responsibility for planning the next move, you're being told what to do. This can be a nice break for those who tend to choreograph sexual encounters, as well as a welcome change for people whose imaginations may need a little jump start. Games also give you permission and guidance when it comes to exploring fantasies you might otherwise be too embarrassed or shy to bring up with a partner. Finally, if you've been intrigued by many of the suggestions for acting out your fantasies but aren't sure where to start, games can be a great way to try on a new persona, practice talking dirty, and engage in a little exhibitionism, among other things.

Concerns about Fantasies

Many of us have an unwritten code about what is appropriate material for fantasy. When our imaginations cross the line, we might feel guilt or fear that something's wrong with us. Remember the beauty of fantasy is that it's all in your head! No one need be invited in that you don't want, so the only judge and jury is you. If your fantasies are bringing you pleasure and not causing anyone else pain, why not leave the thought police out of it?

Nonetheless, the only person who can give you permission to enjoy your fantasies is you. If you are worried about them, you might want to examine the reasons behind your concern. There are a few common anxieties people experience when it comes to fantasies.

Guilt That Fantasies Aren't about Your Partner

I fantasize about people I know giving me oral sex, and about women giving me oral sex while an old flame watches and masturbates in a corner chair waiting to fuck me when I come. Oddly enough I have zero fantasies of my current partner. They are all of other people.

As noted earlier, many people's fantasies don't involve their current partners. There are no rules that say they should. We feel a sense of obligation to feature in our dreams the person we're intimate with in real life. But just because you spend all day working for an auto-body shop doesn't mean your daydreams have to all take place in cars. Perhaps you feel okay fantasizing about someone else while masturbating, but not during sex with your partner. You'll certainly agree that fantasizing about someone else doesn't mean your partner is dispensable or any less desirable, so why not just enjoy the fantasy as you would sex toys or erotic books and videos—as fun and easy ways to heighten your arousal. Trying to restrict your fantasy life only inhibits your experience of sex. If, however, you'd like your lover to figure into your fantasies, try substituting her or him in a leading role (or as a bystander) and see if you can sustain the charge.

If your partner is giving you grief about fantasizing about someone else, chances are he or she isn't being honest about his or her *own* fantasies, or perhaps doesn't fantasize at all. Try explaining that your fantasies aren't an indication that you want someone else, they simply increase your sexual excitement, and in the end you both benefit. Reassure your partner of your affection and ask if he or she has any fantasies to share. If none of this works, you might be better off keeping your fantasies to yourself!

Anxiety Over Fantasies That Stray to Taboo or Forbidden Behaviors

Oh, dear. My sexual fantasies are totally politically incorrect and in the past have caused me to suffer guilt. I often fantasize about being completely under the control of a majestic woman. I also fantasize about multiple sex partners and prostitution.

This is probably the most common, troublesome impediment to enjoyment of our fantasies. Many of our customers punctuated their descriptions of unusual fantasies with the disclaimer "This is only a fantasy," meaning "I would never do this in real life." For most people, this reassurance is what enables them to push the boundaries of the erotic imagination.

Nonetheless, some people fear that if they are fantasizing about some taboo-breaking activity, they must harbor a secret desire to actually do it. There is absolutely no indication that having a fantasy automatically leads to acting on that fantasy. In fact you may fantasize about a specific scenario or activity precisely because it's outside the realm of your experience. When Jack Morin surveyed men and women about their peak erotic experiences and their most arousing fantasies for his book *The Erotic Mind*, he found that power play was a key component in exciting fantasies twice as often as it was in real-life encounters. Certain themes that might be anxiety-provoking or inhibiting to enact in real life can be powerfully arousing in the security of our fantasies.

Taboo subject matter is infused with erotic significance almost by definition. The forbidden, the mysterious, and the dangerous possess a seductive appeal. As behaviors become less taboo, we are less likely to rely on them for fantasy material. Not long ago a woman showing a little leg from underneath heaps of petticoats would send a guy into erotic overload.

Fantasizing Too Much or Too Little

Some folks feel that they fantasize too much. Just as with masturbation, there are no standards against which to compare yourself. If your fantasies interfere with your ability to do anything else, then you'd be wise to seek professional help. If they're not hurting anyone, and you just feel a guilty pleasure for having an active imagination, enjoy yourself—we salute your filthy mind!

If you feel that you don't fantasize and would like to, you can stimulate your imagination in several ways. Focus on an erotic memory or scene from a sexy movie, read some literature, look at a magazine, or watch an X-rated video. Or pay attention to the thoughts and images that pass through your mind when you're masturbating or having sex. You may be assuming that you don't fantasize simply because you don't have a full-fledged erotic movie running in your head, complete with plot and dialogue. Yet any image, memory, or fleeting thought that you use to heighten arousal counts as a fantasy.

There's this guy on my school's hockey team who totally has the Canadian lumberjack thing going on. We had sex once and it broke my bed. Basically, if I want to get off I just replay the fond memories I have of that night, and think about things we could do the next time we meet up.

My lover and I had returned from a weekend in Monterey where we had great sex and made some awesome memories. When I got into bed that night (alone; we don't live together) my mind went back to the room, the hot tub, etc. I was so hot and so wet—it reminded me of the dreams that I'd occasionally have, because at this time, I wasn't masturbating regularly. Looking back, I think this was the turning point in desiring to pleasure myself—I bought the vibrator shortly thereafter!

If you feel that fantasies aren't necessary to your sexual enjoyment, that's fine. Just as there are no rules against fantasizing, neither are there any saying it's compulsory.

Anxiety over Fantasies You Don't Want to Have

You may feel that the fantasy you use to get off is one you'd rather do without. Perhaps you're a survivor of sexual abuse and your fantasy relates to the abuse. Maybe there's an evil ex-lover dominating your erotic thoughts, and you wish he or she would find someone else's dreams to haunt. Our sexual scripts are affected by the major emotional and psychological events in our lives, and it stands to reason that not all of these will be positive.

If you're unable to accept your fantasies, or if they exacerbate a sense of low self-esteem or self-hatred, you can take steps to change your pattern. Attempt to separate your fantasy from your sexual activity. When you're masturbating, concentrate on your physical feelings, and explore a full range of sensuous touch, rather than focusing solely on genital stimulation. If you find your attention wandering to undesirable thoughts or images, consciously guide it toward other less destructive, yet arousing, thoughts and images. Gaining control over problematic fantasies doesn't mean you have to give up having a rich fantasy life. Read a variety of erotic literature or rent some adult videos to discover new images to supplant the old ones. To reprogram your fantasies, you'll need to explore what it is that gives the current, troubling fantasies their erotic charge. Jack Morin's provocative book *The Erotic Mind* has an excellent section devoted to transforming "troublesome turn-ons." We can't recommend this book highly enough to anyone who wants to learn more about the complex nature and power of the erotic imagination. *The Survivor's Guide to Sex* is another excellent book that discusses troublesome fantasies.

What Now?

Perhaps you've been reading this chapter wondering, "How do people come up with this stuff?" Some folks are highly creative and capable of scripting incredible fantasies using only their imaginations. Others draw on dreams or memories of past sexual experiences. You can elaborate on the activity or change the characters, but the plot has already been written. Most of us do all of the above, as well as employing a variety of visual and written materials to fill our fantasy universe and heighten our arousal—a discussion of these erotic materials follows in the next chapter. Remember, the best thing about fantasies is the freedom they give us to be and act any way we want. A creative fantasy life contributes to a fulfilling, arousing sex life.

PROFILES *in* PLEASURE:

Erotica Readers and Writers Association

"The Web's anonymity really freed women to open up sexually. Once women realized that people weren't going to say, 'ooh look, she's such a slut,' they started signing up."

It's late at night, you're in a sexy mood, but you just need a little erotic inspiration to jump-start your motor. Where to turn? If you've got a computer, you're just a few clicks away from some of the steamiest fantasy material around. Surf over to Erotica Readers and Writers Association (ERWA), where you'll find a collection of provocative erotic fiction, suggestions for music to liberate your libido, lively discussions of hot-button sex issues, adult video reviews from fans, and much more.

We've singled out ERWA because it has taken the best of what the Web has to offer—freedom of expression, anonymity, and community—and created a welcoming, interactive site that invites visitors to explore all facets of their sexual selves. Devoted primarily to explicit writing, ERWA is a welcome refuge for anyone looking for alternatives to the run-of-the-mill porn found on most adult sites. Some two thousand readers and writers visit the site daily, devouring the latest fiction, swapping writers tips, sharing fantasies about "sexy occupations," or debating the merits of thong underwear.

Founded in 1996 by two women tired of reading romance stories that stopped just sort of sex, ERWA started as an online reading group offering women a safe place to express their sexuality. "The Web's anonymity really freed women to open up sexually," explains founder Adrienne Benedicks. "Once women realized that people weren't going to say, 'ooh look, she's such a slut,' they started signing up." Before long, women discovered that this freedom, combined with exposure to a range of other sexual tastes, gave them a new sense of sexual adventure and confidence.

Unlike many other tasteful sex sites, ERWA does more than just post good erotica from a small pool of talented writers—it attempts to awaken the erotic muse in all its visitors. Readers are encouraged to tap into their own fantasies and participate in whatever way they feel comfortable: They can critique other writers' erotica, pen a fantasy of their own, or start up a discussion about their favorite sexual practice. We especially like the collection of fans' favorite sexy songs or lyrics—you would never expect to see a print anthology devoted to this topic—yet music, as ERWA points out, is a powerful erotic stimulus: "Music is an aphrodisiac that has an astounding effect on the libido, easily setting the mood for a sweet romantic interlude, or a savage raunchy screw."

ERWA can be found at www.erotica-readers.com.

Books, Magazines, and Videos

I first encountered the wondrous world of graphic erotica as a boy of 10 who filled his bike tires at a neighborhood gas station. The owner and some of his customers constantly played "pick up" games of poker, using one of those decks with amazingly candid black-and-white photographs of sex on the backs of all the cards. That was forty years ago and I still recall, vividly, and with no small excitement, a few of those breathtakingly arousing scenes.

This man eloquently demonstrates the power of visual or written imagery to elicit a sexual response. Not only can we enjoy heightened sexual arousal in the process of reading or viewing sexual materials, we can also store the memory to draw upon at a later time. You don't have to lay in a lifetime supply of nasty playing cards, though; for many people, good fantasy material is as close as the nearest book, magazine, or video. Whether your preference is for romance novels, lesbian erotica, *Penthouse* letters, adult comix, underwear ads, or adult movies, you don't have to look far to satisfy your tastes.

If you already use books or videos to spark your libido, this section may suggest additional materials you might enjoy. If you've never indulged in this pastime, you may end up with some ideas about how to start. If you've ever been surprised to find yourself aroused by something you had no idea was erotic, you may want to try some of the more explicit materials we recommend in this chapter. And if you aren't at all interested in erotic books and videos, that's fine. Porn isn't everyone's cup of tea, and we don't expect it to be. But if you're uncomfortable with the idea of reading or viewing sexually explicit materials, and aren't sure why, you may want to read on.

To get in the mood, think back to your own first sweet encounter with sexual imagery. Many a youth's surprise sexual awakening resulted from exposure to images depicting everything from hints of a sexual undercurrent to explicit behavior.

I remember getting turned on by the first romance novel I bought at a drugstore when I was 13. I think I read it a thousand times and creamed my pants every time. I still love to read about people's (particularly women's) sexual experiences and fantasies.

I saw a Playboy photo with a woman with flour on her pussy; she was supposed to be a cookie going into the oven. I was 11, and I wanted to try this because it turned me on so

I got baby powder and put it all over my pussy. I got so excited by this, I started to explore myself. I played with my cunt until I came. I had no idea what was happening, but it was fun!

It seems as if everyone has a memory of stumbling on a cache of porn or smutty novel under a family member's bed—it almost makes one believe in a porn Santa who delivers little bundles to both the naughty and the nice. Remember the bra ads in the Sears catalog or those passages from dog-eared Victorian novels? Now you're in the proper frame of mind to read about today's options in the world of porn. At the end of this book you'll find a bibliography of erotic books and videos, so you can finally retire that beat-up old copy of the *Sports Illustrated* swimsuit edition and try something new.

Before launching into a description of the various types of explicit material available, we'd like to confess that we find efforts to discriminate between "erotica" and "porn" pointless at best and tedious at worst. The only criteria Good Vibrations has for selecting the erotic books and X-rated videos we carry is that consenting adults produced them with the goal of inspiring sexual arousal. If what you read or view gets you off, you may call it what you will.

While we use the terms "erotica," "porn," and "smut" interchangeably, we frequently refer to written works as "erotica" and to films or videos as "porn." This is purely a convenience, and we certainly don't mean to imply any moral or aesthetic judgment in doing so. Consumers, reviewers, and media people who discuss sexually explicit materials often seem compelled to make distinctions between "good" erotica, which is defined as displaying literary or artistic merit, and "bad" smut, which is defined as hopeless trash. Needless to say, these distinctions are purely subjective—one person's sublime erotic literature is bound to be another's tawdry smut.

The bottom line in assessing the value of "erotica" or "porn" must be: Does it arouse you? People who critique a piece of erotic writing or an X-rated video without divulging whether or not it turned them on are missing the point. Of course, it's challenging to speak openly about our sexual desires and appetites— it's much safer to criticize a story's clumsy plot device or a video's poor lighting than to confess to the fact that it got us wet. It takes courage to recognize and cop to what makes you hot, but once you do you end up with a clear, honest picture of yourself, along with

the ability to name—and claim—your desire. And, your recommended reading/viewing list will be a much-sought-after resource among your friends!

Knowing what turns you on will help if you're searching for "hot" books or videos. Customers often ask us to recommend titles. We ply them with any number of questions in our attempts to discover what they're more likely to enjoy. Refer to our Erotica Shopping Checklist (see sidebar) before you venture into a store.

My sister and I swap erotic literature because any group of thirty short stories will give us each about five winners.

Keep in mind that one person's arousing read is another's certified snooze. If you're not sure what kinds of sexual activities you'll like to read about or see portrayed, think about what sorts of fantasies work for you, or try to recall the last movie or book you read that elicited some kind of erotic response. By all means explore a variety of materials—your libido may be two steps ahead of your conscious mind. Erotic anthologies and compilation videos are great ways to sample a variety of styles, themes, and activities without going broke investing in a library of sexually explicit materials.

Finally, we want to point out that plenty of written erotica, explicit photos, adult video clips, and other forms of sexual entertainment are now available on the World Wide Web. We explore the Web's sexual offerings further in the following chapter, but in this chapter we focus on more traditional media.

Books

Whether you want to read alone to get yourself "in the mood," recite erotic passages to your lover or reenact scenes from what you're reading, the printed word has tremendous potential to inspire our sex lives. It can transform everyday sex into a euphoric communion or fuel your fantasies with people, places, and positions you might never have dreamed up yourself.

A Little History

When Good Vibrations first opened its doors, our erotica selection could fit on one shelf—Anaïs Nin, Henry Miller, and classics of Victorian porn were about all that was available. These days, it's difficult to keep up with the abundance of titles published every year.

The same social changes that allowed Good Vibrations to flourish—the women's movement, the gay right's movement, and increased public discourse about sexuality due to the AIDS epidemic—converged to usher new voices and a diversity of subject matter onto bookstore shelves. The advent of desktop publishing in the early eighties democratized print production, and independent presses and 'zines sprang up all over the country. At the same time, the so-called feminist porn wars were inspiring women on both sides of the debate (is porn inherently degrading to woman, or not?) to identify their sexual desires, explore their sexual fantasies, and produce sexually explicit materials of their own.

Independent presses were pioneers in publishing representations of authentic sexual experiences and creating content for and by previously marginalized communities. Those writers who developed followings appealed to specific audiences appreciating specific themes—for example, John Preston spoke to gay men, Pat Califia explored lesbian and S/M sex, and Lonnie Barbach captured the straight market. As erotica caught on, mainstream publishers wanted in on the action and began offering up rather tame literary collections of sexual passages.

By the late nineties, the Web was facilitating the distribution and marketing of sexually explicit materials. With its anonymity, ease of communication, and largely censorship-free permissiveness, the Web united aspiring writers with voracious readers so that they could explore the depths of their fantasy lives together. As a result, the erotic fiction being written and published by both large and small houses reflects an even greater range of human sexual experience and fantasy, tends to defy stereotypes and expectations based on gender or orientation, and constantly seeks to uncover new ground, rather than repeat formulaic material.

Since we published the first edition of this book, we've seen various themes dominate the erotica market, only to give way to an entirely different fascination a year or two later. The proliferation of online erotica means that thematic trends tend to come and go even more quickly. Susie Bright, who reads thousands of erotica stories a year, describes the popular trends as of this writing: "Uncovering the sexual in communities that have never been treated erotically before. Recalling the sexual identity of young people, at a time when young people's sexuality is so taboo. Stories about working in the sex business. Going to hell and back. Viagra jokes,

antidepressant jokes. Independent women making non-TV type decisions about their sex lives. Stories that aren't easily cast as gay or straight."

The net result for erotica book buyers is greater selection and more diverse content. Whereas once women's erotica might've portrayed a very narrow slice of female sexuality, today you'll find gender-bending, power play, multiple partners, and broken taboos. Whereas once you might've been thrilled to find a single story about bisexuality, today you'll find entire anthologies, even series, devoted to a specific theme, orientation, or sexual activity.

Where to Shop for Books

If your neighborhood bookstore is a chain, they may or may not stock erotica, depending on where you live. Even if your chain carries erotica, the books can be hard to find. We've rarely seen erotic fiction displayed in a section all its own. If it's mixed in with the rest of the fiction, you either have to browse through thousands of titles or know the name or author of a specific book. Maybe the erotica is shelved with the nonfiction sex books, but these are equally difficult to track down. If you're truly lucky, your store will have a sexuality section, which may include erotica. Unfortunately, many stores shelve sex books in their general "health" section and you usually won't find fiction there. One more drawback: Chains tend to carry books published by mainstream houses, which results in a limited selection since most of the more diverse material is published by smaller presses.

If you live in a larger town or city, you might have more luck with alternative bookstores, gay or lesbian bookstores, or sex boutiques like Good Vibrations. The owners are often more open-minded about sex, or at least willing to listen to customer recommendations. And if you want to keep the chains from ruling the book world, it's nice to support the little guys. They also tend to feature titles from smaller presses, so you've got a better chance of seeing a bit more variety in your erotica.

Mail-order and online catalogs and book clubs can be a good source of erotica. Some online book retailers specialize in sex (the Venus Book Club), while others carry such a large inventory (Amazon.com) that you'll have little problem finding something to order. Sites like Amazon.com often post customer reviews, which can help you figure out whether something suits your tastes.

Fiction

There is a wealth of erotic fiction available today in nearly every genre—science fiction, horror, epic romance, among many others. Some folks prefer the subtle or romantic, while others want access to the explicit language of sex; it is the latter that we'll focus on here. The bulk of erotic fiction appears in short-story anthologies (many authors) or collections (one author), though full-length novels are catching up. Some novels claim to be "sexy," but be wary, since this is a common advertising ploy, and in reality the sexual content is often microscopic or nonexistent.

In the following section, we'll briefly identify some notable erotica genres. For specific titles and authors, please see our bibliography. For up-to-the-minute recommendations, contact any of the book catalogers in our resource listings. The following publishers are reliable sources of innovative erotica: Down There Press, which publishes the *Herotica* series; Simon & Schuster, which publishes the *Best American Erotica* series; Cleis Press, which publishes a myriad of erotica series, including *Best Gay Erotica, Best Lesbian Erotica, Best Women's Erotica, Best Black Women's Erotica,* and *Best Bisexual Women's Erotica;* Alyson Publications, which publishes gay and lesbian erotica; Black Lace, which publishes steamy novels for women by women; and Circlet Press, which publishes science fiction erotica.

WOMEN'S EROTICA:

I like erotica written by women, especially if they have the courage to be explicit and the ability to write well.

Erotic fiction penned by women includes stories published by both large and small presses that reflect a variety of themes, characters, and sexual tastes. Tales written by and about large women, stories of lesbians losing their virginity, and erotic musings by women of color are just a few examples of how real-life diversity is finally being reflected in the growing body of sexual literature.

I like reading erotica/porn for women that incorporates all sexual orientations. If it was just for straight women, I wouldn't feel that I exactly related, and ditto books for lesbians. The Herotica *series is good.*

Not surprisingly, you will definitely find greater representation of female sexual experience (that's ladies' orgasms too, please) in women's erotica than you will in some other genres.

I love anything with passionate kissing, romance paired with intimate connection, an element of teasing and unexpected sexual daring, and sauciness and insatiability/eagerness on the part of the woman.

You can also expect more variety in sexual orientation, age, ethnicity, body size, and sexual preferences.

Particularly in the earlier women's erotica from the eighties, the term "erotic" was somewhat loosely applied. Some material billed as erotica is less explicit than a "Dear Abby" column, so browse before buying. However, editors, publishers, and consumers of women's erotica have noticed an evolution in the genre. In its early days women's erotica reflected more of a hearts-and-flowers romanticism, but today's fiction busts out in every direction with no taboo unbroken and no sexual pairing untried. Says *Best American Erotica* editor Susie Bright: "Mainstream publishers still think that women and men's tastes in literature are utterly and eternally separate. Meanwhile, the radicals who started feminist erotica in the seventies and early eighties are bored with the early depiction of their desires…it seems babyish to them now. The hipsters of erotica are really looking for something that is beyond stereotypes."

GAY PORN:

As you might expect, male sexuality is front and center in gay porn, authored primarily by men—but with plenty of women covering this territory as well (Anne Rice and Carol Queen for example). Perhaps because it rarely confuses its priorities—one-handed reading is as important as the quality of the writing (often more so)—gay porn never fails to deliver what it promises: no-holds-barred graphic depictions of sex. Consequently, there has always been a large market for gay male porn (both written and visual), whose fans include a growing number of lesbians and straight women. You don't have to look farther than the nearest gay bookstore to find volumes of gay sex writing featuring surfers, body builders, truck drivers, leather daddies, and urban professionals

I like hardcore sex and gay porn dishes it out reliably.

I like the abundance of sex in gay porn—lesbian sex stories are too focused on emotional conflict for me.

SMUT: At Good Vibrations we've affectionately named this genre "dimestore smut"—inexpensive, devourable, mass-market collections of explicit writing often by anonymous or pseudonymous authors, with roots in classics like *Autobiography of a Flea* and *Fanny Hill*.

Smut doesn't pretend to be anything other than writing about sex—its goal is to get you off. These books specialize in colorful language, meticulously detailed sex scenes, and taboo activities. Smut books tend to favor content over form (that is, no Pulitzer-Prize aspirations), or as one of our coworkers so aptly described them, "They offer little of lasting literary merit but plenty of enjoyable, rambunctious lechery."

Smut books are my choice for a sure-fire turn-on. They skip the flowery euphemistic language that bogs down some women's erotica and describe nasty, naughty sex on page after page.

No, it's not great literature—but I don't care. The erotic exploits of the naughty Victorian lads and ladies are jolly good, spicy fun.

Smut can also be full of stereotypes, so if you're looking for politically correct sex, skip these books. The genre includes an abundance of "Victorian pornography," though many of these supposed period pieces are in fact "unearthed" (that is to say, written) annually. These books are printed by the truckload; they can be as formulaic in style as their tamer sister, the Harlequin romance, but more diverse in theme—you won't find gay priests, sadistic heterosexual twins, or lesbian jet-setters in a Harlequin! The diversity apparent in more mainstream erotica is increasingly reflected in smut. There are spin-off imprints devoted to specific themes, as well as a growing number of talented writers who've elevated the quality of the writing.

Black Lace's erotic novels invariably get me hot and bothered, and I often read them when I am looking for new material. However, the best books for my masturbation purposes are the Marketplace *series by Laura Antoniou. The plot is so good sometimes I forget to masturbate!*

And while there are a large number of anthologies and short-story collections, smut is where you'll find the highest concentration of novel-length works. These books have also found their way onto the shelves of a few airport bookstores, which often give them equal display space alongside the current best-sellers. No wonder so many people fantasize about sex on planes!

AMERICAN MASTERS: A handful of authors have produced such a unique body of erotic work that we've dubbed them "American Masters." Authors like Henry Miller, Anaïs Nin, Marco Vassi, Pat Califia, Nicholson Baker, Aaron Travis, and Danielle Willis have penned sexually explicit literature so forceful and original that they have achieved cult status among many erotica lovers. All are masters of their craft, using their polished, explicit prose to explore the limits of human sexual behavior.

I recently picked up an Anaïs Nin erotica book and started to read some while I was alone. It got me rather hot and bothered and I knew that I must read this with my husband in bed. It proved to be very scintillating fodder.

MULTICULTURAL EROTICA: The explosion in the erotica market has brought a welcome infusion of titles that represent a variety of cultural perspectives. Although erotica is still primarily Eurocentric, you can now find separate erotic anthologies from Asian, Latino, African American, and Jewish communities. Men and women of all sexual orientations are represented.

I like books that reflect who I am whether that is as a large-size woman, black woman, or part of an interracial coupling.

EROTICA SERIES: In an erotica series you can sample high-caliber writing from a variety of authors in a single anthology. Most series publishers release annual editions, which focus on a specific theme, be it as general as "women's erotica" or as specific as "bondage erotica." When you find a series editor whose erotic sensibility matches your own, you're guaranteed a reliable source of pleasurable reading.

SCIENCE FICTION, SUPERNATURAL, GOTHIC, HORROR: Tales of aliens or the supernatural have always tickled our imaginations, so it's no surprise they make good grist for sexual fantasy. Anthologies featuring well-known authors together with little-known writers abound on a variety of subjects—alien sex, lesbian vampires, gay intergalactic hunks, and futuristic stories about prostitution, to name a few.

S/M: The sheer number of titles in print with S/M themes reveals what a powerful hold S/M has on our fantasy life. Nearly all of the genres we've discussed so far include books that deal with various forms of power play. So whether you're looking for women-authored stories of bondage and discipline, gay leathersex encounters, tales of schoolmistresses disciplining impertinent lads and lasses, or otherworldly crimes against nature, you shouldn't have to search very hard to find them.

LITERARY ANTHOLOGIES: There's always an anthology in print of steamy passages culled from the classic and contemporary works of literature. Since you might not otherwise have known your favorite author had a few erotic stories stashed away in the closet, these comprehensive anthologies can be very enlightening and exciting. They should delight any student of literature frustrated that the nasty stuff never made it onto the required reading list. Unfortunately, sometimes the editors stretch the limits of what they consider erotic, but if you cast yourself back to the time, place, and conditions under which the pieces were written, you may just get yourself in the mood!

AUDIO EROTICA: Those of you who want to spice up your morning commute or your next road trip can now enjoy audio versions of erotic fiction from classics of the Victorian age, such as *The Pearl*, to the more contemporary *Herotica* series. Passion Press, now a division of Good Vibrations, specializes in this genre. Audio erotica can appeal to folks who are visually impaired, as well as to those who aren't interested in reading books or watching videos. Many folks claim they'd rather leave the casting up to their imaginations, but discover that a sexy voice will put them over the edge.

In my sixty-seven years, I have never purchased anything that was so exciting, or which had such a therapeutic effect, as an erotic audio. I can't imagine watching a video again after hearing how attractive and graceful the performers sound.

I think I would like listening to well-made, genuine sex noises while masturbating. Or listening to a really hot, genuine BDSM scene on CD.

Erotic Nonfiction

FANTASIES: Nancy Friday broke ground in the seventies when she published a collection of hundreds of women's sexual fantasies. This important work acknowledged the fantasy lives of women but, more to the point, these fantasies were impossible to read without getting turned on.

The threesome I had with two other women was initiated by reading a Nancy Friday fantasy that got us all so hot we could not contain ourselves any longer!

Friday published subsequent collections of both women's and men's fantasies, and these volumes remain some of the best fantasy fuel around. Although other collections of fantasies continue to materialize, Friday's volumes were the most commercially successful and are still in print.

SEX INFORMATION AND HOW-TO GUIDES: If you've gotten the least little bit turned on while reading this book, then you know first-hand what this category is all about. Reading about the sexual practices of others can often be as arousing as any fiction! Many of our survey respondents claimed that sex manuals have inspired their fantasy lives. Recent years have seen a boom in how-to guides on everything from Tantra to oral sex to S/M to anal sex. See our bibliography for specific recommendations of books that are both edifying and exciting to read.

PERSONAL ADS: One cheap way to get off, whether you like your porn short and sweet or short and hardcore, is to place or answer a personal ad. You don't have to look farther than your nearest alternative newspaper or online matchmaking site. Look for an explicitly sexual matchmaking site if you want to cut right to the chase.

Midnight ritualistic phallic worship. Masculine, aggressive masseur seeking similar for heavy mutual dirty talk, jerkoff, showing off, chanting, phallic appreciation, late night my place. Visual/verbal buddy-to-buddy fantasy, not physical.

The schoolmaster provides home tutoring, training, and discipline for the behavior problems of wayward, gum-chewing girls (18) who cannot seem to complete their assignments.

Erotic Art Books

Although erotic art books run the gamut of sexual expression—from collections of fine-art nudes to *Playboy* centerfolds—only you can say what you do or don't find erotic (or what you consider "art," for that matter). But there's no denying the power of a visual image to elicit a strong erotic response, so we encourage you to view a variety of images and learn what pleases you most. Erotic art books tend to fall into the following basic categories, though some combine elements from each. Many are also accompanied by erotic or instructional text. With the exception of truly famous artists, there's a limit to the number of erotic art books you'll find in chain bookstores. You probably have a better chance of locating erotic art books online, in alternative or lesbian and gay bookstores, in sex boutiques, in some mail-order catalogs, and in art collectors' catalogs or shops.

PILLOW BOOKS: The origins of the pillow book date back to second-century B.C. China. These were manuals for married couples, complete with instructions on foreplay, intercourse, techniques, positions, and advice, lavishly illustrated so that one could learn and practice at the same time. The originals no longer exist, but the form has reinvented itself over time and across cultures—the most famous pillow book being the Indian *Kama Sutra of Vatsayana*. This book is almost always in print, but don't confuse the classic edition with more sanitized modern versions. Publishers like to rewrite the text and add lots of softcore photos of happy heterosexual white couples demonstrating the positions. A contemporary pillow book usually features graphic depictions of sex illustrated with drawings or photographs.

EROTIC PHOTOGRAPHY: Perhaps you prefer the work of certain famous contemporary photographers like Robert Mapplethorpe, Herb Ritts, or Jan Saudek, or you're attracted to the star quality of a collection of Betty Page photographs. You might be a fan of collections that focus on a specific activity or lifestyle like S/M, cross-dressing, fetish wear, or sex work:

The S/M photographs in Sexual Magic *by Michael Rosen validated and inspired me. He captures the eroticism, the creativity, and the passion of his subjects.*

The female nude can be found in everything from collections of lesbian sex photographs to art-history tomes and airbrushed *Penthouse* publications. Male nudes are the subject of many gay photography collections. The pictures in some of the historical collections of erotic photography are worth a thousand words—grainy images of spankings, nymphettes, and illicit encounters offer a welcome peek into our prudish past. Fetish photography is also very popular. Taschen publishes a number of beautiful historical and fetish photography books.

FINE ART: Collections of erotic fine art are popping up all over the place these days—there's even a fantastic playing-card deck adorned with fifty-two different fine-art nudes (which we would dearly love to send to the gentleman whose quote opens this chapter). Some books focus on a specific time period, others on the works of different artists, still others on a specific theme such as the nude or previously banned work.

Once in a while we run across a crafty collection of erotic folk art that usually features work spanning several centuries and cultures, such as Victorian canes or Navaho kachina dolls.

Magazines

Erotic magazines are appealing for several reasons: You've got visual erotica at an affordable price, sex information, fiction, the infamous "Letters to the Editor" section, and a new issue to devour every month or two. There are a multitude of sex magazines serving almost every imaginable sexual interest. Whether your tastes run toward bondage and fetish gear, lesbian culture, erotica for eggheads, or more traditional skin magazines, you usually don't have to look beyond large newsstands or adult, gay, and lesbian bookstores.

When On Our Backs *has a butch or FTM on a femme, or on another butch or FTM, I can't get enough of it.*

Gay men's magazines are hot. Those boys are easy on the eye and supply the leading men in my erotic daydreams.

I use magazines of a not terribly hardcore sort to arouse myself, Playboy *and* Penthouse. *I am mostly interested in pictures of women (*Vogue *is often a good choice) who are sophisticated-looking and partially dressed.*

If you want alternatives to the slick, glossy mainstream magazines like *Playboy* or *Playgirl*, try a 'zine. 'Zines are usually low-budget publications (black-and-white, printed on newsprint, or photocopied on inexpensive bond) with a specific theme, often sexual in nature. If you can get your hands on them, you'll find cutting-edge sex writing. Look for these in alternative bookstores.

> *I love the sex 'zines because they fly in the face of conventional sex magazines and cater to a greater variety of sexual tastes.*

Unfortunately, magazines and 'zines are more often labors of love than money-making endeavors. Their creators either burn out or run out of money, so there can be a pretty rapid turnover in this field. However, many of the original 'zine editors have staked out territory on the Web, offering virtual editions of their magazines at little or no cost. The Web is home to many new publications offering the alternative content pioneered by 'zines, combined with colorful sexual imagery. See our resource listings for some recommendations.

Comix

Graphic Novels

Many classic X-rated stories like *Story of O* and *Emmanuelle* have been illustrated in the popular genre known as graphic novels. This genre often appeals to folks who like their exquisite artistry as well as their typically controversial content.

> *I remember getting really hot once looking at an illustrated story involving a stern, domineering woman and her Great Dane. It reminded me of a really kinky version of Cruella De Vil in 101 Dalmatians.*

Adult Comix

Artists and cartoonists often use the traditional comic book format to explore very untraditional sexual themes in the genre known as comix. Look for these in adult comic bookstores.

Videos

Thanks to cable television, VCRs, and DVDs, countless people have discovered the pleasures of watching X-rated films in the privacy of their own homes. The presence of substantial adult sections in video stores indicates that millions of people are indulging in this recreation. An estimated 30 percent of all video rentals are X-rated tapes, and the adult video industry is a multi-billion dollar business.

Who's Watching

> *When I was in high school I came home early from a date one night and walked in on my parents watching an X-rated flick in our living room. They were sitting together about two feet from the TV and looked up at me, mortified at being caught.*

If it's hard to imagine our parents having sex, it's probably even harder to imagine them enjoying porn! But not all porn is consumed by men in small booths in the red-light district. Our parents, siblings, children, friends, coworkers, and anyone else you can't imagine all watch porn. We started carrying X-rated videos at Good Vibrations in 1989 after literally hundreds of women and men asked us to. During her years as a porn critic Susie Bright noted: "Contrary to the stereotype that porn viewers are inarticulate raincoaters who have miserable sex lives, people who watch erotic movies have sex lives and they aren't incapable of getting a date. They like movies and they like sex. Their sexual tastes run from real romantic to the kinkier, the better."

People watch erotic videos for the same reasons they read or view other sexually oriented material—to get aroused, to get new ideas or collect fantasy material, to learn about sexual techniques or behaviors, to get more comfortable with sex. Many couples watch X-rated movies together as a means of igniting sexual desire or sharing with a partner the types of activities they find enjoyable. Later in the chapter we'll share customers' revelations about how they prefer to use porn. For now, let's talk a bit more about the industry.

What to Expect

A VERY BRIEF HISTORY: Porn experienced its Golden Age around the same time the contemporary sex manual hit its peak. The counterculture of the late seventies and early eighties spawned a slew of directors whose films reflected the sexual liberation of the times. Films by the Mitchell Brothers, Radley Metzger, Richard Mahler, Henri Pachard, Robert McCallum, and Anthony Spinelli (among others) were characterized by an unprecedented cinematic quality while delivering hot sex, realistic relationships, and believable story lines. Peep shows, however, continued to be the primary marketplace for porn, creating a demand for fast and cheap production. The talented directors were simultaneously being ignored by Hollywood, and the combination resulted in a loss of incentive to continue making quality porn.

Technology turned adult filmmaking on its ear, and continues to play an important role in its evolution. The invention of the video camera made filmmaking more accessible to a growing number of entrepreneurs with vision (like Candida Royalle). It also resulted in a huge audience of home viewers, and adult producers began churning out volumes of assembly-line porn at rock-bottom prices. Most of the porn that's been released since the mid-eighties is mediocre, formulaic, and sloppily produced.

However, the emergence of digital video has infused adult video with a more professional look, due largely to the facts that it's a more film-like medium and is easier to edit. The popularity of Pay Per View adult TV channels has also spawned a demand for bigger budget films, which usually translates into significantly higher production values. DVDs—in addition to offering "extras" like director's cuts, interviews, and behind-the-scenes material—have also introduced an interactive element to porn viewing. "Fantasex" casts the viewer as director, so you can choose which act the porn star will demonstrate, what angle you'd like to view, and whether he or she appears solo or partnered.

As for content, by the end of the twentieth century, some positive changes were occurring in porn. Once it became clear men weren't the sole consumers of porn—over 40 percent of video rentals are to the "women's and couples' market"—producers released instructional couples videos, such as Nina Hartley's popular series, along with comedies and dramas highlighting authentic female pleasure. Certain contemporary directors broke away from the pack. Andrew Blake's films are praised for their high production values and beautiful casts—they are the ultimate porno eye candy. Paul Thomas's films earn a lot of fans for delivering

strong plots, eliciting compelling performances, and portraying female orgasms. And several other female porn stars have started working behind the camera—some (like Chloe) producing gonzo features every bit as hardcore as what men are doing, while others (like Veronica Hart) mixing suspense, romance, and sex with more compelling storylines. Even in front of the camera, women are coming into their own, with realistic orgasms and women-centered scripts.

Our national "hard-body" obsession has extended to porn, with both positive and negative results. Performers of the seventies looked more like real people, and many contemporary viewers are frustrated by the fact that most of today's porn stars and starlets are walking Barbie-and-Ken doll advertisements for plastic surgery. Those seeking a greater diversity of body types have to rely on women-produced, independent, and amateur videos in their quest for silicone-free breasts.

I like videos that feature women that are not "pros" and don't have fake tits—I like to watch videos where it looks like the people involved might actually be having a good time (gasp!) I often prefer girl-on-girl pornography because I find it more plausible that they are actually pleasuring each other rather than the "jackhammer" videos of male porn stars penetrating females.

On the bright side, viewers who have resented the fact that for years female performers were held to certain standards of beauty, while the appearance of male performers was secondary to their ability to get it up, appreciate the fact that heterosexual porn now features a bevy of beautiful men—from Sean Michaels to Rocco Siffredi. While we resent the plastic-surgery norm, there's no question that the glamorous starlets of the nineties are doing a lot to bring porn into the mainstream, becoming the latest darlings of our celebrity-hungry culture. When the girls of Vivid Video are featured on a billboard dominating Sunset Boulevard, and sexy, articulate starlets pop up everywhere from the *Tonight Show* to the E! Entertainment network, surely there's a sea change in societal attitudes at work.

COMMERCIAL PORN: Even though commercial porn has been around for decades, it rarely rises above a certain level of mediocrity thanks, to the combined efforts of censors and unimaginative filmmakers.

Emphasis is placed on cranking out hundreds of fast-buck films each year, resulting in hordes of barely distinguishable films. Poor sound quality, awful lighting, and faulty tapes are some of the production problems you may encounter. One-dimensional plots, bad acting, and formulaic sexual encounters are among the most common complaints. This doesn't mean there aren't exceptions or that even the bad ones won't turn you on. We're just reminding you, because forewarned is forearmed! If you don't expect Academy Award–winning material you won't set yourself up for disappointment. Your ability to suspend your normal standards will vastly increase your enjoyment.

Commercial X-rated videos follow fairly rigid industry conventions with regard to the activities depicted. You can expect predominantly heterosexual sex focusing on male sexual pleasure, a "girl–girl" scene, lots of fellatio, external come shots, and both anal and vaginal penetration. Sex toys are an ever-increasing presence in porn. Adult toy manufacturers now arrange brand-name tie-in's by featuring certain porn starlets on the packaging for their products and positioning these products in the starlets' videos. In most of the older porn (with the exception of gay porn), there's almost no condom use, but some performers and directors today are opting for safer sex. We applaud this trend—what better way to teach viewers how to eroticize safer sex than to depict a really hot condom encounter?

The appeal of any given porn movie depends on you and your tastes. You might find that just seeing sexually explicit acts performed in your living room is an instant turn-on. Or you may require your porn to meet certain standards for you to feel any erotic charge.

I am interested in videos featuring penetration, where the men don't pull out when they ejaculate. That's how I like it at home.

As these customers illustrate, erotic enjoyment can hinge on a particular star, certain production elements, or a particular theme or plot device:

In one memorable film I saw in Europe, this highly attractive couple did all sorts of amazingly inventive things in and around an enormous corner bath and over-sized shower cubicle. The direction of the movie was slick and professional, the photography stunning, the lighting perfect. The close-ups were sharp and

revealing—you could even see her tightened labia sliding along her partner's cock as he withdrew himself almost completely on each stroke. Orgasms were not faked. Fortunately I had my husband with me for it turned me on hugely (him too). But this quality is rare in such films.

I absolutely need real chemistry between the partners in order to enjoy them, though, and good directing/ cinematography. And either with a plot, or without one, but not with a fake one. Often feature films are more exciting than porn because there is context and psychological tension (though I don't like soft porn— I want to see the fucking and I want to see the genitals).

A particular director or producer's special touch can make all the difference to some viewers.

I prefer the newer videos, which are superior visually and feature good-looking couples. Most films directed by Paul Thomas are, in my opinion, vastly superior to the others. Skin tones are warm, the camera shots are smooth and lingering, and, most importantly, the people in the film are given long and continuous stimulation (i.e., the women actually orgasm).

I am interested in videos that reflect honesty, humor, and emotional reality and are also professional and artistically sensitive. The best example so far is Andrew Blake's work.

One of the best things about Every Woman Has a Fantasy, *which was co-written and produced by a woman, is the very believable storyline. Along with the well-written script and good acting, this made for a refreshingly good and exciting erotic film.*

People's criticisms of pornographic videos run the gamut. Many bemoan the fact that women's sexual gratification is rarely the main event in porn and is sometimes absent altogether (though this situation is slowly changing, perhaps due to the growing numbers of female viewers, directors, and enthusiastic stars). What's more, depictions of female sex can be stereotypical and downright misleading, as this customer points out with the reference to an orgasm-from-thrusting:

The whole video was fucking and come shots. The woman was supposedly just getting off from the thrusting, but it would've been so nice to see her masturbate and to watch the expression on her face as she came.

In addition to equal time for female orgasms, our video customers often ask for sex and storylines that mirror real life.

I very much enjoy the focus on female pleasure and obviously real orgasms. I'm not just saying this to be PC—it really turns me on, much more than most other porn!

Porn that doesn't feature romantic connection, specifically a lot of kissing while in the act, is always very disappointing to me.

I can't believe how ugly some of the men are. Give me a break! Like I believe this gorgeous girl is going to suck him off as he sells mops door to door.

Others are understandably frustrated by the lack of diversity in mainstream porn. If you'd like to see depictions of "natural" women, your best bet is to seek out women-produced, independent, S/M, or amateur videos. If you're looking for porn featuring people of color, you'll find that mainstream tapes that feature casts of color tend to be filled with offensive racial stereotyping and race fetishism. According to Good Vibrations' video reviewer: "Trying to find an authentic film that represents an underrepresented area of the population—and does so in a respectful manner—is daunting, time consuming, and frustrating. Try finding a movie featuring very large women that doesn't have a title like *Chubby Chasers*, or an Asian film that doesn't have a reference to 'fortune cookie nookie'."

There's very little interracial sex in mainstream porn, because this has been enough to get videos deemed "obscene" according to the community standards of certain Southern states. The break-out success, however, of African American performers such as Sean Michaels and Mocha is a good sign. Here again, your best bet is to seek out independent and amateur productions. Lesbian- and feminist-made films tend to have diverse casts. We're hopeful that the success of the growing amateur market will prod mainstream producers into seeking out performers who better reflect the demographics of our multicultural nation.

LESBIAN AND FEMINIST PRODUCTIONS: As we noted earlier, a lot of the criticism of commercial porn stems from viewers' disappointment when it isn't as cinematic, well-acted, or poetically scripted as their favorite Hollywood movies. Efforts to subvert industry conventions have come primarily from independent filmmakers like Candida Royalle (Femme Productions), or production companies that specialize in lesbian-made videos (SIR Videos; see the sidebar), or women-oriented films (Maria Beatty's BDSM films). These alternative producers give long-overdue screen time to the female experience of sex, and also frequently go out on a limb when it comes to presenting sexual activities that the industry shies away from. For example, female ejaculation, sex between interracial couples, and erotic depictions of safer-sex activities can be found in these films. Some independent films are also more experimental in format. As the demand for alternative videos increases, expect their quality and availability to steadily improve. You're unlikely to find these tapes at the local video store, so search for them online, try a sex boutique, or visit a gay and lesbian bookstore.

I watch new lesbian-made videos as soon as they are released. The best part is seeing real lesbians having real sex. The worst part is waiting a year for another one to come out.

I like those Femme videos because the women and men aren't Barbie and Ken types. They're more like your yuppie next-door neighbors.

At Good Vibrations, we've been in the somewhat privileged position of both seeing what customers want in adult films and evaluating what currently exists. True to our motto, "If you want something done right do it yourself," we started producing a line of videos we felt addressed the lack of diversity in contemporary porn.

Our video production company, known as Sex-positive Productions, currently has four titles under its belt, with more on the way. *Slide Bi Me* features an enthusiastic and insatiable bisexual cast devouring each other at a company picnic; *Please Don't Stop* is an educational video for lesbians of color; *Whipsmart* is a beginner's guide to S/M, and *Voluptuous Vixens* features big beautiful women. We try to represent a variety of ages, body types, ethnicities, and sexual orientations in all our videos, in addition to giving sex toys their rightful place in our storylines.

SIR Videos

"We don't show soft core, fa-la-la sex; we have down-and-dirty dykes getting it on in a big way."

"Our movies have real dykes, real boobs, real orgasms, real fun. and real hard-ons (no Viagra needed)," says Jackie Strano, who, along with real-life partner Shar Rednour, has produced and starred in a successful line of lesbian-made videos. That succinctly sums up why SIR Productions' videos are miles apart from the garden variety porn mass-produced by the adult industry.

According to Jackie, the industry's idea of a lesbian film is a "straight girl being a day tripper for hire. When we have two girlie-girls together it is femme on femme. *And* we have butches in our movies." But she adds magnanimously, "Hats off to the industry gals who are fierce and fully enjoy every lesbian role they do; we love 'em!" She also explains that SIR videos are different than some of the other lesbian-produced porn because "We are big on dirty talk and role-playing. We don't show soft core, fa-la-la sex; we have down-and-dirty dykes getting it on in a big way."

You need only check out SIR Productions' award-winning *Hard Love and How to Fuck in High Heels*, or the futuristic *Sugar High Glitter City*, for a glimpse into the world of real lesbian sex, which includes plenty of strap-on sex, female ejaculation, smoldering oral sex, and lots of that naughty talk. What's more, in addition to the diversity in the cast's body size and ethnicity, these girls always seem to be having a damn good time.

And while lesbians are clearly their target market, SIR Productions' subject matter isn't limited to lesbian sex. In fact, their runaway best-seller is what they describe as "educational entertainment"—a beginner's guide for both straight and gay couples to strapping on a dildo and anally penetrating a partner. A best-selling video at Good Vibrations for years, *Bend Over Boyfriend, Volume 1* (written by SIR and co-produced by Fatale) proved that anal sex was a far more popular activity than people were willing to admit.

Look for an upcoming video version of the book *The Survivor's Guide to Sex*, as well as forthcoming films about talking dirty and sex during pregnancy.

Look for SIR videos at www.sirvideos.com. (And for the record, "SIR" stands for Sexual Indulgence and Rock-n-roll!)

GAY MALE PORN: For years gay male porn has been a booming industry, resulting in more diversity in style and content than straight movies, and earning this genre a wide range of fans, including plenty of women. Gay porn features exceptionally attractive men, and condom use is more common in these productions.

I enjoy reading erotica and watching boy-porn films. As a lesbian, I used to feel sheepish about the boy porn, but I find it has the spunk and speed I need.

My boyfriend and I watch male-to-male porn together. We try to emulate what they're doing on the screen.

AMATEUR TAPES: The amateur videos you sometimes find in adult bookstores are actually what's known as "pro-am," or professionally amateur videos. Basically, successful filmmakers shoot real people engaging in real sex—these aren't polished actors or actresses, and there are no scripts. Amateur videos tend to be low on production values and talent, but long on enthusiasm and sincerity. They depict a wider range of physical types than commercial porn does, and multiple-volume series such as *Masturbation Memoirs* and *Screaming Orgasms* depict in loving detail women who are authentically turned on. If you prefer your porn slick and glossy, however, you may not appreciate the real-life awkwardness that's on display in these videos. Amateur tapes appeal instead to the viewer who might be tempted to videotape the couple next door having sex—if only it weren't against the law!

Amateur videos and videos of real partners turn me on. There is nothing more erotic than explicit interesting sex between real lovers.

Never have I seen anything more beautiful, moving, and erotic as these on-screen orgasms. Masturbation Memoirs fulfilled a visual erotic and educational dream, touched me profoundly, and raised my consciousness.

HENTAI: If you think there's nothing new in porn, check out a Hentai video. "Hentai" is the name for a genre of explicit, animated cartoons from Japan that combine engaging storylines, amazing visuals, and explosive sex. Lots of mythical creatures, fantastical sex, and controversial material abound in these films, which tend to focus on futuristic themes. And guess what? Since it's animated, you don't have to worry about bad acting or lousy direction. If you're a fan of "anime"—the Japanese-inspired animation that has enchanted many a child—you're bound to be intrigued by the adult version. According to Good Vibrations' video reviewer, "Animation is the perfect medium to unleash our darkest and most twisted sexual and violent fantasies. It has produced a wonderfully sick, perverted, erotic fuckfest…with very intense visual expressions that one would hopefully never act out, but that can be unbelievably stimulating to experience vicariously."

SEX-EDUCATION TAPES: An increasing number of sex-education tapes are available, from talking-head sex therapy to porno-educational endeavors like porn star Nina Hartley's guides to various sexual techniques (see Nina's profile in the Oral Sex chapter). The videos in the latter category set out to turn you on, and though those in the former category may not intend to do so, you may find yourself aroused by the explicit sex talk or participants' demonstrations. Sex-education tapes are a great way to get no-nonsense, explicit sex education, often on under-represented themes like Tantra or sex and disability. We've listed a few of the popular ones in the videography at the end of the book.

Watching the women in the masturbation circle in Betty Dodson's Selfloving *video made me feel like I was part of a women's jill-off club—I came with the best of them!*

Concerns

I don't want to watch certain activities. If you're worried about viewing scenes you may find disturbing or shocking, review our suggestions on how to choose a video, so that you can get as much information as possible before you rent or purchase a tape. Read the box copy or, if you have the good fortune to be in a store with savvy clerks, ask for more information. If you notice that specific activities or situations make you uncomfortable, read some books that address the topic to gain some outside perspective.

View the video by yourself to freely and honestly explore your range of reactions to the erotic material. This way, you won't be inhibited by someone else's presence, so you'll be able to focus all your attention on what is or isn't turning you on. You may discover that an activity you were convinced was repulsive holds a particularly explosive charge. Sometimes you just have to feel it to believe it!

In my college anti-porn feminist days I stumbled on a cache of Penthouse magazines someone had collected for a term paper. I got so wet looking at those women I knew something was amiss with our rhetoric.

Should women be involved with porn? Some people register surprise when they hear that a feminist sex toy store is peddling pornography. Women's participation in porn, whether as consumers, producers, actresses, or critics, has spawned years of debate in the women's movement. While volumes have been written on all sides of the issue—and we urge you to read them—we'll take just a minute to illuminate our perspective.

Conditions in the porn industry, as in any industry, vary widely. Women are no more exploited in porn than they are in any other industry, and in some ways are less so—they're better paid, for one. Furthermore, women have been taking greater control as producers and performers since the early eighties.

We are opposed to limiting or restricting access to sexually explicit materials. Although it's true that images of women in X-rated films can be as stereotyped and demeaning as in mainstream films, we doubt that eliminating porn would result in the economic and social equality of the sexes. We believe porn reflects the social, sexual mores of our society, rather than creating these mores. Restricting the production and consumption of porn only perpetuates the lowest-common denominator of mainstream X-rated videos. The only way to combat the existence of low-quality porn is not to censor it, but instead to produce more and better kinds. As we've seen from our customers' comments, they want porn, they enjoy porn, they just want better-made porn! Entrepreneurs, are you listening? It's time to get your hands dirty!

And remember, if you're bored viewing a sex-flick, uncomfortable, or just plain in a hurry, you can always use that popular button on the remote control—fast forward!

I can't believe my lover likes that stuff! You may be in a relationship where your partner doesn't exactly share your penchant for porn.

> *She got really pissed when I watched X-rated videos other women. I tried to explain that I think of her when I watch them (and I really do), but she refused to believe it. So I was damned if I did, and my balls would explode if I didn't.*

Attempt to find out what he or she is objecting to. If you find your partner feels hurt that you need outside stimulation to get aroused, perhaps you can read the Fantasies chapter together. Find out what fantasies or images, if any, turn on your partner. Draw a parallel between the images we invent ourselves and those we pick up from books and videos. Stress that you're *not* watching porn as a way of unfavorably comparing your partner to the actors and actresses on screen, you're doing it to enhance the arousal you can share with your partner. Expecting one person to be the sole source of your arousal unnecessarily confines your sexuality and is simply unrealistic.

Perhaps the source of your partner's objections is embarrassment or discomfort with specific activities or behaviors, and therefore a discussion might help you sift out what components of the porn she or he has seen (or possibly only *heard* about) as disturbing. Your partner may have never actually seen an X-rated tape, in which case you can try to find out what you'd both like, and then watch one together. Or, he or she may be more comfortable initially watching it alone. To a certain extent, porn is an acquired taste, and it can take a few viewings to let go of your internalized judgments and just enjoy your visceral responses. If, after all's said and done, your partner simply doesn't enjoy porn, you can politely ask that he or she not rain on your parade, and continue to indulge privately.

Videos always get my girlfriend soaking wet, and she's not a porno fan.

I can't believe I like that stuff! You may have your concerns that porn, while pleasurable for the individual, is somehow harmful to society. Despite the common myth that porn "degrades" women or inspires violent behavior, numerous academic and government studies have been completely unable to demonstrate any causal link between consuming sexually explicit materials and performing antisocial acts. For an excellent overview of this subject, we recommend ACLU President Nadine Strossen's *Defending Pornography: Free Speech, Sex and the Fight for Women's Rights.*

Remember, fantasy is not real life. Images of forbidden, taboo, or degrading activities can excite us even though—or especially because—we have no desire to act them out. Ironically, it is often the acts or behavior we find most disconcerting that are the most titillating; that they are forbidden infuses them with erotic appeal.

┌─ *Erotica Shopping Checklist* ─────

- ✓ *Activities:* What types turn you on? Will descriptions of taboo activities light your fire or douse it?
- ✓ *Orientation:* Are you interested in a specific orientation (straight, lesbian, gay, bisexual, transgendered), or is a mix desired?
- ✓ *Voice:* Are you interested in a specific point-of-view, for instance a woman's perspective, a gay male perspective, a partnered perspective?
- ✓ *Language:* Do you prefer explicit sexual references or colorful euphemisms?
- ✓ *Genres:* What kinds of themes entertain you in other media, for example science fiction, film noir, historical fiction, adventures in far-off lands? Erotic materials are available in a wide range of genres.
- ✓ *Comparison shopping:* Is there a similar title you can suggest to the clerk for comparison's sake?
- ✓ *Format:* With books, would you prefer short stories over novels? With videos, perhaps you'd like a compilation rather than a full-length feature.
- ✓ *Quality:* Are literary merit and high production values priorities?

Shopping for Videos

WHERE TO GET VIDEOS: All adult bookstores and almost all video stores have a video section from which you can rent X-rated tapes. We realize this isn't going to work for all of you—the idea of venturing into the adult section of your local store might be intimidating. We can testify that the clerk probably has as much interest in your taste in porn as he or she does in your taste in cereal, but undoubtedly there are some of you who fear your penchant for dildo-packing cowgirl tapes might make it into Liz Smith's next column. If you're too shy to make your selection from your neighborhood store, you could (a) travel to another town to rent tapes; (b) subscribe to the *Playboy* channel; or (c) rent or purchase tapes online or from mail-order catalogs that promise discretion and confidentiality. Once again, the convenience and anonymity of the Web make it an ideal place to shop for videos. What's more, you can use the search function to compare prices, track down websites of favorite stars or directors, and read industry and customer reviews.

HOW TO CHOOSE VIDEOS: If you've never purchased an adult video or DVD, you may be over-helmed by the volumes of cheesy-sounding titles or rows of seemingly identical boxes. Here are some tips:

- *Think about what might appeal to you in a porn movie.* Are you looking for certain kinds of sexual activities, certain couplings, certain famous porn stars, particular directors whose quality you like, or an interesting plot? If you're clear about your personal criteria, you'll at least have something to look for.
- *Read the box.* While the information on the box is not always helpful or accurate, it may mention or allude to something you're interested in.
- *Read reviews.* Just like mainstream movies, adult movies are reviewed, and reviews can provide some hints about the sexual content, the plot, or the actors involved. Look for these in online and print magazines like *Adult Video News* or *Screw*, though keep in mind that these are trade magazines designed to sell videos, so don't expect critical analyses. For more thoughtful reviews, sex 'zines and online magazines can be a great resource, as can almanacs like *Only the Best* or the *X-rated Videotape Guides*.
- *Look for award winners.* Publications such as *Adult Video News* sponsor annual awards ceremonies, and awards are usually noted on box copy. This can give you a leg up, but bear in mind the disagreements you've had with the Academy Award judges in the past.
- *Ask friends for recommendations.* Obviously not everyone is comfortable quizzing friends about their tastes in porn, but personal recommendations can be invaluable in separating the wheat from the chaff. Surfing websites is an excellent way to learn about other people's porn preferences while maintaining your anonymity.
- *Ask the store clerk.* This isn't always easy either, but if you can muster up the courage, you may tap into a valuable resource.
- *Look for a rating system.* Some retailers and reviewers use rating systems to help viewers narrow down titles of interest to them.

At Good Vibrations we've compiled a selection of adult videos we believe to be a cut above the rest. These are distinguished by at least one of a variety of criteria: good acting, superior filmmaking, unusual sexual activities, sexually explosive scenes, believable or compelling plots, woman-oriented, or educational content. We've listed the most popular of the titles in the videography, so if you're interested in becoming one of the millions of erotic video fans, you'll have a good place to start.

Enjoying Porn

Now that you have access to this plethora of sexually oriented materials, you may wonder what to do with it all. We'll let our customers offer some suggestions.

To Enhance Masturbation

When I was younger I used to read erotica while masturbating. I always liked to have my orgasm coincide with the characters' so I'd reread the same exciting paragraph over and over....

I prefer to lie on my stomach while I'm looking at sexually explicit material and rub my penis against a cushion. I actually buy soft cotton socks so that I can ejaculate into them if I get aroused beyond the point of no return.

I read mostly Penthouse letters to the editor, and Victorian pornographic novels, such as The Pearl and My Secret Life. Also lesbian fantasies. I read them while using my plug-in vibrator. I rarely finish reading more than a page or two before climaxing and enjoy teasing myself by taking away the vibrator to make the good feelings last. I have two magazines from ten years ago that I still use.

I read books to myself silently and then masturbate when I become wet. It's fun to see how long I can keep from touching myself.

So Both Partners Can Get Turned On

If I'm with a partner, sometimes halfway through the film I'll be so horny we'll have to turn it off and have sex.

We often read stories silently at the same time and then focus the arousal on each other when we are done reading. I sometimes read to him aloud. We look at magazines a lot together, but while he is more turned on by Playboy, I am turned on by the more hardcore photographs of actual penetration. Because of this we aren't aroused by the same pictures.

Watching porn with a partner is a good way to start a sexual encounter—then let nature take over. With myself, I read a lot of porno books/magazines and then build up the fantasy with my imagination.

My ex-lover and I would watch gay men's porn every time. It was great. I would watch, and she would fuck me; her back was often to the TV.

To Discover New Ways to Enjoy Sex

I sometimes look at Internet porn (short, very explicit hard-core movies featuring anal penetration and/or double penetration). Doubtless that has fueled my current fantasy of double penetration.

I love many different kinds of videos, but recently I've been watching more videos that feature anal sex or rimming (or "booty-lingus" as I've heard it called).

We use books, movies, and videos, both erotic and nonerotic, as sources of ideas for characters and

locations for our fantasy universe, then we make up our own plots and characters.

I use porn videos for education and anticipation of pleasure while beating off alone. I also use them nonsexually with a partner to actually see examples of things each of us likes so that we can discuss them.

To Learn about Our Own and Others' Pleasures and Desires

I read erotica and fantasize myself with the characters I desire. I prefer lesbian erotica to hetero. I consider myself straight, but I always fantasize, read, and daydream about making love to women.

I love reading/looking at erotica by myself and then masturbating. I enjoy doing this to recharge right before my partner comes home or the baby goes to sleep. I also enjoy doing it with a partner. It keeps communication going sexually, and I sometimes learn new things my partner fantasizes about and vice-versa.

Do It Yourself!

Are you a pornographer? If you've taken your own X-rated videos, penned some erotic verse, or snapped some nasty photos of your sweetheart, you qualify! You can write, direct, and star in your own erotic fantasies, and your partner will probably appreciate the imaginative and personal touch. If you're looking for a place to start, try writing down one of your fantasies. Many of our survey respondents reported getting rather excited as they were describing their earliest memories of masturbating, their favorite sexual encounter, or their experience of orgasm. If you're ready to take your exhibitionism to the next level, you might consider investing in a webcam and broadcasting your antics online to the rest of the world.

I have a video of my current partner and me. In one scene, we fool around and then fuck. The way she kisses me and fondles my dick, more than anything else, makes me feel so tender. In the second scene, she is insatiable, insisting that I let her suck my dick (a rare mood for her), which thrills me to no end.

I'd like to act out a scene from a book or video and then record it for posterity's sake!

I love drawing my own erotica and have been doing it all my life, for the most part attempting to sensitively and beautifully depict hetero, homo, and bisexual acts of oral sex in classic pencil-on-paper style.

A Note on Censorship

Anyone familiar with America's history of prudery won't be surprised to learn not only that many of the materials described in this chapter have been banned from libraries, universities, and stores around the country, but also that their producers have been targeted for store and federal harassment. The practice doesn't stop at our borders either; customs in countries Good Vibrations ships to on a regular basis are always surprising us with the materials they choose to confiscate. We refer you to our Censorship chapter for a summary of attempts to restrict access to sexually explicit materials and for some suggestions as to what you can do to stand up for freedom of expression. In the meantime, we encourage you to actively exercise your right to read and view the abundance of materials presented in this chapter—start your own personal collection of erotica, porn, and smut!

Susie Bright

"The erotica wave blew away the idea that everyone wants to only read reassuring little stories about people like themselves— what a bore."

Imagine getting two thousand erotic stories in your mail box each year. Either you'd feel like every day was your birthday, or you'd vow never to have sex again. But for Susie Bright, editor of the annual *Best American Erotica* series, looking for that erotic diamond in the rough is all part of a day's work. "I never get burned out reading, unless you count eye strain," says Susie. "I can ID bad stuff quickly and move on. But good material nails you to the spot until you finish the last line."

When you're committed to publishing the best, you've got to put in the time: finding talented writers, reviewing stories, and editing the cream of the crop. Should you think reviewing volumes of erotica is akin to working in a candy shop—you lose your appetite after a while—Susie is quick to dispel this notion. "This is a really common assumption about erotica, and it needs to be questioned. Is Julia Child sick of cooking? Are all those painters at the museum sick of painting? Are art critics and all those people at the *New York Times* just sick to death of reading books and looking at movies? Of course not! But everyone is sick of a bad movie, a badly told story, from the moment it begins. Inspiring creative work is always…inspiring, and banal work is always alienating."

This response comes as no surprise from the woman who's made a career out of sex. Susie has worked at Good Vibrations, launched the lesbian magazine *On Our Backs*, worked with the pioneering lesbian porn video company Fatale, edited dozens of erotica anthologies, and written countless books and magazine articles about sexual politics, technique, and erotic writing (see the bibliography). Sex is not a hobby for Susie, it's both her passion and her life's work.

She's now working on a tenth anniversary edition of *Best American Erotica*, which will feature erotica, author interviews, and a listing of readers' favorite stories. What type of story makes the cut? "I look for great storytelling with a compelling erotic component or flavor that makes the piece sexually provocative and memorable. It should be arousing, but it doesn't have to be a 'stroke yourself to the finish' type story. It should say something about sex and the human condition that everyone hasn't heard a million times—a new voice, a new style, a candor you don't expect. It can be funny or tragic. It can be one paragraph long or many many pages."

Susie Bright's stint as an erotica editor began in the eighties with the publication of *Herotica,* one of the first anthologies of erotica by women. As editor, Susie helped smash the stereotype that good girls don't fantasize or write naughty stories about sex. This genre quickly became knows as "women's erotica." Since then, she's witnessed (and contributed to) an explosion in the erotica market. "The erotica market expanded like a hot air balloon. It changed the notions of what women will read—and write," she explains. "The erotica wave blew away the idea that everyone wants to only read reassuring little stories about people like themselves—what a bore. Sci fi, mystery, crime, romance, historical adventures—is that about real life? Of course not!"

Of course, this boom means that today's bookstore shelves are jam packed with erotica titles. How to choose? Susie encourages readers to get to know different editors' styles and tastes. Ask friends, ardent short-story fans, or erotica writers about the books that turn them on. If all else fails, pick up the book and read the first and last stories. "Those are usually indications of stories the editor thinks will seduce you at the top, and blow you away at the end. If you don't like the first and the last, you probably won't find paradise in the middle."

To learn more about Susie Bright's current projects, visit her website, www.susiebright.com.

CHAPTER 16

World Wide Web

When the first edition of *The Good Vibrations Guide to Sex* came out in 1994, this chapter was titled Hi-Tech Sex and focused on promising technological innovations in sexual entertainment. Over time, most of these innovations either have failed to live up to their hype (adult CD-ROMS) or have yet to materialize in any user-friendly way (teledildonics). One breakthrough, however, has so completely captivated the public's attention that it's now as ubiquitous as television: the World Wide Web. Given how integrated the Web now is in most of our daily lives—whether it's being used to check stock options, research homework, or buy groceries—that it has also sparked a sexual revolution should come as no surprise.

The Web allows you to explore just about any of the practices or sexual subjects discussed in this book. Curious about sexual anatomy? Go to Annie Sprinkle's personal website to see her cervix, or visit Jackinworld to view pictures of uncircumcised penises. Looking for some tips on oral or anal sex? Dozens of websites feature first-hand accounts along with detailed instructions on technique. Wondering if anyone else out there enjoys S/M? The Web easily connects you to a community of like-minded folks—and you never have to leave your chair. Want to read erotica but never had the nerve to buy a dirty book or magazine? The anonymity and easy publishing tools on the Web make it convenient and exciting to explore or share sexual fantasies, techniques, or information.

We freely admit to our own love affair with the Web. Its sexual charms so captivated us that we published our own primer, *The Woman's Guide to Sex on the Web*. Despite all the positive ways in which the Web can impact our sexuality, it's still often stigmatized as a sleazy haven where perverts and porn proliferate. Yet once you scratch the surface, you'll see that the Web's potential to inspire and transform our sex lives is much greater than any perceived harm. We're happy to point the way and encourage you to log on and have fun!

For the Newcomer

Even if you don't own a computer or you've never been online, we know you've heard of the World Wide Web by now. For those of you thinking about diving into the virtual world, here are some tips on getting started.

The Internet and the Web

While the Web may seem like a relatively recent phenomenon, it's actually a subset of the Internet, which was developed in the sixties by the U.S. Defense Department as a military communications tool. Basically, the Internet connects a vast array of public and private computer networks via phone lines; it was originally federally funded to link a global community of government agencies, scientists, research institutions, and universities. When the military moved on to establish its own high-security networks in the late eighties, the public gained unrestricted access to the Internet, though its use was limited to those well-versed in UNIX-based code.

To make the text-based Internet more accessible and appealing, a British physicist developed technology to create the user-friendly interface known as the World Wide Web. As its name implies, the Web attempts to organize and provide access to the amazing tangle of information available on the Internet by weaving together sites with related content. Thanks to graphics interface programs (known as "browsers"), which allow users to simultaneously display and access textual, visual, and audio information, Web "sites" present information in an attractive, accessible format. The Web also makes it easier to jump from one topic or site to another through a system of "hypertext links"—users simply click on a highlighted word or phrase on one screen, and they're immediately transferred ("linked") to a new screen. One second you're reading about a sex club in San Francisco and the next you're shopping at a toy store in Denmark. The Web's popularity has flourished because:

- There are no restrictions on who can create Web pages, and they aren't difficult to produce.
- It's relatively inexpensive to create a Web page, which means that everyone from Joe hobbyist next door to the large commercial interests can get in on the action.
- It's an extremely affordable way to communicate with people worldwide.
- It offers a tremendous source of information on almost every conceivable subject.

Getting Online

To access online activities and resources requires:

A COMPUTER: A fast computer with a sizeable hard drive will make it easier to take advantage of the Web's multimedia capabilities. A color monitor is essential for viewing the Web's visuals.

A MODEM: Most computers today are sold with internal modems, but you can always purchase an external one if necessary. This device connects your computer to other computers through your telephone line. Speed is an important consideration—the faster your modem, the less time you'll spend waiting to receive images and information over the wires—so we recommend investing in the fastest modem currently available. We won't bother listing today's current modem speeds, since they'll be obsolete in no time. Higher-speed modems like DSL or ISDN require use of a separate phone line, but are becoming increasingly affordable.

Slow speed is one of the biggest complaints of Web surfers, so you can rest assured that the phone, cable TV, and high-tech companies are all working on ways to speed up access. One other thing to keep in mind: If you plan on spending a lot of time online, you may want to invest in a second phone line for your modem, otherwise incoming calls will get a busy signal.

SOFTWARE: Your modem or your ISP (see below) will provide you with software that will activate your computer's dial-up, cable, or DSL connection to the Internet. You'll also need browser software, which is what transforms the Web's programming language into a visual delight, offering options for navigation, editing, organization, printing, etc. The most common browser today is Microsoft's Internet Explorer, but Netscape Navigator has many loyal fans. Browser software is available for free on the Web, and is often supplied by your ISP as part of the start-up package.

INTERNET SERVICE PROVIDERS: To explore the vast resources of the Internet, you usually gain access through a local Internet Service Provider (ISP). You sign up with a single ISP, which charges either monthly or hourly fees—you then access any part of the Internet you desire by calling up the ISP's central computer system. The beauty of this set-up is that you pay no more to surf a Web page maintained by someone in Zimbabwe than you do to read a news group posting from someone right in your own backyard. Your Internet account serves as your personal "on-ramp" to the information superhighway.

Quality of customer service and reliability varies widely among ISPs. Some are user friendly, providing easy-to-install software packages. Others are expert-friendly, and prioritize maintaining a fast infrastructure to minimize noticeable delays or service interruptions. You can find information on ISPs in your local phonebook, in computer magazines, or from friends. Many local and long-distance telephone companies now provide ISP services as well. Try speaking to the technical support personnel of any prospective ISP to help determine whether its services and software can accommodate your level of expertise and computer hardware.

COMMERCIAL ONLINE SERVICES: For many years, large commercial online services like Prodigy, CompuServe, and America Online (AOL) dominated the world of online services. They distanced themselves from the "chaotic" Internet by creating their own communities—an orderly, menu-driven world where chatrooms, stock tips, and weather updates could all be accessed with a simple click of the mouse. Each of these commercial online services used exclusive proprietary software and created much of their own content—online interaction between users of different systems was limited to exchanging email at best. Now that the Web has captured the global imagination, most commercial online services have responded by providing universal Web access for their users, while still retaining their own sense of community. Their convenience and offers of free introductory periods make these fine places to start out online. Unless you are in a remote area, most of these services can be accessed from a local telephone number. Some commercial online services, however, take an active role in protecting users from "objectionable" material within their domain, and you may want to ask about their use of filtering software before signing up.

The Lay of the Land

If the Web is one large directory, the individual addresses or listings are the "sites." Within each site there can be an infinite number of pages. Since you can hop around within or between sites rather than travel in a linear fashion, it's easy to lose your focus. That's why all sites have a "home page." This is the first screen you'll see when you link to a new site, and it often serves as a table of contents page for the rest of the site. It becomes valuable as a home base, since it's very easy to get lost in the site. Most pages offer an easy link back to their home page.

The URL (Uniform Resource Locator) is simply the address for a website. When you're looking a site up by its URL address, make sure to type in the address exactly as written.

How do you find websites? If you know the URL address, you simply type it in and off you go. Most folks, however, discover websites simply by clicking on the hypertext "links" that allow you to jump from site to site. For example, you could be reading a sex therapist's advice column extolling the merits of vibrator use, and the word "vibrator" might be linked to the Good Vibrations website. If you click on the colored link, you'll find yourself on Good Vibrations' home page. Many sites contain a page of recommended links; if you like the site you're on, these suggestions can be valuable signposts.

A search engine offers another useful way to find websites. Consider it the directory assistance of the online world: It helps you locate specific subject matter as well as specific sites. Type in a word or series of words and a search engine will find all the sites containing these words in their name or site description and bring them up in a list. There are numerous search engines; many are accompanied by directories that try to categorize subjects to help focus your search. Once you start using search engines, you'll quickly discover the importance of precise vocabulary. Searching on the word "sex," for example, will yield a daunting number of entries (unless you're simply curious about the sheer volume of sex-related sites). Narrowing down your search if you have a specific interest—for example, typing in "BDSM clubs" or "safer sex for lesbians in Minneapolis"—will save time.

Be warned, though, that it's easy to get so sidetracked by all the intriguing-sounding links you encounter that you lose sight of your original mission. Most browsers have a "bookmark" or "favorites" option that will record an address for you to return to later. Or if you find yourself deep into a chain of links and you want to go back to an earlier site, most browsers will show a history of your travels and allow you to return to any point along the way.

Now that you've got the basics covered, you're ready to go online. You may find the whole notion of surfing for sex on the Web a bit overwhelming, but most sexual content falls into a few basic categories described below.

Since there are literally thousands of sex-related sites, your quest will take you on a unique path reflecting your own interests. To help you get started, we've included some of our favorite websites in the resource listings at the back of the book. These sites represent just a slice of what's out there, yet they provide a good jumping off point for a variety of interests.

Sex Information and Education

Sex Information

It's safe to say you won't find such easy access to so much sex information anywhere else as you do on the Web. If you've ever tried to find a sex-related book at a public library, you probably discovered that it was lost, stolen, defaced, or mysteriously missing. Even if you were lucky enough to find the book you were looking for, you may have been too embarrassed to check it out. Although you may not find the text of this same sex book online (we believe you will some day), you're likely to find sample chapters and a company to buy it from. You're also bound to locate more on the same subject somewhere on the Web. For example, you'll find sex magazines, advice columns, archival collections of research materials, resource listings, and chapters from sex books devoted to every conceivable sexual topic.

There are several advantages to this hodgepodge of sex information, not the least of which is the tremendous variety of perspectives you will be exposed to as you roam. You may have started with a visit to Parents Place looking for tips on nutrition, dropped in on their chat group on gay parenting, read about a great sex education book for kids, which then linked you to the sex shop selling the book. There you're intrigued by a link to the Feminists for Free Expression, and soon you're reading about women defending pornography. We can only hope that this exposure broadens individual understanding and tolerance of alternative sexual viewpoints.

The Web offers a unique culture of information-sharing. Bookstores and libraries naturally only carry work by published authors, and to be a published author (at least when it comes to sex writing) usually requires that you have some professional credential or specialized knowledge. Since anyone can make a Web page, you can find out what the people next door, who love talking about sex, are really doing! Jane Doe enthusiastically writes about her personal

---

As Time Goes By

Every new technological development in art or communication is seized upon almost immediately for use in expressing sexual ideas or creating sexual materials. From Stone Age carvings, to the printing press, to the development of films, to the video revolution, to the design of DVDs and the Web, sex has been the subject matter of each new medium. It's widely taught in literature classes that the first novels were composed in eighteenth-century England. It's less widely noted that *Fanny Hill*, one of the first novels ever published, is a piece of classic porn that's been setting readers' pulses racing since 1749. Among the earliest film reels available are clips of the gay ladies and gentlemen of the twenties having amorous escapades. It's a chicken-and-egg conundrum whether VCRs became must-have appliances due to their convenience for viewing X-rated videos in the privacy of one's home, or whether adult video became a multi-billion dollar business due to the advent of video technology. And from the time of the very first Usenet newsgroups, sex has inspired online communication around the world.

Some might argue that the inevitable use of each new technology for erotic expression is proof that we're a nation of techno-nerds who feel more comfortable with impersonal gadgets than with face-to-face communion. We at Good Vibrations prefer to see the link between sex and technology as proof that most creative impulses are intimately linked to sexuality—humans instinctively seize upon each new medium as a way to explore our boundaries, to add excitement to the human experience, and to reach out and touch someone.

requirements for satisfying oral sex while John Doe shares what he looks for in his favorite pornography. Some of these virtual sex pioneers develop quite a following, their opinions trusted more than a professional's. In addition to individual Web pages, the discussion boards, forums, or mailing lists on many sites are great resources for peer-based information, advice, or opinions about sex.

The Web may do more for our sexual literacy than any other medium that's come before. People are often too embarrassed to buy sex books or ask their doctors about sex. But visit Go Ask Alice, a site run by health educators from Columbia University, and you'll see just how much sexual curiosity is out there. The site administrators answer sex-related questions from readers—now numbering in the thousands—about everything from contraception to self-esteem to technique. The Society for Human Sexuality (see sidebar) archives the largest collection of sexuality materials online. And SIECUS, the Sexuality Information and Education Council of the United States, offers fact sheets, bibliographies, and provocative discussions of contemporary issues in sexuality.

Keep in mind that if you're seeking advice for a specific medical problem, you should always consult with a health professional. The Web can be a great source of information, but don't rely on it for the diagnosis or treatment of medical conditions. For example, one of the many excellent sites on STDs may help you determine that you have contracted an infection, but a health professional should evaluate your personal health history and help you set up a proper course of treatment.

Sex Education

Educational sex sites aren't for adults only—we like to remind people that the Web can be a wonderful resource for parents and children too. Parents can find expert advice on talking to kids about sex, can locate other parents with similar questions and concerns, and can tap resources that will help answer their children's questions about sexuality. Teens can get answers to crucial questions about sex and sexuality that they might not get from schoolteachers, parents, or other adults. Sites like the Coalition for Positive Sexuality and one called Sex Etc. are run by youth who explore issues of sexual responsibility, safety, and health with refreshing candor and openness. Some excellent adult

sites also sponsor teen-specific sites, such as Scarlet Letters' Scarleteen.

Unfortunately, when it comes to kids, sex, and the Internet, the media tend to focus on the importance of protecting children from a vast online wasteland of porn and predators. We're the first to admit that there's a lot of tasteless porn online, but we'd rather parents take an active role in steering kids to quality educational materials than avoid the Web altogether.

And while creeps can be found online, they aren't the pervasive presence you might fear. Teach kids online safety just as you would water or car safety, and they'll be well equipped to surf responsibly. Make sure they know not to give out personal information, including pictures, without your permission. If they want to meet a cyber friend in person, accompany them and arrange to meet in a public place. Encourage your children to bring to your attention any site or email that makes them uncomfortable. Adopting these common sense practices will minimize the risk of harassment, and helps create a positive learning environment for you and your child.

As part of our national preoccupation with "protecting" kids from sexually explicit imagery, parents are often encouraged to install filtering software, which blocks access to adult websites. Unfortunately, filters are problematic, as they can block access to health, sexuality, and First Amendment sites as well as to X-rated material. Rather than restricting access wholesale (most tech-savvy kids can circumvent filters anyway), we encourage parents to take a proactive approach to their children's online sex education. Bookmark sex sites you find appropriate, discuss surfing habits with your kids, and talk to them about sites that make you or them uncomfortable (a useful way to teach about sexual stereotypes at the same time).

We make no bones about our belief that kids have as much right to accurate sex information as adults. After all, they are sexual beings from birth, and we owe it to them to foster a healthy and happy sexuality. Children are naturally curious, and unless you address their questions, they'll seek answers elsewhere—with potentially harmful results. In the past, well-intentioned parents who couldn't bring themselves to discuss sex left educational sexual materials on the family bookshelf for kids to read in private. Today it's even easier; parents can point kids toward online resources.

Community

Maybe you just had a baby and want to find other moms who will share their experiences about post-partum sex. Perhaps you're contemplating sex reassignment and need advice on hormone therapy. Or it could be you're moving to a new city and wonder what businesses in the area are queer-friendly. You can find special-interest websites, which offer a host of valuable resources, provide a place to ask questions, and sometimes allow you to chat with other users. Anyone who's ever tried to get sex-specific information, resources, or advice offline knows the search can be frustrating and difficult. The Web offers discretion, up-to-date referrals and a non-judgmental embrace from other folk with interests like yours.

One of the most powerful contributions the Web has made to individual sexual exploration is its ability to unite sexual communities. If you thought you were alone in your preference for BDSM or polyamory, simply log on and discover what a welcoming and diverse community awaits you. If you've been frustrated by the lack of sex information or support as a person with a disability, check out the growing numbers of sites that disseminate relevant information. No longer do queer teens growing up in small towns need to feel isolated when they can log on and exchange Instant Messages with like-minded youth around the world. Finding your desired community involves some simple investigation. Use search engines and directories, check out discussion boards, ask for recommendations in chatrooms, subscribe to mailing lists (see the Chatting in Delayed Time section below), or check out your favorite sites' links.

The wondrous fringe benefit to all this is that the Web more accurately reflects the diverse sexual spectrum than any other medium today. It doesn't matter what the church, your mother, the latest women's magazine, or the president decides is "normal sexual behavior"—all you have to do is go online to discover that people's sexual tastes and genders cannot be neatly categorized. Not only does the Web offer refuge for people who might have been considered on the "sexual fringe," it inspire's people to push the envelope of their own sexual fantasies and activities—and could ultimately serve to make us all more tolerant and sexually free.

Shopping

It didn't take long for commercial interests to discover the sales potential of the Web, which has been a particular boon for sex-related businesses.

Benefits of Shopping Online

For the thousands of people who have no access to a store like Good Vibrations, for those too embarrassed to shop in one anyway, or for those who'd rather not have adult catalogs sitting in their mailboxes, the Web is the ideal solution. It's a discreet, easy, and convenient way for folks to order from the privacy of their own homes. You can shop at any time of the day or night, without anybody seeing you, and without speaking to a soul.

It's true that nothing quite compares to picking up a product and holding it in your hands. But online retailers can provide far more detailed and up-to-date information about products on a website than in a paper catalog, so shoppers can do their homework before buying. Not sure what a G-spot vibrator is supposed to stimulate? Perplexed about how to size up the right dildo for you? Wondering why some butt plugs flare in the middle and others don't? All these answers are online. And let's face it, most people shopping in a retail store won't ask their most explicit questions of a store clerk, but they are more likely to send a query through email.

Happily, online consumers enjoy a few extra perks as well. Discounts, freebies, sales, and other ordering incentives are common: Many companies want to divert retail or catalog customers to the Web since it's a cheaper way to do business. Search engines make price comparisons easier, though bear in mind that many companies rename products, and one company's G-spot Vibrator might be top-of-the-line while another company's might be junk.

Finally, since Web surfers are accustomed to unlimited amounts of free information, most commercial businesses who hope to succeed will offer information, services, or resources in addition to their product line. For example, visitors to the Good Vibrations website will find replicas from our antique vibrator museum, sex trivia, information about our cooperative business structure, a lively magazine, answers to customers' most frequently asked sex questions, and much more. This abundance of information produces savvy consumers and allows potential shoppers to become more familiar with a company before they decide to patronize it. It's worth noting that word travels fast on the Internet, so a company that treats customers poorly or engages in bad business practices can lose its reputation overnight.

Finding Good Companies

If you'd like to start shopping online, we hope you'll make Good Vibrations your first stop (if you haven't already!). But we also encourage you to see what else the Web has to offer. Whether you're looking for fetish wear, sex toys, educational sex videos, or lingerie, you'll find it online. Online shops resemble those you'll find in the real world—generic adult bookstores exist, but so do a plethora of more unique boutiques. Folks who may not be able to afford the start-up costs of a retail store in their town's commercial district (or who might be run out of town even if they could) can still do a brisk business out of their home with a Web page attracting customers from all over the world.

While it can be hard to differentiate legitimate businesses from those out to make a fast buck, these tips should help you weed out less reputable sites:

- *Get site recommendations from friends.* Word-of-mouth referrals are priceless.
- *Go with recommendations from sites you trust.* If you like a particular site, check its links page or find out if it's affiliated with any stores.
- *Look for the "about us" page on a site.* Try to determine who's behind the site so that you can assess whether they seem above board or not.
- *Verify a company's legitimacy.* Call its toll-free number, request a paper catalog, or send snail mail (ordinary postal mail) with your questions. Since email can be easily manipulated, don't rely on that for confirmation. You can always check with the Better Business Bureau if you're skeptical.
- *Check out a company's policies.* If it has a generous return policy and clearly stated policies on confidentiality and privacy, there's a good chance it's not out to scam you.

Fear of Fraud

The primary reason people cite for not shopping on the Web is fear of fraud. The truth is that your credit card number is no more at risk of being stolen online than when your card leaves your hands, even briefly, in day-to-day use. The majority of the online fraud that does exist is similar to credit card fraud offline: A company employee steals your card number off your order, or your next door neighbor pilfers receipts from your trash and goes joy-surfing. In the event something does go awry, credit card companies usually cover fraudulent charges over fifty dollars if you report your loss promptly.

Most reputable sites will process your credit card information using what's known as "encryption software." Basically, you input your data on a "secure" page, the data is scrambled as it travels from your computer to the company's, and upon arrival it is deciphered. Your information is only at risk during its journey between the two computers, and breaking the encrypted code is extremely difficult and time-consuming for a hacker, all for relatively little reward. Some sites will tell you when you're about to enter a "secure" environment, but not all will. It's best to ask before ordering, look for a stated policy, or call the company and ask what it can do to protect your credit card.

Erotic Entertainment

If you thought the Web made shopping for sex products easier, just imagine what it's done for erotic entertainment. Before the Web, "erotic entertainment" pretty much consisted of going to strip clubs, renting adult videos, or buying X-rated magazines from the newsstand. Now you can enjoy the visuals of all three, without leaving your house. And if you prefer the written word, the Web not only saves you the trouble of aimlessly wandering the aisles of your local chain bookstore in search of sexually explicit fiction, it houses the largest collection of erotic writing in existence.

Visuals

Regardless of whether your tastes lean toward *Playgirl* or *Fat Girl*, countless sites offer the opportunity to view erotic pictures, watch video clips, or access live-action video. The majority of material mirrors what you'll find on the newsstand: unrealistic-looking women in unnatural poses engaged in all manner of sex acts.

I find most online sexual content literally unbelievable, and therefore no fun. For example, I don't want to see pictures of women pointing vibrators at their pussies, I would like to see them using the vibrators. Also, the people (women especially) in most online porn don't seem to be enjoying themselves. Where is the fun in that?

Unfortunately, the worst of what's available on the Web is most aggressively thrown in your face—whether you get trapped in an endless loop of raunchy porn pop-up frames during an innocent visit, or your mailbox fills up with HOT TEEN VIXEN spam because you once registered for a mailing list. Sadly, this just reinforces the stereotype that when it comes to sex, the Web is full of nothing but testosterone-fueled, trenchcoat-wearing geeks who jerk off incessantly to these pictures.

In fact, if you dig a little deeper, you'll find the Web offers a much wider range of erotic imagery than your typical adult newsstand. If you're fond of historical erotica, visit sites that catalog museum-quality images from antiquity on. If you prefer contemporary fine art or photography, look up individual artists or search on your preferred genre. Websites devoted to a particular theme or practice (large women, S/M, celebrities) often maintain a picture gallery. Many of today's online sex magazines (or "e-zines") combine cutting edge or envelope-pushing erotic imagery with written erotica.

Although still photographs provide the most visual diversity in online erotica, you can also indulge your voyeuristic side by viewing adult video clips or what's called live "streaming" video—the Web equivalent of watching a peep show or going to a strip club. Most of this material is produced by the adult industry and is available either pay-per-view or by paid subscription.

I get off intensely on the little video clips of penetration—vaginal, oral, anal, or some combination thereof.

We set up the office as a sex-room and drank wine and played with each other's private parts while watching some perverted video clips. It was hot fun.

Amateur video clips and webcams provide the most realistic peek into the bedrooms of average Joes and Janes. Anybody with an exhibitionist side can hook up a webcam and launch a website, inviting the world to voyeuristically drop in on them throughout the day. So if the thought of watching the girl or guy next door take a shower turns you on, then this may be the medium for you.

My most memorable masturbation experience was actually one where I was being watched. I became a bit more intimate with an online friend via our webcams. He watched and told me what he'd be doing, and that's what I did to myself. His voice was mesmerizing and the experience was unbelievably arousing.

I love looking at amateur online porn—women and couples that look "real"—no silicone, shaved bushes, etc. Especially when the women are smiling or looking very aroused, or when there's clear signs of sexual satisfaction, such as money shots.

When it comes to sexual entertainment for women, the Web offers a mixed bag. On one hand, women now have easy access to the provocative imagery they might have been too embarrassed to seek out offline. Not too many women are comfortable buying a porn magazine in a typical adult shop, but it's easier than ever to view nude photos of your favorite celebrities, hunky men in (largely gay) magazines, tasteful porn in e-zines, lesbian sex magazines, or explicit couples' photos. On the other hand, most online porn still caters to a primarily straight or gay male aesthetic. However, as more women create and gain access to visual representations of their desires, they're disproving the stereotype that "men like visual porn, women like written erotica." We can only hope that women's increasing demand for equal representation, along with the relative ease of publishing on the Web, will result in a greater variety of imagery both online and offline.

Written Erotica

If you think the pen is mightier than the sword, you ought to see what a keyboard can accomplish when the results are posted to the Internet. Aspiring writers and professionals alike have found a welcome and appreciative fan base, after years of having traditional publishers reject their work for reasons having little to do with the quality of the material. Readers and writers with very specific sexual tastes have found each other thanks to the convenience and anonymity of online publishing, which provides a safe forum for expression.

I'm not into visual stuff—to me, sex involves the mind as much as, if not more than, the body. Words give a better view of the mind, and also allow me to visualize the participants as I see appropriate, whereas visual stuff is all about casting what they think people want to see (skinny, long hair, lots of makeup—ugh).

Particularly for women, who traditionally have shied away from sexually explicit entertainment, the opportunity to explore fantasies, craft a few of their own, and share these with others can be sexually transformative. According to Adrienne Benedicks, founder of the Erotica Readers and Writers Association, women simply need permission to let their inner bad girl out, which is liberating in itself. From there, it's a short hop to writing fantasies and exploring new ones, which ultimately leads to greater sexual awareness.

I love to write erotic stories, I use them as a way to let my partner know what I would be interested in trying or doing. If he is interested then we can try it, but if he is not we can just enjoy thinking about the fantasy I have written out.

I absolutely adore reading erotica online. I probably spent more time reading Elf Sternberg's stories than all my class work combined in my first year of college. I love the vast collections of good, free stories, on any subject imaginable.

In some cases, the discovery of shared fantasies has led to the development of an entire genre of online erotica, as is the case with slash fanfiction, erotica featuring sexually explicit (often S/M-themed) stories about characters from cult TV shows.

For online sexual entertainment I—and I blush to say this—read Buffy the Vampire Slayer erotic slash fanfiction, mostly about the character Spike.

I have recently gotten into X-Files slash. I became a fan of the show just before the plot fell off the edge of a cliff, and naughty stories starring my favorite characters are a great way to get thrills on all sorts of levels.

You can find written erotica in a variety of places online. Individual authors post popular stories, online magazines regularly serve up varied pieces, erotica sites like Adrienne's offer anyone with a story to tell a place to post, and sites devoted to sexuality often maintain an erotica section.

To many, that the Web offers a place where erotica can flourish is both a blessing and a curse. Yes, there's an abundance of material that's varied in both content and style, but there's also very little quality control. So if you've got specific literary standards, your best bet is to develop a relationship with an e-zine or an author you like, and go from there. And just like anything else on the Web, finding erotica that suits your tastes involves a bit of sleuthing: Search by genre, author, story title; get recommendations from friends or other sites; try online magazines that regularly features a mix of styles.

I spend a few hours a week looking for "sophisticated pornography" online. I write erotica and my wife proofs it. On several occasions we have ended up acting out some of my fictional stories, making them true stories after-the-fact!

Chatting, Cybersex, and Romance

Do you enjoy reciting your sexual escapades for friends or lovers? Do you fantasize about having an alter ego of a different gender or sexual orientation? Do you wish for sexual adventures that are entirely risk-free and turn out exactly as you imagined? If you answered yes to any of these, you're a good candidate for hooking up with someone online for a little virtual sex play.

What differentiates this category from the others we've discussed is that it's strictly about communication *between users*, versus a site operator or Web host who posts information that you read at your leisure. It's simply a convenient way for users to hook up and talk. Chat usually takes two forms: real time, in which the conversation happens instantaneously, and delayed time, in which messages are posted and received sequentially over time.

Chatting in Real Time

On most systems, you can engage in "live" chats with other users, that is, typed conversations taking place in real time. Chatrooms are usually devoted to a specific topic and proceed like cocktail parties where guests mingle in groups or pair off for more private conversations. Each line you type is displayed, along with your handle (your online pseudonym) to everyone in that room, though most chat programs have a way for individuals to exchange private messages. Although AOL's popular chatrooms pioneered the chat craze, many websites today offer chat functions and sometimes feature special guests or events.

Web-based chats (like Yahoo, MSN, or site-sponsored chats) are usually fairly easy to access, and the site provides the necessary software for free. These are a good way to get your feet wet in the chat world, as they don't require much technical expertise and are fairly intuitive. A bit more complicated is IRC (Internet Relay Chat), which uses shareware to connect you to many different Internet channels with chatrooms galore on every conceivable subject. If you're new to chat, we recommend visiting one of the excellent websites devoted to chat basics to get tips on technical aspects, "netiquette," and privacy.

Chatting in Delayed Time

The most popular methods of delayed chat, in which users post and read messages sequentially, are commonly known as discussion boards, forums, or conferences. These are public discussions on topics of shared interest, but unlike live chats, each message is saved on the site so that users can track the thread of a discussion as it progresses. Groups are identified by very specific topic headings, to keep all participants "on the subject." You can exchange ideas on sexual politics, technique, and pornography with hundreds of other users. Sample topics range from "how to give/receive a good rim job" to "where to see authentic female orgasms in porn."

Discussion boards existed before the Web and were organized into a huge hierarchy known as Usenet News, which is now accessible through Web browsers. Usenet News is organized into general categories, and the "alt" category (short for "alternative") houses an infinite number of sex discussions. There is a group somewhere in the alt.sex hierarchy for nearly any sexual specialty you can think of. The longer the group name, the more specific the topic, so whether you'd rather chat about *Star Trek* or sheep you can log right in to alt.sex.fetish.startrek or alt.sex.sheep.baaa.baaa.baaa.moo!

Mailing lists (also known as listservs) are an email-based variety of discussion boards. Members subscribe to a website's mailing list on a specific topic, and each member's email commentary is forwarded to the entire group. This can save you the trouble of constantly logging on to a discussion board and is a good way to stay informed of late-breaking news or events. Mailing lists tend to attract a group of more committed participants, and can have a real family-like feel.

Finally, private email provides a simple, direct method of communication. You can use email to exchange sweet seductions with a trans-Atlantic pen pal you've never met or to spice up your lover's boring day at the office. You don't need the Web to send email, though many websites and ISPs do provide free email services.

Surfing Tips

Safety

- Don't give out personal information in chatrooms or in your member profile.
- Use anonymous email to protect your privacy.
- If you get unwanted messages, ignore them; simply don't respond. If they persist, see whether your software allows you to block mail from a specific sender, or complain to the site administrator.
- If you plan to meet your online pal in person, take some precautions: Meet in public, tell a friend where you're going, bring cab fare and a cell phone, practice safer sex.

Netiquette

- If you're a new user (a "newbie"), read for a while to learn protocol before joining chats and news groups.
- Read a website's FAQ (frequently asked questions) to reduce unnecessary questions.
- Be brief in your comments and give others a chance to speak.
- Practice good spelling and grammar.
- Refrain from making moral judgments or proselytizing.
- Stick to the subject and avoid redundancy.
- Be polite, greet newcomers, avoid foul language (unless you're talking dirty!).
- Avoid uppercase, it's the equivalent of SHOUTING.

Cybersex

This is the term most people use when referring to a sexual act that takes place online between two or more people. Each party sits at a computer and pounds away at the keyboard (and other sensitive areas), until the desired climax is achieved.

WHAT'S THE APPEAL? As with phone sex, the appeal of cybersex has to do with anonymity and the interactive fantasy component. You can be as nasty as you want to be with other users—sharing erotic stories, describing sexual encounters, initiating virtual sex acts—either publicly (which has the appeal of exhibitionism and group sex) or privately. Because no one ever sees you, you can try out different names, personalities, genders, or sexual preferences.

Cybersex is great because you really get to use your imagination and yet you know (or think you know) that someone else is getting off right along with you.

There is an anonymous quality that allows one to be a bit of a voyeur without any involvement, and that is kind of fun.

Perhaps because you may never see the other users, a particular type of intimacy and conversation develops. Shy people often feel freer to assert or reveal themselves in this faceless format; a strong sense of community often results.

The Net allows an unguarded level of conversation that I would never, or only rarely, be able to engage in with women I meet every day. I find that informative, fun, and stimulating intellectually as well as sexually.

With electronic sex you don't have to worry about catching a disease or being rejected. I can experiment with all kinds of sex because there are no consequences.

As this woman points out, cybersex can also be a great stand-in for couples who don't live together:

When my lover and I were living a thousand miles apart for a year or so, we would often chat with each other privately on the Net, and exchange long, involved fantasies with each other—usually one-handed! At the moment of climax each of us would pound the

keyboard with our free hand, letting our partner know by the spray of gibberish what had just happened. Sounds corny? That's love in the time of the Internet for you.

There are some downsides to cybersex. Some find it hard to masturbate and type at the same time (may we suggest a strap-on vibrator?). Others find cybersex unsatisfying after the novelty wears off. And many women complain about having to fight off a barrage of sexual solicitations in their efforts to find someone worth cybering with.

I find the lesbian chatrooms boring! I am always accused of being a man because I want to talk about sex. This is ridiculous. As if "real" lesbians don't fantasize or have sex.

I engaged in cybersex for a short while but ultimately found it dull, redundant, and inefficient (too hard to type and masturbate at the same time...for this woman, anyway!). I also found it to be too anonymous for me. I like to make real, genuine person-to-person connections and that is a huge challenge when staring at a computer screen.

IS CYBERSEX CHEATING? THE GREAT DEBATE: People tend to fall into two camps when it comes to this issue. In one camp are the folks who feel that, yes, cybersex is cheating if you're in a monogamous relationship.

Now that I'm married, I very much believe in keeping my activities strictly monogamous. I don't have interactive sexual communication/relations with anyone.

In the other camp are those who feel that cybersex is simply another form of sexual exploration, no different from reading erotica, fantasizing, or masturbating. We fall into this camp, and we'd encourage you to look at cybersex as a sexual enhancement tool, which—at its best—provides the opportunity to explore your fantasies, learn new techniques, and adopt a bolder communication style. Sure, if you're cybering to avoid, replace, or hurt your partner, that's a problem (and not one caused by your computer), but if you're just experimenting for fun and pleasure, cybersex might actually enhance your sex play with a real life partner. As our friend Michael Castleman likes to say, "Who cares how you get your appetite as long as you come home for dinner?!"

Cybersex led me to some AMAZING phone sex encounters that have been very powerful...and also resulted in meeting some very wonderful people.

I love to have cybersex with my husband. I travel on business a lot, so there are times when we are apart for a week—and sometimes even two. So having cyber and phone sex helps. It's one big sex-fest when I get home, though!

I see cybersex as a very abstracted form of mutual masturbation combined with intermixed fantasies.

Romance and Dating

Plenty of people go online in search of real life partners. Matchmaking sites have proliferated, taking personal ads to a whole new level of detail and sophistication. Members can maintain detailed profiles of their physical characteristics, social preferences, and partner requirements, and can then search on many of these same features when looking for a potential mate. Some people like to post photos with their profiles, others wait till they've made contact before sending one out.

I've found online dating services (Yahoo, etc.) to be really refreshing. I live in a small college town without a lot of dating possibilities. I've been able to hook up with a number of folks in nearby metropolitan areas. Particularly since my last long-term relationship ended, I've found it really empowering to know that I can always find people to date.

While there are plenty of generic matchmaking/personals sites online, there are also a growing number of sites that focus on more sexually explicit subject matter. They take the same basic personals concept, but allow members to detail specific sexual activities, techniques, or interests. These sites are great for folks who just want to cut to the chase—no essays about long walks on the beach or candlelight dinners. They can also provide a more direct way to simply engage in a bit of cybersex with people you've screened beforehand—a nice alternative to the cattle-call atmosphere of chatrooms.

Privacy

At Good Vibrations we've always recognized the importance of respecting our customers' right to privacy, which is why we've never sold our mailing list, sent unsolicited catalogs, or emblazened the company name all over our packaging. But with the widespread popularity of the Web, more and more people are worrying about whether the sites they patronize care at all about privacy.

Data Tracking

Yes, it's true, computer technology makes it easier than ever to track, retain, and traffic in all kinds of information about you and your surfing habits. But most sites aren't out to scam, harass, or bombard you with junk mail. As with anything, the few who exploit the system tend to give it a bad name.

If you're concerned about what people can find out about you online, go see for yourself. Do a search on your name, look yourself up in the online yellow pages, and check the user profiles you've filled out to see if you're carelessly divulging unnecessary information. Delete what you don't want known yourself, or ask your ISP to do so.

Think twice before giving out information. Lots of sites take advantage of promotions, contests, or "free registration" to capture your email and demographic information. In most cases they're just trying to determine how best to market products to you in the future. If you're worried about unwittingly signing up for a lifetime of spam, read the fine print before signing up. Many sites have an opt-out clause if you don't want to receive their marketing literature. If you're uncomfortable providing any of the "required" information, check the site's privacy policy first, or simply don't sign up.

Many sites track your surfing habits with a device known as a "cookie"—a piece of data about your visit that the site stores on your computer's hard drive to access upon your return. Cookies are often a necessary part of a retail site's shopping cart system, but the data can be compiled and sold to other companies. Some excellent websites explain "cookies" and how to disable them.

Reputable sites are aware of consumer privacy concerns and will post privacy policies or join organizations like TRUSTe, which require members to follow certain standards when gathering customer data.

And then there's spam. Anyone who's ever received a trickle of spam in their in-box knows that with time the ensuing onslaught makes paper junk mail seem like child's play. At least we can all relax that no trees were killed in the process. Sadly, once your email address gets out there, it's really hard to prevent spam, unless you close that account and start all over again with a new address. If you find spam unbearably annoying, visit an antispamming site for tips on minimizing its flow. As of this writing, spam-blocking software is available, though it may not block all spam.

Stalking

The media loves to pick up on the occasional online stalker story and use it to frighten the wits out of unsuspecting surfers. Yes, you should know that it is possible for virtually anyone to read your email, impersonate you, access the personal information you provided when you signed up with your ISP, grab your password, or track all of your online activities. This, however, is rare. Bear in mind that it's also possible for someone to tap your phone lines and bug your house, but this has probably never happened to you. It's good to be aware of potential risks, but this shouldn't prevent you from exploring or having a good time. People's fear of online crime has more to do with ignorance of this new technology than with

any statistically greater threat. The Web hosts some of the friendliest, most accessible communities you could ever hope to join, so our advice to you is to log on, exercise common sense—and enjoy.

The Communications Revolution

Change rarely comes without controversy. The information superhighway, with its free-flowing exchange of sex information and erotica, has naturally become a fertile breeding ground for legislative interference. Check out our resource listings under "Freedom of Expression" for a list of organizations dedicated to defending your right to online sexual materials.

Many people harbor the anxiety that technological advancements like the Web only make us more dependent on machines—who'll bother to have sex with a real person if virtual sex is so safe and satisfying? It's worth bearing in mind that even the most realistic simulation is still only a simulation, and could never replace the real thing. Cybersex doesn't satisfy the need for physical stimulation or companionship, and vibrators don't diminish the desire for a big kiss on the mouth. The primary appeal of any high-tech toy is its potential to stimulate our most powerful low-tech toy—our erotic imagination. With each new technological innovation, we can expand our fantasy realm and learn more about pleasure.

PROFILES *in* PLEASURE:

The Society for Human Sexuality

"I think that the Internet provides a type of 'emotional safety' for folks who want to explore ideas that they might be too embarrassed to bring up in real-life."

Spend just a few minutes online researching sex and you will inevitably wind up at the granddaddy of sex information sites, the Society for Human Sexuality (SHS). Home to one of the largest online collections of sexuality materials, SHS contains articles on hundreds of subjects—from aphrodisiacs to handballing to vibrators—along with how-tos, interviews, transcripts, and FAQS as well as reviews of books, toys, and videos. Archives of out-of-print sex publications and the work of many excellent sex writers reside here, along with resources and instructions for sex activists and community organizers.

What began as a University of Washington student organization that sponsored sex-positive events on its Seattle campus soon blossomed into an online resource. Russell, one of its founders, currently maintains the site, which attracts well over fifty thousand visitors per day. Imagine that many people showing up at your neighborhood library or bookstore, and you get an idea of the service SHS provides.

All the information is free, and readers are not subjected to any advertising or promotional gimmicks. This is just one among several key reasons Russell believes the site has been so successful. "I'd say persistence, not going commercial during the dot-com bubble economy, always assuming the reader doesn't mind reading, and sticking with the core value of respect for the broad range of consensual adult sexual expression. These are the main reasons for our success."

SHS attracts a lot of Web newbies, who find the site helpful and nonthreatening. "I think that the Internet provides a type of 'emotional safety' for folks who want to explore ideas that they might be too embarrassed to bring up in real-life," says Russell. "It's an easy 'first step' for many people!"

Longevity also contributes to the site's popularity. Having launched in 1995, SHS qualifies as one of the oldest sex sites on the Web, earning much of its audience through extensive links—the online equivalent of word-of-mouth recommendations. Although Russell maintains that the site's first webmaster didn't even know what a Web page was when they began, the group quickly discovered the advantages of the Internet. According to Russell, "The Net's strong suits are helping you find initial pointers to books, classes, and ideas on subjects that you don't yet know anything about; finding information about topics too exotic to merit publication in a book of their own; getting free information quickly and privately regardless of where you live and who you are; and finding 'communities' of people who share your interests."

Russell believes that the Web has barely begun to fulfill its potential as a sexuality resource. Meanwhile, SHS serves as a model, publishing only material that demonstrates or advocates thoughtfulness, tolerance, consensuality, and sexual responsibility. One need only read a few of its popular pieces on erotic massage, the G-spot, sexual positions, or safer sex to appreciate the contribution SHS continues to make to sexual understanding and acceptance.

The Society for Human Sexuality is located at www.sexuality.org.

CHAPTER 17

S/M and Power Play

My favorite thing is when my lover takes total control, dominates me, doesn't ask what I need or want because she knows already; she just goes right ahead and takes me, talking to me the whole time.

Holding my partner down is fun when I'm so hungry I can't stand it and want to devour him and make him surrender to my touch. I love the power I feel in taking control of the situation and possessing another person.

Do either of these sentiments ring a bell for you? We think it's a safe bet that you're aroused by both the thought of being overpowered by a partner and the idea of overpowering a partner. Sexual power play has always had a near-universal appeal, but many of you who readily incorporate aspects of dominance and submission into your sex lives might be surprised to learn that these could be described as S/M activities.

The term *S/M* or *S&M* evolved from abbreviations of the word *sadomasochism*, which the dictionary defines as the "perversion" of deriving sexual pleasure from either the infliction or the experience of pain. Popular misconceptions about S/M can be traced to this dictionary definition and are aggravated by the fact that *sadomasochism* is frequently used to describe the *nonsexual* dynamic between people involved in coercive or abusive behaviors: For example, a bullying boss or battering husband is referred to as a "sadist," while anyone physically or emotionally self-destructive is referred to as a "masochist." Hollywood and TV moviemakers have done their bit to exacerbate stereotypes about S/M by spicing up their thrillers with plots involving murderous practitioners of "S&M." Talk about having your cake and eating it, too—the public is invited to revel in titillating images of spike-heeled dominatrixes or leather-clad masters, but by the final reel, all the evil sadists and pathetic masochists have been incarcerated or killed, and kinder, gentler virtue triumphs.

In fact, S/M has nothing to do with coercion, either sexual or nonsexual. The common denominator in all S/M play is not a violent exchange of pain but a consensual exchange of power. The distinction that S/M is about eroticized power play, not about physical or emotional abuse, is crucial to understanding and demystifying the subject. Some people in the S/M community feel that "sadomasochism" is therefore an inaccurate and inappropriate word to describe their experience, preferring terms such as dominance and submission, sensuality and mutuality, sexual magic, sensual magic, radical sex, or power and trust. You'll also frequently encounter the acronym BDSM, which encompasses a variety of sexual practices or fantasies involving power exchange: B/D refers to bondage and discipline, D/S to dominance and submission, and S/M to sadomasochism.

As the definition of S/M has broadened to include any eroticism that revolves around role-playing, power exchange, and heightening sensation, there's been a notable upsurge of interest in the topic. With growing awareness of the risks of sexually transmitted diseases, many people are intrigued by the prospect of sexual play that is highly arousing yet doesn't presume genital sex. S/M clubs and organizations across the country offer lectures, workshops, and play parties enabling participants to explore power play in a safe, structured context. The negotiation and communication required before two or more people embark on an S/M session can improve your chances of achieving sexual satisfaction, whether you're relative strangers meeting up for a one-night adventure or you're a long-term couple looking to break out of the rut of predictable sex.

When you factor in the popularization of fetish items such as leather, lingerie, collars, and corsets as seen on MTV and in fashion magazines, you have the phenomenon our friend Susie Bright dubs "S/M lite"—S/M imagery that has permeated mainstream culture. The Internet—which allows those curious about power play to access accurate information, resources, and a global community of like-minded enthusiasts—has played a huge part in bringing S/M out of the closet.

Of course, there's nothing new under the sun, and power play has been a compelling aspect of human sexuality from the get-go. One archeologist has even theorized that one of the Ice Age Venus figurines depicts a woman whose wrists are bound together by bands of fur (see the entertaining chapter "S&M on the Steppe" in Timothy Taylor's *Prehistory of Sex*). If erotic bondage was good enough for our ancestors some 25,000 years ago, why shouldn't it be good enough for us today?

The following chapter briefly introduces you to an erotic style enjoyed and explicated by a wide range of articulate spokespersons. If what you read here sparks your curiosity, we encourage you to contact one of the numerous social and educational organizations available to people interested in exploring S/M—

national organizations may be able to refer you to a group or chapter in your own town. Check out our resource listings for referrals to S/M organizations as well as a selection of the many excellent books, videos, and websites devoted to power play.

Let's Define Our Terms
About Power Exchange

In S/M play, one partner assumes the dominant or "top" role, while the other assumes the submissive or "bottom" role in a prearranged encounter that is commonly referred to as a "scene." This role-playing can take subtle to elaborate forms, and scenes may last for a few minutes or a few days. At the subtle end of the spectrum, you might play a dominant role by directing your partner to wear a particular item of clothing or to assume a particular position in bed. Or you might play a submissive role by agreeing that you won't allow yourself to reach orgasm until your partner gives you permission to come. At the more elaborate end of the spectrum, you can make an erotic contract with your partner in which one of you serves as obedient sex-slave to the other. A day later, you might each switch roles.

The bottom line is, you can't dominate your partner unless he or she allows you to take control, and you can't submit to your partner unless he or she accepts control. The interdependency and fluidity of the power exchange implicit in S/M is expressed by the slash between the letters S and M—the two poles of the S/M experience are connected. One can't exist in isolation from the other.

I love giving up control! Being made to hold back my orgasm until I have permission to come makes my orgasms stronger and more intense. I feel so taken care of.

Why, you may be asking yourself, would anyone want to take a dominant or submissive role during sex? To which we would respond: Have you taken a look at your own sex life lately? Sex between two people rarely proceeds along a strictly egalitarian path of mutual arousal to a simultaneous orgasm—more likely, each partner takes turns controlling the sensations the other is feeling. An ever-shifting power dynamic is fundamental to any human interaction. The range of feelings that arise during sex are hardly restricted to hearts-and-flowers sentimentality—protectiveness, vulnerability, abandonment, selfishness, curiosity, spite, pride, and love are all emotions that may ebb and flow in an intimate encounter.

Sometimes I'm almost frightened by how determined I am to make my partner come purely for my own selfish pleasure, just to hear her scream and watch her lose control.

You might recoil at the thought that humiliating a partner could be arousing, but who hasn't enjoyed teasing a lover in the manner described below:

I like to rim my most recent male partner or lick his butt, because he moans a lot when I do. He hates to be involuntarily demonstrative, yet he finds it pleasurable, so he's in this quandary. He usually makes me stop because he's embarrassed about moaning.

Perhaps the gentleman described in this quote might benefit from a stern mistress or master who'd tie him down, lick him to distraction, and refuse to release him until his moans of pleasure were fully audible. After all, he's withholding pleasure, not only from his partner, but from himself—perhaps if someone else takes over the task of "punishing" him for his demonstrative ways, he'll no longer feel compelled to punish himself by censoring his responses. Abdicating control and putting your partner in the driver's seat is a highly effective way to make an end run around your own sexual shame and self-denial.

The Fantasy Connection

A closer look at your own sexual fantasies may give you some further clues as to the appeal of power play. Many people enjoy fantasies that break down into one of two categories. One popular fantasy theme is that of being completely subjugated by kidnappers, rapists, aliens, etc.

I fantasize being forcefully "taken" with one or more men watching and waiting their turns, while my partner directs the action.

The complementary and equally popular fantasy theme is that of being in complete erotic control of a stable full of love slaves, some real-life authority figure, a celebrity, etc.

In my fantasy I'm dominating a man and a woman who are completely at my disposal for any activity I plan for them, i.e., bondage, spanking, anal penetration with dildos.

Power play is central to our erotic imaginations, and practitioners of S/M often argue that consciously addressing this fact has brought a heightened self-awareness, honesty, and integrity to their sexual life that so-called "vanilla" (non-S/M) sex simply cannot provide.

I have fantasized about S/M for most of my life, and have just started exploring my fantasies in the flesh. My new lover is FTM. Being with transfolk involves learning about how potent a sexual organ the mind is. Power play just expands that awareness, and it amplifies excitement, experience, and satisfaction. It requires a trust more overt and profound than that generally experienced in life, and that trust provides the foundation for unparalleled intensity.

Who's on Bottom?

What, specifically, is the appeal of taking a submissive role? In many ways it mirrors the appeal of subjugation fantasies. The implication that you are so desirable and alluring that an overpowering dominant will stop at nothing to possess you is the crux of time-honored fantasies ranging from ravishment by bodice-ripping pirates to prison-yard gang bangs. The fantasy that you inspire overwhelming desire frees you to be swept away by your own sexual desires—at the same time, you're released from responsibility for anything you might say or do. This surrender can be a particular relief to those who feel guilty or ambivalent about sex.

I've just recently begun experimenting with dominance and submission—seems to free me up to "lose control" more easily.

It can also be liberating to those who crave lots of sensation to reach orgasm. Whereas you may feel embarrassed by your own high tolerance for stimulation or for being a "hard come" in vanilla sex situations, as a greedy, "insatiable" submissive you can be an object of pride and respect.

I like being bound and teased—I'm excitingly embarrassed by how kinky I can get when provoked or manipulated to respond sexually. It lets me be free to enjoy sex deeply.

I like it when someone else uses the vibrator on me. It's a power thing. When I'm controlling the vibrator, I have the power to slow down when I think it is too much for me or if I want to savor the sensations. But if someone else is controlling it, then I am at their mercy. I like having my partner see what makes me go wild.

Submissive scenarios can also be a pleasant relief to individuals who have plenty of responsibility in their daily professional lives and yearn for the opportunity to relinquish control in their personal lives.

My most rewarding experience of power play was with a guy who tended to get really stressed about his work and would go crazy trying to overanalyze everything. When he really started freaking out, I'd tie his arms and legs to the bed, blindfold him, and just toy with him for hours until he could clear his mind and get a fresh start on whatever had been bothering him.

The popular misconception that S/M is somehow sexist or demeaning to women has its roots in the presumption that the dominant in any S/M scene will necessarily be that individual who has the greatest economic and social power. Yet, there's no direct correlation between an individual's actual socioeconomic status and her or his preference in sexual role-playing—many wealthy, powerful executives of both genders quite fancy a spanking in their off hours. Furthermore, this "S/M is demeaning" model implies that the submissive is viewed as the partner of lesser value, which isn't the case. After all, as we've said before, it takes two to tango—we'd hate to see anxiety over political correctness inhibiting any of our readers' pleasure in taking a spin around the dance floor.

As a man committed to feminism and equality, it took me a long time to discover that I might want to try playing with power dynamics in sex, but now that I have, it is a major turn on for me. I like to be bossy and forceful, and, after careful negotiation, my partner and I regularly incorporate forced-sex fantasies into our sexual repertoire. The emotions that can be brought out during this kind of play are strong, and experimenting with them seems to be a way of taking sex to a deeper level.

A few years ago I started doing some exploration into my submissive side. There are so many areas of my life that I have to keep under control that I was looking for one area where I could relinquish control and just do as I'm told. Unfortunately, hubby doesn't understand this. He was raised by a raving feminist so equality is very important to him. He thinks that if I do something just because he's ordered me to, then I'm not enjoying it as much as he is. I've tried to explain that there's just as much enjoyment in the submission as in the act, but he hasn't bought into that yet. I'm still working on him.

The classic contradiction of being a submissive is that while you are ostensibly subservient to your dominant, in fact you remain the center of attention, which implies that you are very valuable. This promotes a pampered, childlike security that counterbalances the vulnerability involved in expressing your craving for subordination. In childhood, we all experience a painful sense of powerlessness. Willingly relinquishing control as an adult can give you a paradoxical sense of power—after embracing weakness and dependency, you can come out of the experience reassured of your strength and autonomy.

Who's on Top?

What, specifically, is the appeal of taking a dominant role? The appeal is that you're on top!—your partner has entrusted you to run the show. You control what happens and who gets off when. You also have the responsibility for your partner's safety and enjoyment. Ideally, you shouldn't do unto your submissive anything that hasn't at one time or another been done unto you. You may want to focus on your partner's pleasure.

S/M is something I'm doing with my current partner. I find tying her up and having her "at my mercy" while I'm playing with her nipples, pussy, etc. is very erotic and also quite fun.

I tied her up and went down on her for an hour or so— she was so swollen and sensitive. Then I used her vibrator directly on her clit and gave her at least ten orgasms.

You may want to focus on your own pleasure.

My partner goes down on me while I whip her with a crop. Her pain is commensurate to my pleasure.

I strap a dildo onto my partner and order him to lie back while I ride him. He's not allowed to move, to touch me, or to touch himself. It makes him crazy to have my breasts right over his face, and my ass bouncing right over his cock without his being able to touch me.

Just as being a submissive frees you to yield control and embrace vulnerability, being a dominant frees you to both take control and embrace authority. The dominant can explore feelings frowned upon in our society—selfishness, cruelty, superiority, and lust for power—and can act these out in the context of pleasing a partner. Your partner's trust can be highly intoxicating, and the experience of tapping into your own "dark side" can be quite liberating as well.

The flip side of this freedom is the responsibility for maintaining complete focus on your partner, ensuring that his or her physical or emotional limits are not transgressed, and being the one who's taking care of the situation. It can take courage, especially for the novice dominant, to muster up the self-confidence and panache necessary to carry off a scene. Willingness to assume this responsibility and to expend the energy involved in sustaining a scene is a gift from the dominant to the submissive.

I really like S/M role-playing games. I'm a top. I find pleasure in creating a scene for my lover. It's a custom-made gift created with the deepest of love.

In return, the dominant may acquire a newfound sense of confidence:

When I was growing up, women were taught to be passive, to keep sex from happening so we wouldn't get pregnant. It was an interesting challenge for me to learn to initiate sex and direct the action. What I found was that when I started exploring dominance in the bedroom, it gave me a great deal more confidence in everyday life.

What about Pain?

While it's true that S/M is not fundamentally about pain, it's equally true that some S/M activities—such as whipping or applying nipple clamps—may sound pretty darn uncomfortable. It's more accurate, though, to describe these activities as producing sensation than producing pain. Think about it. If you were from

another planet and you walked into an aerobics class, you might be astonished to learn that the students had paid to undergo this torture. We live on the beautiful California coastline, and every weekend the coastal highway is filled with bicyclists pedaling their way to the top of each hill with grim expressions that hardly seem to denote recreational bliss. Yet, if quizzed by an alien, both the aerobics students and the bicyclists would likely say that they were proud to have worked their way up to this level of exertion, and that actually their physical activities serve to pump intoxicating levels of endorphins through their bloodstreams. Even when physical exertion is painful, there's a big subjective difference between pain that you're controlling and training yourself to surmount and pain that you didn't expect or request.

Similarly, if you were to walk in on a scene of a man being flogged, you might assume that he was in great pain, but he would probably describe himself as being in an altered state of heightened sensation. Sexual arousal affects how we perceive pain. You've doubtlessly had the experience of enjoying certain types of stimulation during sex—hair-pulling, nipple-biting, scratching—which you wouldn't enjoy in the slightest once your arousal had subsided. It's a bit arbitrary to coo proudly over the scratches and bites you've received during passionate lovemaking and then pass judgment on the crop marks somebody else received during his or her passionate lovemaking.

I have always incorporated elements of S/M into my sexual experiences. I remember a boy kissing me at a party when I was 14. I wasn't really that interested in him until he started clawing my back with his nails. He made me bleed and I wound up dating him for years.

I love to be on the receiving end of domination. Not that I can't enjoy sex without it, but it takes things to another level. Pain brings things into focus, heightens my senses and reactions, and underlines the intimacy of the experience. Anticipation does the same thing. For power play to work, though, it definitely requires a few things. Trust is one, probably the biggest. And it has to be a mutual activity.

It's also worth noting that individuals with neurological disabilities that dull their perception of physical stimulation sometimes experience pleasure exclusively from the intense sensation provided by certain S/M activities. And some able-bodied individuals who pursue intense sensation do so as an almost meditative discipline, a way of triumphing over and transcending the flesh.

What about Fetishes?

Certain objects, materials, or body parts can trigger sexual desire in individuals who fetishize them. Clothing fetishes are probably the most common, and many people harbor fetishes for uniforms or lingerie, or for materials such as leather or latex. A fetish can be mild (the object or material helps enhance a sexual scene) or extreme (the object or material is essential to sexual arousal).

> Power and uniforms turn me on a lot. My favorite thing to do is to make a partner take off my boots— which are laced up to my knees—and give me head the whole time she's working on the boots.

We are mentioning the topic here, as folks with fetishes sometimes become part of their local S/M communities principally to have a chance to dress up in and be close to the material or clothing they love. The point is, don't assume that because somebody loves leather, she or he necessarily enjoys S/M play. Likewise, someone who enjoys S/M doesn't necessarily love leather. Dressing up in fetish clothing, be it lacy lingerie or studded leather, is one of the most universal ways of being sexually adventurous, but while costuming may be part of an S/M scene, it doesn't serve as a signpost.

> I joined the Outcasts, the lesbian S/M group, so I could meet women who'd appreciate my wardrobe. Now I'm thinking of starting a group called the Outfits, especially for girls who like to dress up.

What's the Appeal of S/M?

It's Exciting

Few things are as dampening to sexual excitement as predictability. Eroticism thrives on drama, particularly the drama of surmounting obstacles, whether these obstacles are long distances, family ties, or religious proscriptions. In his groundbreaking book *The Erotic Mind*, psychotherapist Jack Morin suggests that the equation for unforgettable sex is "attraction + obstacles = excitement." He lists four "cornerstones" or common contributors to sexual arousal: longing and anticipation,

violating prohibitions, searching for power, and overcoming ambivalence.

Half the thrill of sexually engaging with a new partner is the thrill of the unknown: the myriad possibilities of seduction, the opportunity to present whatever side of yourself you choose, the mystery of your new partner's responses. Hot sex requires an "other" to react against, and sustaining your identities as separate individuals is crucial to sustaining a sexual spark. Many long-term couples know that the key to keeping their sex lives fresh is to take neither each other nor each other's availability for granted. The common experience of having passionate sex after a big fight is just one example of how asserting differences or raising a temporary obstacle can stoke the sexual fires.

S/M play incorporates these erotic "cornerstones," and can reintroduce the thrill of the unknown into even the most familiar of relationships. Preparing for an S/M scene involves building anticipation, exploring taboos and prohibitions, negotiating power, and defining limits of physical and emotional resistance. S/M combines the drama and unpredictability of seduction with the security of prearranged boundaries. The heightened mutual awareness you must bring to an S/M encounter is what makes S/M play so much more memorable for its practitioners than vanilla sex.

It's Dramatic

S/M involves accessing your imaginative, playful side. In preparing for S/M play, you are essentially preparing for erotic theater—you choose to incorporate whatever dramatic tension, aspects of your fantasies, props, or costumes you find most arousing. Role-playing, as anyone who ever played cops and robbers as a kid can testify, is both fun and liberating. You are freed to express parts of yourself that you don't express in daily life, and you can play-act frightening or dangerous situations while remaining completely safe. The use of the word "scene" to describe an S/M encounter is in keeping with this theatrical metaphor.

It's Safe

S/M play is safer sex, in the same way that playing with sex toys is safer sex. Both these sexual variations deemphasize genital intercourse or the exchange of bodily fluids and emphasize a full-body approach to sex. The S/M community has been active in advocating safer sex through its organizations and classes and in upholding safer sex guidelines at parties, events, and workshops. The one creed linking the vast variety of S/M activities is that all S/M play must be "safe, sane, and consensual." According to this maxim, no one should embark on an S/M scene without clear communication of each party's physical and emotional limits plus a certain level of mutual trust. Excessive drug or alcohol consumption, which could impair a dominant's judgment while blunting a submissive's awareness of having exceeded physical limits, is also discouraged.

It's Inclusive

The S/M community is somewhat unique in including and incorporating individuals of different ages, backgrounds, and sexualities. While there are and always will be specific organizations for gays, lesbians, or heterosexuals involved in S/M, the community as a whole tends to be inclusive on the basis of a shared interest in power play. It's also worth noting that the S/M community puts a high premium on experienced practitioners, and that this is one sexual subculture in which age and maturity can be seen as a turn-on, rather than a turn-off. How refreshing.

Of course, as this survey respondent indicates, no community is perfect!

> In truth, I got fed up with the S/M community in my town and turned my back on it. Sometimes I miss some of the people, but I'm not sure it's worth it to go back and hear all their silly rules: "You're a submissive. Why are you capitalizing your name?" "A dominant shouldn't behave that way!" and perfectly idiotic prejudices: "Dominants are smarter than submissives." "People into S/M are smarter than people into vanilla sex." "Why can't switches make up their minds?" Gag me!

Getting Started

Defining Your Desires

If you're intrigued by the thought of experimenting with sexual power play, you may be wondering, where do I go from here? First, examine your own desires and expectations. Your sexual fantasies can reveal a lot about what aspects of power exchange you find most exciting and what types of role-playing appeal to you. Of course, it's possible that your most exciting fantasies are those you have no intention of acting out. Some people's fantasies are in counterbalance to their actual sexual behavior.

> Even though I define myself as a top, my fantasies are as a bottom. I have straight fantasies, which freaks me out. I only think this way while fantasizing. Once sex is over, if I think of men, I'll be nauseated!

Many people enjoy two types of fantasies: the "I'd never do this in a million years, but I sure get hot thinking about it" fantasy and the "I'd leap at the chance to make this one come true" fantasy.

> I want to be topped by five or six butch leather dykes. I want an enema. I want to be whipped and pierced. Those are the ones I want to actually happen. The fantasy that makes me come the fastest these days is of getting fucked by men in hotel rooms for money. But I don't necessarily want that to actually happen.

Think about what key elements inspire your hottest fantasies: Is it certain positions, certain words, the idea of being spoken to in a certain tone of voice, certain items of clothing, certain locations, certain smells? Identifying these elements could help you identify the components of a satisfying scene.

> I like the idea of being super cozy and in those full-length zip-up pajamas with the plastic white feet and sucking each other's thumbs. I have this idea of a giant regression playground where we just enjoy sensuous activity without any orgasmic goal, like someone rubbing my asshole with lube, or sliding around in oil, or kissing forever, or role-playing that we're children playing at grown-up sex who don't know what we're doing.

Get specific about what activities you do and don't want to explore. An excellent exercise is to make three lists: one list of all the erotic activities you've tried and know you like; one list of all the erotic activities you're sure you don't want to try; and one list of all the erotic activities you're curious about possibly trying. This will give you a frame of reference for how to proceed. You'll probably find it interesting to do this exercise once a year to see what activities move from one list to another over time—so much more functional and so much less discouraging than dusting off that list of New Year's resolutions!

Finding a Playmate

Suitably armed with all this self-knowledge, it's time to broach the topic with a partner. We know, this is the scary part. You could bring the matter up in a general way, by asking what he or she thinks of erotica such as *Story of O* or by describing that sexy panel of dominatrixes you saw on a daytime TV talk show. You can comment that you've had S/M fantasies and are curious whether he or she does too. Don't be disheartened if your partner's first response is a nervous joke about "whips and chains." There's a lot of misinformation generally available about S/M, and it's likely that the same person who expresses discomfort with the idea of whips has a fantasy bank full of army sergeants, schoolmistresses, and prison matrons. It may just take time to tease out the details of what types of role-playing might appeal.

Sometimes it's easier to discuss your fantasies with someone you've just met than with a long-term partner or spouse. Unfortunately, the more attached to someone you are, the more afraid you can become of revealing information that you fear your partner might find off-putting or silly. In either case, it helps to be as specific, nonthreatening, and nonjudgmental in your language as possible—for instance, "Sometimes I pretend that you own me, you've kept me locked in my apartment all day, and now you're coming over to have your way with me," as opposed to "Why don't you ever take charge in bed!" Or, "Yesterday, I imagined tying your hands to the bedposts and taking an hour to go down on you," as opposed to "You never let me take as long as I want!" Whatever response you get, remember that naming your own sexual desires is a brave act and you deserve a respectful response. By the same token, you should make every effort not to respond to any of your partner's suggestions or counterproposals with defensiveness or hostility.

Despite the most tactful communication on your part, you may find your proposal rejected. You have the option of seeking other like-minded potential partners at S/M classes, at social events, through personal ads, or in online chatrooms. You may consider employing the services of a professional, or you may decide to restrict your interest in S/M to fantasy and solo sex.

If you're in a monogamous relationship, you'll probably want to discuss your partner's reservations on more than one occasion, to see if you can reach some common understanding. Ideally, you'd be able to compromise on activities that would satisfy your curiosity without making your partner feel badgered or bullied into trying something against his or her will. It's possible that your partner has leapt to the conclusion that your interest in trying something new implies dissatisfaction with your current sex life, and that he or she just needs some reassurance.

Some people think sex should always be spontaneous and may protest that planning a sexual scenario seems cumbersome and artificial. You can remind your partner that in your courting days, both of you probably put plenty of time into planning your every encounter, yet your romance never suffered for it.

Negotiating a Scene

If you've both acknowledged interest in exploring power play, it's time for some fun research. Here's where those lists you wrote—detailing activities you've tried, ones you haven't tried but are curious about, and ones you have no interest in trying—come in handy. You and your partner could each draw up a set of lists and swap them as a basis for discussion. If either of you draws a blank at possible activities, you may find books and videos helpful and inspirational.

I watch porn videos nonsexually with a partner to actually see examples of things each of us likes. Then we discuss what we'd like to do.

Perhaps the first thing to agree on is who'll take the dominant and who'll take the submissive role. This decision can be based on anything from personal preference, to who has more experience, to flipping a coin. You should then clarify what activities you're each interested in trying and which you absolutely do not wish to try—for instance, "I'd like to be tied up and spanked, but I don't want to be blindfolded at any point." You should each know the other's level of experience with those activities on the "done this" list, as well as with any sexual activities you wish to incorporate into the scene. If you'd like to beat your partner with a crop, he or she may be understandably curious to know just how many times you've wielded a crop before. If you'd like to be tied up and anally penetrated with a dildo, your partner should know whether or not your previous experience of anal penetration has involved anything larger than a pinkie finger. The fact that you have the opportunity to enact some of your fantasies does not mean that every activity you undertake will flow as pleasurably and effortlessly as it does in your fantasies. Don't throw common sense out the window with your inhibitions.

TIMING: If you're at a play-party or negotiating with someone you've just met, your negotiation may serve as the foreplay to your scene. You might step right into your respective roles and work out the details, with the dominant adopting a top persona to interview the submissive. Or you may prefer to stay out of role during your discussion and to set a future date to play. There's certainly nothing wrong with giving yourselves time to let some anticipation build.

Couples who've been enjoying power play for some time probably won't need an elaborate negotiation before each scene. Advance notice could simply take the form of telling your partner over breakfast that you've got something planned for her when she comes home that night, or leaving explicit invitations on his voice mail. You may have developed your own personal ways of signaling your intentions—putting on a particular collar or wearing a special pair of boots.

You'll need to know how much time you've got together, as the pacing of your scene will vary depending on whether you have an hour before you have to get home and pay the baby-sitter, all night before you have to get to work, or an entire carefree weekend ahead of you.

LOCATION: As with any kind of date, the classic inquiry "my place or yours?" is a relevant consideration, and your decision may be dictated by any number of things: who has more privacy at home; who has more toys; who has eyebolts screwed into the wall; who has a four-poster bed; who has to get up early for work, etc. If you and you partner live together, you may wish to escape your daily routine and situate your scene in a hotel room or at a play-party.

Will it be a public scene? If all or part of your scene takes place at a restaurant, bar, or public space, you need to be discreet to avoid harassment or intrusion. You may, however, each have different ideas as to what constitutes "discreet." Set your guidelines ahead of time—how are you willing to be addressed and treated in public? Maybe you're willing to wear a collar, but not to be led on a leash. Maybe you're willing to be addressed as "Mistress," but not to have your partner sit at your feet in the taxi. It can be extremely arousing to be out on the town with your scene—don't let a misunderstanding ruin the mood.

Nothing excites me as much as secret public sex. I enjoy being ordered to wear butt plugs, vibrators, ben wa balls, or bondage under my clothes and then to be covertly disciplined in public.

If you're planning to get together at a play-party or with more than one person, you should negotiate how you're both going to interact with other people. Is there one particular person or several people who are welcome to join you? To what extent are you willing to have others participate in your scene: physically, genitally, voyeuristically? You can avoid a lot of unnecessary jealousy or bad feeling if you think things through ahead of time.

PERSONAS: You may be perfectly content simply to define your roles as dominant and submissive, without any further elaboration. Or you may want to establish some parameters. Is the top to be referred to as "Mistress," "Master," or "Sir"? Is the bottom allowed to make eye contact with the top? Should the bottom speak only when spoken to? You may want to assume very specific roles, which will determine what kinds of things you wear, say, or do. This is where you can let your creative juices flow. Now's the time to unlock your fantasy treasure chest and release a character or two. Perhaps you've always longed to play Roman senator and slave boy; Catherine the Great and stable hand; priest and nun; schoolmarm and student; doctor and patient; inquisitor and P.O.W.; parent and child...the list is endless.

I like to act out being some hot daddy's sex slave. I am kept naked and servile.

My partner pretends to be a bad little girl, and I'm the teacher giving her a bare-bottom spanking.

I like to pretend to be corrupting or initiating a much younger man who is inexperienced, but very interested in exploring sex with an older woman.

Whether or not you adopt specific characters, you'll probably find it both helpful and fun to dress up for your scene. You may well have a greater sense of conviction as a dominant when you're clad in leather, boots, or spiked heels. Your feelings of vulnerability and helplessness as a submissive could well be enhanced by revealing or restrictive clothes. Clothing can add a sensual impact, not to mention sound effects, that greatly enhance a scene—the sounds of stilettos clicking, leather creaking, zippers being forced open, and fabric tearing can be highly arousing. You don't need a celebrity diva's income to afford this kind of disposable wardrobe either—trips to the Goodwill can keep you costumed in style, and you may find that shopping becomes its own form of foreplay.

HEALTH AND SAFETY GUIDELINES: A top should make sure to get basic medical information from the bottom, so as not to endanger her or his health during the scene. Someone wearing contact lenses should not be tightly blindfolded. Someone with asthma or a cold shouldn't be gagged. You should both communicate about back pains, joint troubles, heart conditions, epilepsy, diabetes, high blood pressure, or any other conditions that could affect tolerance of pain, range of motion, and flexibility.

It's also crucial to discuss safer-sex guidelines and what genital sex, if any, you are willing to have. An S/M scene doesn't necessarily include sex.

I really love S/M as a turn-on prelude to sex, but also S/M can be a complete sex act in itself. With a good spanking, I can feel as good as if I had sex.

You should be very clear in advance whether or not your scene might include masturbation, oral sex, penetration of any kind, or sex toys, as well as which safer-sex precautions you choose to follow in each case. While this negotiation is particularly important when you're playing with a new partner, even long-term partners might find that they have different limits or desires around genital play during an S/M scene than during vanilla sex.

SAFEWORDS: Both partners need a way to clearly communicate if they are feeling overwhelmed and want to slow down or stop the action altogether. Safewords afford a quick and easy way to alert your partner to the fact that you need a break. Usually, couples agree on words or signals that will be completely unambiguous. *No, don't,* or *stop* are inefficient safewords, as you may well find yourself deep into role-playing and crying out these words without the slightest desire for anyone to

stop doing anything. *Yellow* or *red* are frequently used to mean "slow down" or "stop." Some couples agree to use the top's first name as a signal to ease up, or you can simply say, "safeword." The bottom line is, select a word that's easy to remember. It's also helpful to have a safe signal, such as snapping your fingers, in the event that one of you is gagged.

Expectations

S/M involves exploring fantasy and playing with illusion. As with any case of bringing a fantasy to life, you're far less likely to experience a disappointing discrepancy between dream and reality if you try to clarify your expectations and motivations ahead of time. Power play is a blend of mental, emotional, and physical stimulants, and simply going through the physical motions will probably not be particularly arousing in and of itself. Ask yourself what feeling you want to get out of your experience. Do you want to feel powerful, awe-inspiring, vulnerable, frightened, taken care of? Once you have a sense of the emotion you're seeking, you can figure out how best to go after it.

The same physical activity will be appealing to different people for different reasons. It helps to figure out not just what you like, but why you like it. You might want to be tied up because you like the sensation of immobility or because you like being exposed or the illusion of being someone's property. Is it important that you are being punished for an invented infraction, humiliated by a cruel dominant, trained by a loving master? The distinctions are crucial to the success of your scene. Neither you nor your partner can expect to intuit what intangible components will provide satisfaction and enhance sensation. Talk about it—S/M play provides a unique opportunity to get specific about naming your desires.

Finally, be realistic. Bear in mind that you can't do everything you've ever dreamed of in one session. If you leave each other wanting more, you're far more likely to play together again than if either one of you feels overwhelmed by what happened between you.

Toys and Techniques

For simplicity's sake, much of the following section is addressed to the top in a scene on the assumption that she or he will be the one wielding the toys. As you read on, please keep in mind that just as clothes don't make the man (or woman), toys don't make the scene. Although there's a tendency to equate S/M with the use of equipment, many people incorporate power play into their sex lives without a single prop. That you're intimidated by whips and can't tie a knot to save your life doesn't mean you can't be a thrilling dominant. Anyone's flair with toys can be enhanced if she or he has played without them first. The power of the human voice and an authoritative manner are greater than any ropes and chains.

I find the deepest pleasure in the trust aspects of intense sex. There is huge power and eroticism in giving your body to a sexual experience because you trust someone. I was once nervous about allowing a lover to penetrate my vagina with his cock and my ass with a dildo at the same time. His soothing voice assuring me that it would be OK and I could handle it almost sent me over the top before we even attempted it. It was heavenly.

Imagine ordering your partner to keep her legs spread wide open while you tease her clit, or directing your partner to keep his hands clasped over his head while you go down on him—if the punishment for disobeying is that you'll instantly stop what you're doing, chances are good that you will be obeyed to the letter.

Bondage

Restraining your partner or being restrained is a highly popular activity—many of our survey respondents listed bondage among their favorite sex games.

Once I put handcuffs on my boyfriend and sat him on the couch so I could play with him. I kissed him and touched him all over. It drove him nuts. He kept begging to be let free and stretching out his neck as far as he could to kiss me. I just kept pushing him back and telling him no. Then I started riding him and I loved feeling him strain against his bonds. He didn't have any control over what was happening. I think that's the closest I've ever come to losing it.

I'm both afraid of and fascinated with bondage. I tease and chide my partner until she ties me to the bed. And then I am faced with an urgent fear that I will be left there…. The combination of that loss of control and the faith I am putting in my partner to respect me is really trippy. I like it.

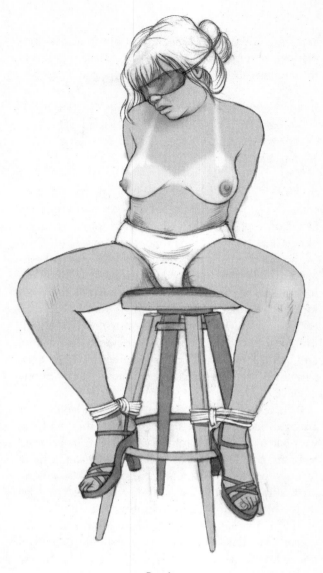

Bondage

I like being tied up and teased or even left for a while. I like to play the helpless wench (maybe if I were helpless in real life, I'd be a dominatrix). I like to be forced to think about it until I'm in a frenzy of desire and begging for it.

Bondage can be appealing for many reasons. You may be inspired by the idea of rendering your partner helpless, so that you can tease and torment her or him at your leisure. Or you may like the idea of erotically displaying your partner spread-eagled on the bed and exposed to your merciless scrutiny, posed gracefully with arms overhead, strapped to a chair, or just plain hog-tied. You may want to dress your pet in a collar and leash and do some obedience training. Cock-and-ball toys provide a specific type of bondage that serves to simultaneously restrict and display a man's genitals.

I've had fun being handcuffed, tied up, etc. One of the most fun sex-plays I've had was when I allowed a partner to tie up my cock and balls and pull me by this "leash."

SAFETY TIPS: Whatever your pleasure, bear in mind some basic safety guidelines. One commonsense rule: Don't do anything that will constrict joints or cut off circulation. If you're tying rope, cords, or a scarf, don't use any knots that tighten with resistance—slip knots are bad, bowlines are good. If you're knot-illiterate, it's time to dig up that old Boy Scout manual or to look for a similar reference guide. A lot of people tie each other up with thin scarves or stockings, not realizing that the soft, slippery material is hard to untie and can tighten, resulting in pinched nerves or even permanent nerve damage—the same is true of phone or electrical cord.

Whatever material you use, make sure you've left enough room to fit one finger between the bond and your partner's wrist or ankle (and two fingers between a collar and your partner's neck). You'll also feel more secure if you keep within arm's reach a pair of scissors, preferably bandage scissors (these have a blunt edge on the blade that would rest against the body).

No one should be kept completely restricted for longer than half an hour, and you should be careful not to let your partner's arms or legs fall asleep. You're both responsible for regularly monitoring bound body parts for cooling or numbness—signs that blood has stopped flowing into the extremities. Be particularly attentive to someone in standing bondage or who's holding his or her arms overhead—your partner's elbows should be slightly bent to reduce stress on the joints. Never suspend anyone by his or her wrists, ankles, or neck. Never tie anything around someone's neck or otherwise restrict breathing—if you're using a gag of some kind, check regularly to make sure it's loose enough that your partner can breathe and make noise. And, finally, don't ever leave someone who's bound or gagged alone in the room—this is no time to go answer a phone call. Sure, you may want to pretend to "desert" your bottom for several minutes at a time, but you should keep an eye on him or her from wherever you are hiding.

PROPS AND PROCEDURES: It can be intimidating to hop into the driver's seat and tie somebody up if you've never done so before. Take your time and enjoy the sensuous feel of whatever bondage material you're using. You can entertain and distract your partner with a running commentary on exactly what you're going to do next. This may be the perfect occasion to whip out a blindfold or to wrap a scarf over her or his eyes—you won't feel scrutinized, and your partner will feel vulnerable and filled with anticipation.

Supplies: Bondage materials run the gamut in texture and price range. Rope, clothesline, and scarves are all cheap and readily available. Just keep your safety precautions in mind when using these materials. A trip to a hardware store is something of a field day for a bondage fan—you'll find snap hooks, double clips, chain, and eyebolts at bargain prices. You can screw eyebolts or hooks into your bed frame, walls, baseboards, door frame, or ceiling—hang that macramé plant-holder from the ceiling hooks when your mom comes to visit, and no one will be any the wiser. Mountaineering or backpacking stores are also great resources and carry panic snaps: clips that release easily even if weight is pulling on them—these should be used for any standing bondage.

Restraints: Some people really like the idea of co-opting household supplies for their sex scenes, while many others prefer to buy something designed especially for what they have in mind; therefore there's a thriving industry in restraints, bonds, and cuffs (we'll use these terms interchangeably). While it may seem like a bit of an investment to buy restraints, consider the advantages: They are wide, padded, comfortable, and much safer than thin cords. Furthermore, many are so beautifully crafted they can double as accessories.

Less-expensive restraints are made of nylon webbing or fabric—they wrap around the wrist or ankle and fasten with either a buckle or Velcro. You can find varieties that have a long lead, which you then tie wherever you please, or that are set with *D*-rings. The advantage of the *D*-ring variety is that you don't necessarily need to tie any knots, provided you purchase a little hardware. You can fasten the restraints together with a double clip, slip a leash clip over the *D*-rings, or use chain to fasten the restraints to an eyebolt in your wall. Of course you can also just tie a rope or scarf to the *D*-rings and fasten the other end wherever it suits you.

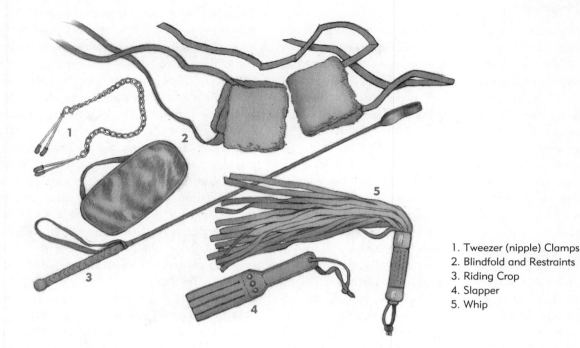

1. Tweezer (nipple) Clamps
2. Blindfold and Restraints
3. Riding Crop
4. Slapper
5. Whip

Various styles of S/M toys

You can buy fabric bonds in every color of the rainbow. Their quality and sturdiness can vary quite a bit, and the ties of some of the cheaper fabric varieties rip off the body of the restraint with a simple tug or two. If you do have the chance to shop for restraints in person, rather than by mail, check how well the fastening is reinforced, and make sure the leads are sewn down securely.

On the luxury end of the scale are leather bonds. Most leather bonds are padded, and some are fleece-lined, for a plushy, snug fit. The buckling variety fasten with wide buckles—some buckles are designed so that you can slip a padlock through and lock the restraint shut. These buckling models are all fitted with *D*-rings. If tying restraints onto your partner strikes you as a bit intimidating, you'll appreciate how easy it is to be suave and commanding with buckling bonds. If you're shopping in person, check that all rivets and snaps are secure and that the restraint fits comfortably, but not so loosely that it could slip off.

Handcuffs: These have a certain classic appeal, but they should be used with caution. Make sure the cuffs you purchase have a safety catch that locks them into position, so that they won't tighten further after being fastened—and make sure the safety catch works with a pin, not a lever. Don't even think about buying hand cuffs unless you're willing to pay top dollar. Be careful in positioning those wearing handcuffs so that they're never lying with their body weight on top of all that sharp metal. And, as with any locking toy, keep the key handy! If you like the idea of playing with locks, your best bet would be to key all your padlocks and cuffs to one standard key.

Accessories: You have a number of options for mixing and matching bondage components, from straps fitted with *D*-rings that buckle around the mattress to elaborate Velcro sheet sets. Bondage belts are wide leather or fabric belts fitted with *D*-rings. You fasten the wearer's wrist restraints to the *D*-rings on the belt, creating a fetchingly submissive look. Bondage belts also provide a great way to tug your partner back and forth during intercourse.

For a spread-eagle effect that doesn't require a lot of effort, you might want to try a spreader bar—an adjustable metal bar with cuffs on either end. You can fasten the cuffs around your partner's wrists or ankles and adjust the bar to spread the wearer's arms or legs as far apart as you'd like. Just the thing for those Scarlet Letter, Puritan-in-the-Stocks fantasies.

Flagellation

Slapping, spanking, whipping, and paddling all fall into the category of flagellation. From a casual smack on the butt during intercourse to an all-out flogging, flagellation runs the gamut of sensation. As an activity that inhabits the fine line between pain and pleasure, flagellation inspires a good deal of judgment and disapproval in those who've never experienced its charms.

If you're on the receiving end, you may enjoy enacting a fantasy role-play: naughty child receiving a spanking; unruly student getting rapped across the knuckles; P.O.W. being tortured; mutinous sailor undergoing a flogging. You may want the flagellation to be largely play-acted, with more bark than bite. Or, you may want to test your own limits of physical endurance, whether to prove your devotion to a dominant, to earn a certain reward, to feel completely present in your body, or purely to attain that endorphin buzz. Either way, you're bound to experience a certain amount of fear, a rush of adrenaline that only serves to heighten and intensify sexual arousal.

Sometimes all I want is more sensation. I get greedy to have my cunt filled, my face slapped, my nipples bitten—all at the same time in order to get that "fucked into oblivion" feeling.

If you're on the administering end, you'll want to keep up your end of the fantasy role-play. Tailor your actions and comments to the story behind your scene: Are you punishing your partner for wrongdoing, indulging your bottom, or testing limits? You get to enjoy the excitement of performing a forbidden activity, the rush of displaying physical strength, and the challenge of coaxing your partner into accepting ever-increasing levels of sensation.

When I take a crop to my partner's ass, I feel as though I'm feeding him. It's a strangely tender act.

SAFETY TIPS: In general, aiming for fleshy areas is safe, while hitting bone, joints, or over any internal organs is not safe. This means you should avoid the head, the neck, the spine, the area between the rib cage and pelvis, the shins, and the backs of the knees or elbows. This leaves you with the well-padded butt, upper thighs, upper arms, and shoulders. Hitting breasts in moderation is okay, unless your partner is pregnant, is nursing, is prone to cysts, or has silicone implants—these can burst if struck directly.

If you're slapping someone on the cheeks (the only part of the face you should be hitting), support the head with your other hand so as not to jerk the neck or jaw. Be careful not to box the ears—a blow over the ears can cause dizziness at best or a burst eardrum at worst.

When using an instrument such as a whip, crop, paddle, or cane, you should be aware that the tip of the instrument carries the greatest force. When wielding a whip, aim it so that the tips of the tails land first, to avoid the "wrap" effect, in which the tips wrap around and hit the side of your partner's body with considerable speed and impact. Until you've developed your aim and perfected your technique, it's a good idea to put pillows on either side of your partner to absorb the wrap.

You should follow safer sex precautions with your S/M gear, just as you would with any toy. If your instrument has come into contact with bodily fluids, such as blood or ejaculate, you should clean it thoroughly before using it again. In a perfect world, we'd all have separate toys for each of our partners, but most of us can't afford not to share. Clean your instrument with soap and water, then apply a disinfectant, such as rubbing alcohol or Betadine. Diluted hydrogen peroxide or bleach make good detergents, but they can be hard on leather. Clean each tail of a whip individually. Rinse thoroughly and dry. With leather products, it's a good idea to use a conditioner after your cleaning routine to keep the leather supple.

PROPS AND PROCEDURES: The key to safe and pleasurable flagellation is a gradual buildup. The strength of your blows should escalate in time with your partner's mounting arousal. Don't rush it. The more turned on someone is, the higher the pain threshold. You should start with very light blows and only increase their intensity as your partner indicates she or he wants more. Contrast the slapping, spanking, or beating with other types of stimulation. Kisses on a freshly slapped cheek or feathery touches on a newly spanked butt can feel exquisitely sensitive and tormentingly good. If you're using a specific instrument, such as a crop or whip, you can alternate your blows with teasing the instrument around your partner's body—for instance, gently poking the tip of the crop against her clitoris or softly brushing the strands of the whip across his thighs.

You'll need to find out whether or not your partner objects to any marks, as this will affect how light or heavy your touch should be. The narrower the instrument you use, the more likely it is to leave marks.

An excellent guideline is not to try any technique on a partner that you haven't experienced yourself. Test that crop on your own inner arm, thigh, or shoulder before you swing it toward anybody else's back. We hope it goes without saying that you should not hit a human being with any implement before practicing your aim and finesse on an inanimate object, such as a pillow. Bear in mind that the shorter an instrument, the easier it will be to control, and the longer, the more difficult.

Plenty of household objects lend themselves to flagellation scenes, from the classic belt (watch out for the buckle) to hairbrushes to rulers. Different shapes generate different kinds of sensation. A thin, round object, like a ruler, hairbrush, or cane, will produce a sharp, biting sting and can cut the skin, if you wield it with a heavy hand. A broad, flat object, like your hand, a belt, or a paddle, will produce a dull, penetrating thud that's spread over a wider surface area. Again, the greatest force of any instrument is at its tip.

Obviously, the lighter and softer the material, the harder you can hit with it without causing pain. Given a doeskin whip, you can pretty much whale away with impunity, but you'd better lighten up quick if you switch to latigo leather or neoprene rubber. By and large, the more tails a whip has, the more diffuse its impact—a single-tailed whip, like a bullwhip, can do the most damage, and is no toy for an amateur.

Implements designed especially for flagellation fall into several categories. Slappers are slim paddles made of two flaps of leather, sewn together at one side. The cracking sound of one flap hitting the other creates a dramatic effect, while the actual sensation produced varies from mild to heavy, depending on how stiff and thick the leather of the paddle is. Straps and paddles are easy to control and produce a wide range of sensations, again depending on the materials used. Thin straps or those encasing flexible steel produce more of a sting, similar to getting smacked with a ruler. Riding crops are usually made of flexible fiberglass rods encased in leather with a leather flap at one end. These are about two feet long, easy to maneuver, and quite versatile.

I went into this equestrian store once and got incredibly turned on by all the sexy equipment. I was sneaking a peek at the display stand of riding crops, when the nice elderly woman who ran the store came over and said, "I see you're admiring our whips!" I got so flustered, I nearly knocked over the stand.

Whips are made of nylon, suede, leather, or rubber in a variety of lengths—different materials will create different sensations. Canes are usually made from thin, supple wood, though you can find canes and rods out of synthetic plastics. Given their thin, flexible design, canes can deliver a highly cutting sting.

Whatever you choose to use will depend both on the sensation you're looking for and the scene you're creating—a cane will be just the thing for those English schoolboy fantasies, while whips are ideal for a flogging scenario.

Senses and Skin

SENSORY DEPRIVATION: One popular way of enhancing an S/M scene is sensory deprivation. When one sense is restricted, all the others become heightened and more sensitive. The classic example of sensory deprivation is using a blindfold—with vision removed, suddenly every sound, smell, and touch is intensified. Once blindfolded, you feel completely at the mercy of your partner, wondering what's about to happen next. For the novice dominant, blindfolds are an invaluable tool for creating suspense.

I blindfolded and tied my boyfriend up for the first time last night. I was shocked at how much this aroused me and how much freer I felt. I loved being the one to allow or deny sensations.

Blindfolds can be homemade out of scarves, bandannas, ties, and so forth, or specially purchased. The sleep masks sold in drugstores work fine, or you can spring for a sexy black leather-and-fleece blindfold from a leather specialty store. Of course, this particular form of sensory deprivation won't be appealing to people who derive much of their sexual arousal from visual stimuli.

I'm paraplegic and have no sensation from the chest down. I get my pleasure largely from what I see, smell, and taste. I don't like to have sex with the lights out, because I won't get aroused unless I can see my partner.

You can restrict your partner's hearing by using ear plugs, or simply control what she or he hears by using headphones. Some people enjoy exploring near-total sensory deprivation through mummification, a process whereby the bottom is completely encased in a material such as plastic wrap (with holes left for breathing). On a less elaborate level, you can control the sounds, smells, and tastes your partner is allowed to experience during a scene as one more way of emphasizing your overall control of the situation.

PLAYING WITH TEMPERATURE: Perhaps you remember that scene in 9 $\frac{1}{2}$ Weeks where Mickey Rourke slid ice cubes down Kim Basinger's silken shoulder. After all, it spawned a slew of derivative ad campaigns for everything from perfume to liquor…and with good reason. Ice has an immediate erotic appeal, whether it's applied to cool an overheated body, dripped teasingly onto nipples, slipped startlingly into a vagina, or contrasted with heat. Imagine trailing ice along a warm, freshly spanked butt—the contrast of extremes can feel torturously good.

If ice is the time-honored cold toy, candles are the classic hot toy. Dripping melted wax on your partner's skin is perfectly safe, provided you use plain, paraffin candles. Scented, colored, or beeswax candles melt at a higher temperature, and could burn or blister your partner's skin. Before you drip wax onto your partner, test a drop on the inside of your own arm. You might want to start by holding the candle high, so that the wax will be cooler before it hits the surface of your partner's skin, and gradually move the candle closer. Try dripping hot wax and cold ice in rapid succession for maximum sensation.

I love sensual massage with oils and hot candle wax followed by kisses all over. The wax is exciting because it is shocking, warm, sensual. I sometimes like to have it scraped off with a dull knife.

Clamps

You can use clamps to create sensations ranging from a slow, dull ache to a mean bite. So what's their appeal? The same as that of having your skin pinched, bitten, or otherwise tightly grabbed onto. As always, the pleasure this type of intense stimulation can produce is in direct relation to how sexually aroused you are at the time. Although people can—and do—put clamps almost anywhere on the body, we're going to focus on the most common erotic sites: nipples and genitals.

SAFETY TIPS: Apply the clamp slowly and gently, gradually releasing the tension. When you first put a clamp on, you'll probably experience a sharp bite for about thirty seconds. This will gradually subside, as blood flow to the clamped area is cut off. Unless you flick, tap, or pull on the clamps, you'll be feeling a dull ache and pressure, rather than a sharp pain. If you jostle the clamps in any way, the sharp sensations will return—this may be exactly what you want, and certainly plenty of people enjoy these surges of sensation. Inevitably, when you remove the clamp, the blood flow back into the numbed tissue will produce a brief, intense pain. You can reduce this pain by releasing the clamp slowly and delicately. The longer the clamp has been on, the more it will hurt to remove. A good rule is not to leave clamps on for more than about twenty minutes at a time.

PROPS AND PROCEDURES: Clamps are the ultimate in inexpensive toys. From clothespins to office supplies, there are countless everyday objects that can be co-opted for this kind of play. Test any clamp on the crease between your thumb and forefinger first to get a sense of what it will feel like on other tender areas of your body. You can adjust the tension of clothespins by wrapping rubber bands around one end or another. The more skin being held in the clamp and the wider the object you're using, the milder the sensation will be—for instance, a loose wire office clip will feel like a massage tool as compared to the nasty pinch of a miniature clothespin.

Nipple clamps are generally made of metal, have padded vinyl tips, and are frequently attached to each other with a length of chain. When Good Vibrations first started carrying nipple clamps, they flew out the door, and we had to wonder why we'd taken so long to add them to our product mix. After all, we've heard countless people over the years express their enjoyment and appreciation of intense nipple play.

Due to my having very responsive nipples, I like rough nipple play and also like to pinch and lick my own nipples, either during or outside of having sex with a partner.

Nipple stimulation is very, very exciting and also very relaxing. I feel it tingling in my cervix. And if it were being done to me for long enough, I think I could get to an orgasm from this alone.

I love nipple pinching, pressing, and sucking. Love breast stimulation even to the point of it hurting— that actually really gets me hot.

Alligator clips have broad, flat pincers and tighten with a screw adjustment. These fit better on men than women, as they don't expand enough to stay on larger nipples. Alligator clips are named for their serrated metal pincers, but you should never apply one to your skin unless the pincers are well padded with vinyl. Tweezer clips have two long, slim pincers that slide shut—they are highly expandable and versatile. Japanese clover clamps look something like a metal figure eight with small rubber pads for pincers. Clover clamps are designed so that when you tug on them, the pincers tighten, intensifying sensation. Skirt-hanger clips have wide padded pincers and distribute an achey sensation over a wider surface area.

If you're experimenting with nipple clamps for the first time, wait until you're so aroused that pinching and tugging on your nipples with your fingers feels tantalizing, rather than unpleasant. Position the clamp behind the tip of your nipple, rather than right on the tip, where it not only will feel quite uncomfortable, but might fall off. If you're playing with miniature clothespins or other tiny clamps with a ferocious bite, you might want to position these around the aureola, rather than directly on your nipple. Once your clamps are in place, you make the call as to whether to leave them alone or to mess around with them further.

Nipple clamps—what a turn-on! When they're flicked, my switches go off!

Women with cystic breasts and women with silicone breast implants should be cautious about using clamps, and all women should be aware that their sensitivity levels may fluctuate with their menstrual cycle, so that a pair of clamps that feels delightful one week could well feel unbearable the next. Similarly, pregnant or nursing women may feel disinclined to play with clamps.

All the nipple clamps described above can easily double as labia, clitoris, foreskin, penis, or scrotum clamps. You'll probably encounter more people who enjoy having clamps placed on their outer labia or scrotal sac than the more sensitive, nerve-rich clitoris or glans of the penis, but anything's possible.

A nipple clamp on my clit can be exciting.

Piercing

Although piercing is not an S/M activity per se, there's some overlap between the S/M community and the body modification community. "Body modification" is the term used to describe the act of creating permanent adornments such as tattoos or piercings. These types of adornment are found in tribal cultures all over the world and have existed since the beginning of recorded history, which is why the term "modern primitive" is often used to describe someone who is exploring body modification today.

Throughout history, piercings have been done for ornamentation, as a rite of passage, to convey status, and to augment erotic sensations. The Apadravya, a vertical piercing through the glans of the penis, is mentioned in the *Kama Sutra* as a means of providing additional stimulation during intercourse. Today, people's motivations for getting piercings can range from the playful to the spiritual. Some people get piercings as a way of claiming ownership of their own bodies; some as a rite of passage; some as a way of heightening consciousness of their bodies; some as an endurance test; some for sexual stimulation; and some for purely decorative purposes. The traditional sites for piercings are nipples, genitals, ears, face, tongue, and belly button.

Nipple piercings are common among both men and women, and nipple rings may be used to enhance sensation in the same way that nipple clamps are. You may find that nipple piercings enhance your awareness of your nipples as well as their sensitivity.

Since getting my nipple piercing, I like the fact that I can get really turned on by having something other than my dick played with. Having a woman tug on the ring with her teeth and tongue feels indescribably good.

Women can opt to get one or more labia piercings, to pierce the clitoral hood, or to pierce through the base of the clitoris. Clitoral hood piercings are frequently ring-style piercings with a ball bearing positioned to rest strategically against the clitoris.

Men have a variety of penis piercings to choose from. A Prince Albert is a ring-style piercing that extends along the underside of the glans from the urethral opening to where the glans meets the shaft of the penis. A frenum piercing is usually a barbell-style piercing along the underside of the shaft of the penis. Some men get a frenum ring-style piercing, so that the ring can be swung up to encircle the head of the erect penis, creating a modified cock ring effect. All but the largest and most obtrusive penis piercings can be left in during intercourse, for extra stimulation. Many people comment that their piercings have enhanced their awareness of their genitals in a way that augments sexual feelings.

Permanent piercings should only be performed by professionals working with sterile tools and sterile jewelry. This is not a do-it-yourself kind of activity.

Emotional Issues

Power play offers a unique blend of physical, mental, and emotional components, and the result is that S/M games can be frightening. For one thing, you're experimenting with activities that many people you know might casually label "sick" and "perverted." For another, you're exposing some of your deepest fantasies to a partner and, in the process, you're expressing feelings that aren't as "nice" or "loving" as you've probably been taught sexual feelings should be. S/M can bring up strong emotions, painful memories, shame, and surges of anger and guilt. It's important to honor the fact that you're getting in touch with feelings that may not be pretty, but that are nonetheless real. You and your partner should trust each other enough that you can discuss what emotions are coming up for you, both during the scene (if necessary) and after.

It's always a good idea to spend some coming down time with your partner after a scene. Whether you're feeling purely positive or somewhat ambivalent about what just happened, you owe each other positive reinforcement for the energy you each put out, the risks you each took, and the experience you shared. Discuss

what thrilled you, frightened you, turned you on. How do you feel about yourself? What might you do differently next time? Keep your focus on feelings and the overall impact of a scene. There's no need to do a play-by-play or to critique technical details.

If you or your partner is a survivor of sexual assault or abuse, a lot of powerful feelings can come up in the context of a scene. You'll both need to be extra respectful of emotional danger zones and communicative around them. Some survivors have found S/M to be helpful in the healing process, but the ways in which this is true will vary greatly from person to person. In any case, remember that S/M isn't therapy and be cautious about overstepping your boundaries.

At first my experiences at sexual power play disturbed me. I thought it stemmed from being a sex abuse survivor. It disturbed me that I enjoyed it and that I enjoyed playing a submissive. I also thought that as a feminist, it was in direct contrast and opposition to everything I believed in and practiced in my daily life. But then I started thinking that one of the delicious things about sex is fantasy—that you can be whatever you want to be without the retribution or punishment you would normally experience if you practiced this behavior out in the open. That's when I realized that being submissive sexually actually makes sense for me and I started to relax and enjoy it more.

I like for my lover to spank me, but sometimes it brings up bad memories of my assault. Being pinned down or otherwise restrained can get very unsexy and very scary very fast. So, in power play, I'm usually the one in charge.

Ultimately, S/M wouldn't have the potential to be frightening if it didn't also have the potential to be an exhilarating, empowering way to play. We placed this chapter near the end of our book, because the subject of power play brings together much of what has gone before. S/M blends communication, touch, fantasy, and sex into an eroticism that can be as exciting, creative, and highly pleasurable as you want to make it.

CHAPTER 18

Where Sex Toys Come From

Now that you've read through several chapters describing sexual products, you may well be asking yourself, "Who comes up with this stuff, anyway?" And how could you be expected to know? It's highly unlikely that *Fortune* magazine will ever do a cover story on dildo manufacturing. There are no Dun and Bradstreet stats on vibrator sales. Yet despite the invisibility that cloaks the industry, sex toys are practically a billion-dollar business in this country, and sales are only increasing.

According to a 1997 National Sexual Health Survey, still the most recent study to date, an estimated 10 percent of sexually active American adults—approximately 14 million people—report enjoying sex toys alone and with their partners. Survey researchers interviewed more than 7,000 adults between the ages of 18 to 90 and found that the enjoyment of sex toys is impressively widespread—sex toy users were equally likely to live in rural areas or big cities. We'd like to pull back the curtain and tell you what we know about the designers and manufacturers responsible for the quiet buzz of satisfaction that's rising from bedrooms all across this great land of ours.

When Is a Sex Toy Not a Sex Toy?

The earliest vibrators were marketed as cure-alls for any number of bodily ailments and advertised as contributing to the "health, vigor, and beauty" of men and women. This disingenuous marketing strategy continues today.

Vibrators sold in drugstores or discount chains are marketed exclusively as massage tools. Product illustrations show models running massagers up and down their aching necks and shapely calves, while packaging inserts refer to "facial attachments" and "foot attachments," as though there were no possibility of placing these appliances anywhere between your navel and your knees. You've probably seen advertisements for phallic-shaped battery vibrators featuring a female model who presses the tip of the vibrator against her forehead or cheek to massage her migraine—putting a new spin on the old standard, "Not tonight dear, I've got a headache."

The Prelude 3 is the only quality electric vibrator ever marketed for sexual purposes, and it was promoted with mail-order ads in men's magazines throughout the seventies.

By 1978, realizing that it would be impossible to break into a mainstream retail market with this truth-in-advertising approach, the Prelude marketers dropped all sexual references from their packaging and promotion, and the Prelude took its place next to all the other "housewares" and "personal care products" in drugstores across America.

While brand-name appliance companies make no reference to the sexual possibilities of their massagers, tips from the instruction booklets such as "Always ready to help you in providing refreshing relief at the end of a busy day" or "Removes everyday dullness" are certainly evocative to the initiated. Unfortunately, the only exception to the See No Evil, Hear No Evil marketing strategy is a caution found in some package inserts that "This unit is not intended for use on the genital areas of the body." Over the years, Good Vibrations' sales clerks have had to field many an anxious call from customers panicked by this decidedly inaccurate warning.

The advantage to this camouflaging of electric massagers is that their distribution isn't restricted to sex stores and, unlike cheaply made novelty vibrators, massagers are subject to the same kind of consumer scrutiny and standards as any other type of appliance. The disadvantage is that customers can't get honest information and advice about using their products and may fear that they're the only perverts in Sears' history to consider slipping that handy back-massager south of the tailbone. Mainstream appliance companies dare not risk the wrath of the Religious Right or the threat of potential legal liabilities by acknowledging that their products make great sex toys, and consequently they miss out on the possibility of creating even more pleasing and functional toys.

As in most areas related to sexuality, Web retailing is pushing the envelope. You can find insertable vibrators for sale on drugstore.com's "sexual health" page. Although product descriptions are vague and sanitized of specific sexual details, references abound to "sensual massage," "soothing tired muscles," and adding "bliss to the bedroom." Clearly, the merchandisers are doing what they can to fly beneath the radar of corporate sponsors.

Adult Novelty Manufacturers

First, let's dispel a popular myth. The people who manufacture sexual novelties are neither cigar-puffing Mafiosi dedicated to the destruction of our nation's moral fiber, nor sexually insatiable swingers dedicated to spreading the gospel of hedonism. In fact, the women and men who work in the adult industry are, by and large, a conservative bunch, chock-full of family values, and dedicated to making a living. While a handful of manufacturers are educated consumers of sex toys, we've always been astonished at how few novelty packagers or their sales reps have even tried their own products or have any interest in doing so. They are equally bemused by our sincere enthusiasm for sex toys and our concern for product quality, function, and appearance. In the adult bookstore business, products sell based on packaging alone, and many of Good Vibrations' sales reps can't quite understand why we're so fixated on what's actually inside their boxes.

Novelty toys hail from all over the globe. Certain products are made in the United States, primarily rubber dildos and plugs, because they can be produced as cheaply here as overseas, if not more so. Most vibrating novelties are made in China, Taiwan, Korea, and Hong Kong, where battery packs are produced much more inexpensively than they would be here. Many of these overseas factories produce novelties purely as a sideline. For instance, a doll factory might also manufacture blow-up dolls. A factory producing hair dryers and small massagers might also produce battery vibrators. Historically, novelty toys have been manufactured with no more concern, attentiveness to detail, or loving craftsmanship than the toy you fish out of a Cracker Jack box, and the kindest way to describe their quality would be to say that they have a built-in obsolescence.

The Sad History of Toy Design

The low sexual literacy rates in our American culture have made it all too easy for sex toy manufacturers to market products with dubious claims and minimal regard for the facts of human sexual response. In some cases, manufacturers just aren't particularly well educated about human sexuality themselves. In others, they're actively exploiting people's sexual insecurities for the sake of selling products. After all, it's quite common for people who find a sex toy disappointing to assume that something must be "wrong" with their own responses, rather than with the design of the toy itself.

By and large, the adult industry still perpetuates a distinctly retro and inaccurate view of female sexual response. In the world according to novelty manufacturers, women crave penetration from a penis above all else, and bigger is always better. Battery vibrators are insertable and phallic in shape. In adult novelty-land, women require only the mildest form of clitoral stimulation to be slingshot to the heights of orgasmic bliss. The classic example of this less-is-more approach to clitoral stimulation is what we call the "the nub syndrome." Over the years, adult novelty manufacturers have saluted the existence of the clitoris by decorating the base of many dildos with little rubber bumps; adorning French ticklers with rubber fronds; and covering the surface of clitoral vibrators with vinyl spines. Sure, some women may actually enjoy the extremely subtle massaging sensation provided by these nubs, just as some women enjoy ribbed condoms or ben wa balls. We, however, have encountered far more women who find the nubs pointless at best and annoying at worst.

While women who buy adult novelties may wind up feeling inadequate in terms of their sexual responses, men are likely to feel inadequate in terms of their sexual prowess. Novelty manufacturers take advantage of time-honored male insecurities about penis size and "potency" to sell a plethora of "penis extenders" and "erection prolongers." Penis extenders are hollow, vinyl prosthetic devices that fit over the head of the penis. Other such prosthetic devices fit over the entire penis, whether it's erect or not, and are held in place with elastic straps. Erection prolongers are usually numbing creams. Both types of products perpetuate the questionable notion that it's better for a man to avoid feeling any sensation than for him to "perform" as anything less than 100 percent stud.

Never mind that not all women crave long, thick penises; that a man who wishes to penetrate his partner when he's not erect could easily and pleasurably do so by wielding a dildo; or that numbing your penis and distancing yourself from the sensations you're feeling is probably the single worst way to gain control over your sexual responses and the timing of your orgasm. People in the adult industry live in the same sex-negative society as the rest of us, and if manufacturers discontinued all merchandise that plays on people's sexual insecurities, they'd have to abandon factories full of molds and throw out warehouses full of products.

Medical professionals are the latest to throw their hats into the three-ring circus of sexual mystification, dubious claims, and outsize hype. Perhaps you've read about the Eros vibrator? This tiny, battery-powered suction device retails for well over $300 and can only be prescribed by a doctor. It was approved by the FDA in 2000 to treat "female sexual dysfunction," a catch-all label for women whose experiences of desire, arousal, or orgasm don't fit the current medically defined norm. Yet there are countless ways to heighten arousal and sexual response—fantasy, massage, masturbation, oral sex, playing with sex toys, and using a lubricant, to name just a few—that cost far less and are far more effective than the Eros.

Positive Trends in Toy Design

On the brighter side, by the end of the twentieth century, novelty toy-making was showing major signs of improvement. Fueled by escalating consumer demand, the adult toy industry has grown by leaps and bounds. To stay competitive in a crowded marketplace, manufacturers have had to take steps to improve the quality and packaging of their toys. Like any other American industry, the adult industry is one in which money talks. Over the years, businesses like Good Vibrations have begun to have a greater impact on adult manufacturers—not because manufacturers have a deep-seated yearning to support our sex-positive, educational mission, but rather because we speak for a "sophisticated" clientele that increasingly makes up the consumer base for adult products.

We happily acknowledge the many positive changes that have taken place in novelty toy design since Good Vibrations first opened its doors. For one thing, color has come to the world of battery vibrators. Once available only in hospital white or pseudo-skintone-peach, battery vibrators are now produced in a dazzling rainbow of colors. Interior designers take note—you can match a vibrator to the decor of every room in your home. This may seem like a minor development, but simply offering a greater color selection bespeaks an acceptance of sex toys as consumer products. As former retail clerks, we can testify that nothing normalizes a purchase for a nervous customer better than weighing the decision as to which color to choose.

The materials out of which sex toys are made have been evolving constantly since the mid-eighties. Recent years have seen the advent of supple, colorful materials such as jelly rubber and ever-more realistic materials such as cyberskin. The motors used in battery vibrators are undergoing a serious upgrading as

American manufacturers work to compete with higher-quality Japanese vibrators. Microchips and watch batteries allow for small, strong, and silent motors, leading to greater versatility in product design.

In 1996, several adult-toy manufacturers organized the first annual Adult Novelty Manufacturers Expo, where manufacturers could network with distributors and retailers about product quality and design. A growing number of adult manufacturers are gearing products toward the so-called "women's and couple's market," while a growing number of adult bookstore owners are steering clear of the legally (and physically) sticky realm of onsite video viewing booths in favor of creating "upscale" shopping environments that will have greater appeal to women.

Several states criminalize the sale of products "designed or marketed as useful primarily for the stimulation of human genitals," defining these as "obscene devices." As a result, adult toy manufacturers tend to position themselves as being in the "novelty" business, and their packaging emphasizes the "fantasy" value of their products, rather than their function. It would be much easier for an upscale adult establishment to challenge zoning restrictions and other obscenity laws than it would be for a "dirty bookstore" to do so. It requires considerable financial resources to take on the legal system. Just as the owners of the Adam and Eve mail-order catalog successfully challenged federal indictments for interstate trafficking in obscene materials (see the Censorship chapter), a major adult retailer with deep pockets and his or her eyes on the prize of mainstreaming sex toy shops might be able to overturn antiquated state statutes. Meanwhile, you can do your bit to revolutionize the adult industry by seeking out those businesses whose approach to presenting sexual materials best fits your personal politics.

Entrepreneurs

We readily admit to a bias in favor of other small businesses—Vibratex is one excellent example. This second-generation, family-run import company—owned by the husband-and-wife team of Dan and Shay Martin and founded by Shay's Japanese parents—has been supplying Good Vibrations with a unique line of Japanese vibrators since the mid-eighties.

Vibratex is justifiably famed for its high-quality dual-action vibrators such as the Rabbit Pearl—

GV Tale: Joni's Butterfly

As proof of the "make-a-quick-buck" manufacturing philosophy of the adult industry, consider the tale of "Joni's Butterfly." Joani Blank, the founder of Good Vibrations, knew that a no-hands, wearable clitoral vibrator would be a highly popular and sensible design, and she mentioned this to one of our novelty distributors. He took her rough sketch of the idea off to Hong Kong, and came back with a finished toy. Joani had several improvements to suggest: The vibrator was too bulky to wear during intercourse and the elastic leg straps were too flimsy to hold it firmly in place, but the molds had already been made and production was under way. To Joani's dismay, her name (albeit misspelled) was permanently attached to just the type of shoddy battery toy she's spent her professional life decrying. Since very few novelty manufacturers get patenting or trade protection on their products, countless Butterflies flooded the market, and Joani received no royalties for any of these.

The moral of the story is, if you have an idea for a sex toy that you'd like to see realized exactly as you envision it or if you'd like financial compensation for the idea, your best bet would be to produce and patent the toy yourself. If, however, you'd just like to get your idea on the marketplace in some form, and you aren't attached to being paid for it, you should definitely consider forwarding a description of your better mousetrap (in writing) to one of the adult manufacturers in Southern California. Now that manufacturers are required to attach a disclosure label to any packaging that features sexually explicit imagery, you can easily find the address of companies such as Doc Johnson, California Exotic Novelties, and Topco on their product boxes.

knocked off by every other novelty company around, the Rabbit Pearl features a rotating, insertable figurine and a vibrating clitoral attachment shaped like a bunny. Lore has it that General MacArthur's postwar legacy to Japan included laws forbidding the manufacture of sex toys resembling genitals. Although you can now find Japanese vibrators or dildos that resemble penises, you'll also find the inevitable smiley face etched on their heads, indicating "I am a toy, not a sex device!" Vibratex products cost more but are of significantly better quality than most other battery vibrators.

Many of our favorite suppliers are the owners of cottage industries. Some got into sex toy production purely by chance, some found that what started as a hobby turned into an occupation, and some are former customers who became convinced they could design a better mousetrap and went into business for themselves.

By far the most beautiful dildos in existence are produced by small manufacturers. Wooden and acrylic dildos are often sculpted by craftspeople who enjoy this erotic outlet for the imagination. Silicone dildo production was invented by Gosnell Duncan of Scorpio Products. After attending several workshops on sexuality and disability in his capacity as president of his local chapter of the National Spinal Cord Injury Foundation, Gosnell became intrigued by the challenge of creating a more pleasing dildo than was generally available. He worked with a chemist friend at General Electric (apparently, G.E. *does* bring some good things to life) for several years before developing his final formula. Gosnell hadn't intended to sell his dildos outside the disability community, but by the early eighties, word had spread to the sex boutiques… and an industry was born.

Other silicone manufacturers followed suit because they enjoyed Scorpio's products, appreciated silicone's superiority to other materials, and knew that Scorpio's limited supply of silicone dildos was not satisfying the growing demand. Silicone molding is an exacting and labor-intensive process. Many people have claimed, "I could do that," but only a handful have had the tenacity to follow through. These businesses may be small, but they've made a huge contribution to the pleasure experienced in bedrooms around the world.

Leather work is another field that's full of entrepreneurs. Many of the most beautifully crafted whips and restraints in existence are handmade by individuals who were inspired to go into business because they couldn't find the products they craved in any stores. Stormy Leather, now a major wholesaler of dildo harnesses, restraints, and fetish clothing for men and women, was founded in the owner's bedroom with one sewing machine and a commitment to creating comfortable, functional dildo harnesses for women to wear.

Over the years, Good Vibrations' suppliers have included a woman who imported and hand-dyed ostrich feathers, a Berkeley couple who made wooden massage tools, and a local designer who whipped up latex hot pants on request. These entrepreneurs will never be able to command the resources, the marketing power, or the gross sales of Doc Johnson or Hitachi, but we'd like to salute them for doing their bit to make the world a more sexually fulfilling place.

Susan Colvin

"Toys were most interesting to me because each toy is unique. I liked that there were unlimited opportunities, unlimited ways to make changes."

When Susan Colvin began working for an adult toy company in the early eighties, she was one of only two women in management positions industry-wide. Today, her company, California Exotic Novelties, is one of the top three novelty companies in the United States. After fewer than ten years in operation, Cal Exotics boasts a 100,000-square-foot warehouse, more than sixty-five employees, and a product line sold around the world. Known as "the best marketer in the business," Susan is a shrewd businesswoman who had the vision to recognize the women's market for sex toys long before many of her peers.

In the early nineties, CPLC's video production arm was one of many adult companies hit with an obscenity indictment during sting operations by the Justice Department. As CPLC's general manager, Susan was held personally liable and convicted of interstate distribution of obscene materials. She and the CPLC management team decided to disband the company and sell off its video arm. Susan purchased the name of CPLC's novelty line, Swedish Erotica, and launched her own toy company in 1994.

After years in the industry, Susan knew the niche she wanted to target: "When I visited adult stores, I saw that they were only geared to men. And I talked to women who said they didn't want to walk into adult stores even though they were interested in the products. I felt that if changes were made, people would come." From the very beginning, she had a vision of how California Exotic Novelties could stand out from the pack: "My concept was that we should come out with higher-quality items and better packaging. I was sure that couples and women would be more interested if toys weren't marketed just to men. Most people just laughed: They said, 'the consumer doesn't care; they're not going to pay for higher quality.'"

It turns out, of course, that the consumer *did* care. California Exotic's rise has coincided with the explosive growth of the adult toy industry. When Susan started out at CPLC, videos ruled the shelves at typical adult stores, and novelties made up only about 10 percent of their inventory. The market has broadened in recent years, as lingerie stores, specialty shops, and countless websites have all added adult products. Although Susan modestly attributes her success to luck and timing, it has probably had more to do with her drive, business acumen, and willingness to take risks. And she never gives up on what she knows to be a good idea: Susan championed the development of remote-controlled vibrators and rechargeable battery vibrators, despite considerable start-up expense. Cal Exotics gets product ideas from consumers, from retailers, and at trade shows—if they hear the same request from enough different people, they'll work to create a prototype.

A lot has changed since Susan started out in the industry, not least of which is attitudes toward her profession. Always candid about the work she does, she's noticed that people respond much more favorably now than in the past: "When I meet people at parties, I tell them that I manufacture adult novelties. Years ago, they would clam up or change the subject. Now most people are just fascinated and they want to know where they can get a catalog or the latest toy!"

Check out Cal Exotics online at www.calexotics.com.

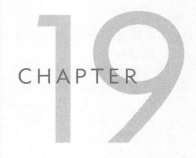

Safer Sex

"Safer sex" is the term used to describe sexual activities that minimize the risk of spreading sexually transmitted diseases. This chapter may seem redundant since many of the activities you've read about so far qualify as safer sex. Masturbating, playing with sex toys, massage, sharing fantasies, and erotica are all safe and creative ways to enjoy sex. One of our motivations in writing this book was to illustrate the dozens of ways one can enjoy sex without engaging in high-risk activities. In chapters where we describe somewhat risky activities, we've incorporated easy ways to practice them safely.

Nonetheless, we would be remiss in omitting basic information about sexually transmitted diseases, since the more information you have, the better able you are to make decisions regarding your own sexual health. What's more, we jump at the opportunity to get excited about safer-sex accessories. Too often they are treated purely as a necessary evil—weapons and armor in the war on disease, rather than as sex toys, deserving the same enthusiasm we lavish on vibrators and dildos.

The definition of safer sex can be expanded to include another area that directly impacts our sexual health: contraception. Although we consider birth control an important responsibility in a sexually active person's life, we have chosen not to enumerate the many forms of contraception in this chapter. There are entire books and websites devoted to this subject alone; most treat the issue with the attention, thoroughness, and respect it deserves. Keep in mind as you read, however, that condoms are a reliable method of contraception when used correctly.

Just the Facts, Ma'am

Sexually Transmitted Diseases or STDs

One in five people in the United States has been infected with a sexually transmitted disease (STD) at some time in his or her life. There are over fifty known diseases that can be transmitted through sexual activity; chlamydia, gonorrhea, genital warts, genital herpes, hepatitis B, syphilis, and AIDS are among the most common. Itching, nausea, painful urination, vaginal discharge, fatigue, skin changes, rashes, and sores on or near the genitals can be signs or symptoms of an STD, and you should visit your doctor or a health center immediately if you suspect you may have contracted one.

If you're sexually active, it's a good idea to get tested regularly for STDs. Chlamydia, for example, is the most common STD in the United States largely because up to 40 percent of men and 85 percent of women show no symptoms when they contract the infection. Although chlamydia is easily treated with antibiotics, if a woman's infection remains untreated, it can lead to Pelvic Inflammatory Disease, possibly resulting in infertility or ectopic pregnancies. Women who have been treated for chlamydia should get rescreened within a few months because of the high rate of reinfection.

If you're diagnosed with an STD, your doctor will give you specific guidelines for treatment. STDs are either bacterial or viral. Bacterial infections, such as gonorrhea, chlamydia, and syphilis, can be treated with antibiotics. Viral infections like hepatitis, HIV, genital warts, and herpes aren't necessarily curable. If you haven't been vaccinated for hepatitis B and become infected, your initial infection can be treated with gamma globulin, but the disease may remain in your system and you may remain a carrier. Both herpes and HIV infection are incurable at this time, though antivirals can suppress the severity of herpes outbreaks, and ongoing breakthroughs in the treatment of HIV/AIDS are increasing the chances of long-term survival for HIV-positive individuals.

An estimated 80 percent of the population has been exposed to genital warts. These warts are caused by the human papillomavirus (HPV) and can be transmitted by skin-to-skin contact. There are up to a hundred different strains of HPV, which cause warts all over the body, and about twenty of these strains cause genital warts. External genital warts can be removed via lasers or freezing, but this does not eliminate the virus. Most strains of genital warts are harmless, though certain strains produce cancerous cell changes that result in cervical or anal cancer. Not only can you have the virus and show no symptoms, but the strains of HPV that cause cervical or anal cancer aren't visible to the naked eye. The best protection against cancer-causing genital warts is for women to have regular vaginal pap smears. With rates of anal cancer on the rise in the gay community, doctors are recommending regular anal pap smears as well.

I'm very concerned about STDs and HIV not for myself but for my daughter, who is 12. I did catch herpes and venereal warts having unprotected sex in my twenties. I have had many long talks with my child about the topic, and even when she was only 9. I showed her a condom and told her why she must always use one.

HIV/AIDS

WHAT IS IT? AIDS stands for Acquired Immunodeficiency Syndrome. The "acquired" means that the HIV virus must be transmitted to you somehow; "immunodeficiency" refers to the virus attacking your immune system. The HIV virus destroys your immune system's ability to combat disease. The person who dies from AIDS actually succumbs to an opportunistic infection (such as pneumocystis or Kaposi's sarcoma) that a healthy individual's immune system would fight off.

TRANSMISSION: The virus known as HIV (Human Immunodeficiency Virus) is transmitted when an infected individual's bodily fluids—most commonly blood and semen—enter another person's bloodstream via open cuts or mucous membranes. Unprotected (no condom) penis-vagina and penis-anus intercourse are the most common methods of transmission. Sharing blood, such as when intravenous drug-users share needles, is another common method of transmission. The virus cannot be transmitted by mosquitoes (or other insects), a handshake, toilet seats, clothes, phones, food handlers, or sneezing. HIV is only present in high enough concentrations to be transmissible in blood, semen, vaginal secretions, and breast milk. While it's present in trace quantities in sweat, saliva, urine, or tears, there's no evidence that it can be transmitted via these fluids. Although studies have yet to be done on HIV levels in female ejaculate, it seems likely that female ejaculate is a low-risk fluid.

GETTING TESTED: You can take a blood test at any medical facility and at many free clinics that will indicate whether you have been exposed to the HIV virus. Currently there is only one FDA-approved home test (called Home Access), which is available at drugstores. It comes with instructions and tools for you to take a blood sample and return it to a central lab. You can call a few days later to

Basic Safer-Sex Guidelines

- Viruses and bacteria cannot pass through latex.
- Use condoms every time you have either vaginal or anal intercourse. You may want to use unlubricated (or try flavored) ones for oral sex as well.
- Put condoms on sex toys used by more than one person for any type of penetration or on toys that go from anus to vagina.
- Use dental dams or a cut-open condom or glove as a barrier during oral-vaginal or oral-anal sex.
- Use only water-based lubricants with latex (including condoms, gloves, dams, cots, and diaphragms). Never use oil or petroleum-based products with latex.
- Never reuse latex.

hear the results. The home test is anonymous and convenient, and the results are delivered to you by phone counselors. You may prefer, however, to take an HIV test at a clinic where counselors will be on hand to advise you should the results come back positive.

If you've had unprotected sex, you should be aware of the so-called "window period." This period is the amount of time your immune system takes to produce HIV-antibodies in response to infection. While healthy individuals usually develop antibodies within two to twelve weeks after infection, it can take as long as six months to develop levels of HIV antibodies that will be detectable in a blood test. Therefore, you should either postpone your HIV test until six months after the incident of unprotected sex, or repeat the test then to make sure previous testing hasn't produced a false negative result. False positive test results are also not uncommon, so if you test positive once, your doctor or clinician will administer a second, more sophisticated blood test to confirm your HIV status. While there's no cure for AIDS at this time, an HIV-positive diagnosis is *not* an automatic death sentence. An ever-widening range of treatments can keep the virus in check and significantly extend life expectancy.

A Word About Latex Accessories

Introducing latex barriers—condoms, gloves, dams, cots—into your sex play is the easiest and most effective way to minimize the risk of transmitting bodily fluids or of otherwise coming into contact with the viruses and bacteria that cause sexually transmitted diseases. These supplies are inexpensive, reliable, and easy to find. Between 2 and 4 percent of the population, however, is allergic to latex. We'll discuss the alternatives—polyurethane or lambskin condoms, nitrile gloves, and plastic coverings like Saran Wrap—later in this chapter.

We know that whatever barrier you choose, with a little practice, you'll be snapping on the gloves and lubing up those condoms as if you'd been doing it all your life. You can find latex condoms, cots, and gloves in pharmacies, medical or dental supply houses, and sex boutiques. You're more likely to find dental dams at dental supply houses or sex boutiques than at the local drugstore.

When I lost two close friends to hepatitis C and AIDS, I realized how real the safe-sex issue was. Since then, I've helped my friends understand it, and have become the "condom/lube/dental dam/latex glove bank" for them. I haven't done this at all begrudgingly, since I might well save their lives.

A Word about STDs, Lubes, and Latex

As you'll recall from our Lubrication chapter, we think lubes are an essential ingredient in all your sexual encounters, and they are certainly indispensable when it comes to safer sex as well. Recent studies have revealed some interesting relationships between certain lubes and STDs.

First the bad news. Nonoxynol-9, a spermicidal ingredient commonly added to many condoms and lubes because it has been shown to kill viruses in a laboratory setting, has proven to irritate mucous membranes to such an extent that it can cause vaginal or rectal lesions, thereby creating greater opportunity for infection. The Centers for Disease Control now officially discourages the use of products with nonoxynol-9. It is gradually disappearing from condoms and lubes, but you would do well to check any listing of ingredients.

On the bright side, a recent study revealed that out of twenty-two lubes tested, three (of which Astroglide is the most popular) contain unique compounds that were 99 percent effective in killing HIV in a laboratory setting. Further field tests are being done, and we certainly aren't suggesting that you consider Astroglide a tool for preventing HIV transmission. Obviously, you should not forgo the use of condoms and other latex barriers. But this study does provide one more excellent argument for using lube!

Finally, keep in mind that latex products like condoms, dams, and gloves should only be used with water-based lubricants. Oils and oil-based lubes will destroy rubber and render latex barriers utterly useless. Make sure you use water-based lubricants, and don't be confused by lubes labeled "water-soluble"—these often contain oils. When in doubt, read the ingredients.

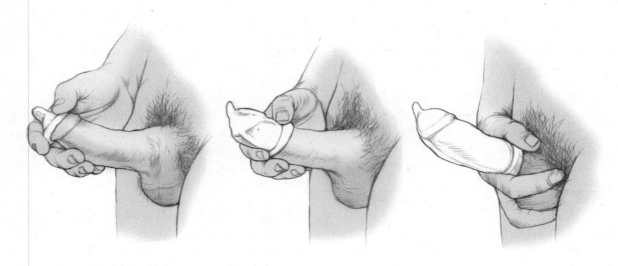

How to put on a condom

How to Put on a Condom Correctly

- Use condoms that have been stored in a cool, dry place. Check the expiration date printed on the package. If the condom looks brittle, sticky, or discolored, throw it out.
- Open the package gently. You don't want to puncture the condom in your hurry to liberate it!
- Put a drop or two of water-based lube inside the tip of the condom. This aids in the unrolling and increases sensation for the wearer.
- Before you start unrolling the condom, squeeze the air out of the receptacle tip, since air bubbles can cause condoms to break. Condoms without a reservoir tip require about one-half inch free at the tip to catch the come.
- An uncircumcised man should pull his foreskin back to help prevent the condom from slipping.
- As you're holding the tip of the condom over the penis or dildo, check to make sure the latex

will be emerging from the inside of the ring as you roll down.
- Unroll the condom down to the base of the penis. Pull back the foreskin of an uncircumcised penis before covering the glans. Apply generous amounts of water-based lubricant to the outside of the condom as well as to your partner's genitals before penetration. Condoms are easiest to apply when the penis is hard, but can be applied to a soft penis—just continue to roll the condom down the shaft as the penis hardens.
- Remember to hold onto the base of the condom when withdrawing so that the condom doesn't slip off from the penis. Withdraw before losing your erection.
- Throw used condoms away. They are not reusable. Use a new condom for each act of penetration.

Condoms

You're probably thinking, "Oh no, not another lecture on using condoms." Actually, we're more interested in singing the condom's praises than in wagging our fingers at anyone. After all, condoms are the most widely available, inexpensive, well known, and oldest sex toy in existence, and these days they come in almost as many sizes, colors, and flavors as ice cream.

Who wouldn't be proud to use a toy with such a colorful history? Apparently you could have found one over 15,000 years ago, as a French cave painting of a man wearing a sheath suggests. Egyptian men wore condoms as a sign of rank 3,000 years ago, while tribeswomen in South America fashioned themselves a female condom made out of a cut-off seed pod. Before lambskin and latex condoms, the Chinese made condoms out of oiled silk paper, the Egyptians used papyrus soaked in water, and the Europeans used fish bladders. Our favorite legend credits the Greek's mythical King Minos with the invention of the condom. Apparently the king had a tendency to ejaculate scorpions and snakes into his partners, so his right-hand man, Daedalus, invented a female receptacle into which the King could shoot his deadly semen. From scorpions to venereal disease to HIV, the condom has a noble history of protecting our sexual health.

If you're planning to sweet-talk your sweetie into using a condom, why not try another name? At one time or another, condoms have been known as diving suits, phallic thimbles, life-savers, dibbers, preservatives, gloves, letters, hats, and johnny bags. Remember to use your "frog-skins" during vaginal or anal intercourse, oral sex, and on any shared sex toys.

I've only used condoms. I have all kinds of condoms. When I was young it was embarrassing and only "boys" got them. I learned that I have to protect myself and that you should be embarrassed if you don't have them. I always have condoms with me, in the car, in every room in the house.

Latex Condoms

There's a reason drugstore shelves overflow with latex condoms in every size, thickness, and color—they're a convenient, affordable, highly effective barrier against disease transmission, as well as a popular contraceptive. Most latex condoms break because they're used incorrectly. The typical failure rate is about 12 percent, but researchers contend that if used correctly and consistently this would drop to about 2 percent. One British study revealed that out of three hundred men asked to demonstrate how to put on a condom, 20 percent failed because they tried to unroll it from the inside out. Another reason for high breakage rates involves the use of oil-based lubes, which are incompatible with latex.

So even though you might have the instructions memorized, if you're blaming faulty condoms, you may just need more practice. Both men and women can enjoy this homework exercise: On your next visit to the drugstore pick out an assortment of condoms, go home, and play with them! If you don't have a willing penis handy, try putting them on a vibrator, vegetable, toothpaste dispenser, bedpost, anything that grabs you. The idea is to practice putting them on and to test their durability, so don't be afraid to get rough with your condoms. Take different sizes, colors, and flavors, either lubed or unlubed, on a test drive to find the condom that's right for you—you might find that one particular brand feels better, tastes better, or is just easier to use.

I always carry several condoms in my car, my wallet, and my Day Runner Organizer (and to think people think I'm anal because I like being organized)!

I always put a condom on my dildo when I use it on someone else and almost always when I use it on myself. I like the texture.

I once used a cut-open condom to lick my girlfriend's newly pierced nipple. That was great because it was so sensitive and erotic for her.

If you're afraid the condom might slip off, pull it down so that it fits over your testicles. A little too much lubricant inside the condom could be causing the slippage. If you're worried about a condom breaking, try wearing two thin condoms at once for extra protection, and don't forget to use lube. If a condom breaks while you are having intercourse, don't panic. Simply stop what you're doing and apply some contraceptive foam—the spermicide in the foam may also kill any viruses present. Don't douche or otherwise attempt to "wash out" your vagina or anus, as this will only push pre-come or semen further inside.

Polyurethane Condoms

Until polyurethane condoms hit the market at the end of the twentieth century, there hadn't been a major breakthrough in condom technology since the debut of latex condoms in the nineteenth century. The Avanti male condom and the Reality female condom were the first condoms made out of poly-urethane, a plastic material twice as strong as latex (now there is also a TrojanSupra male condom, but it contains nonxoynol-9). Check out all the features of this wonder material: It's thinner than latex, which means greater sensitivity for users. It's compatible with oil-based lubricants, so people who can't distinguish between water-based, water-soluble, and oil-based lubes don't have to worry about their condoms break-ing down anymore. It's odorless and doesn't contain the proteins that cause some individuals to be allergic to latex. It transmits heat better and is more resistant to damage from heat and light. People seeking an alternative to latex condoms have by and large expressed great satisfaction with the polyurethane condoms.

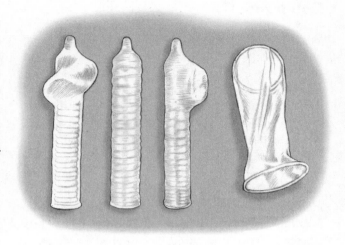

Various styles of condoms
(In Spiral, ribbed, Pleasure Plus, and Reality Female)

I always wear condoms because I have genital warts. (Even treated they come back.) Not practicing safe sex is what gave them to me. I always use polyurethane condoms, though, because they're the only kind with which I can feel anything.

Ready for the caveats? The FDA has not officially approved polyurethane condoms for contraceptive or STD prevention. Studies, however, indicate that the plastic provides an effective barrier to viruses, bacte-ria, and sperm, so it's probably just a matter of time before the FDA puts its seal of approval on them.

A much muddier issue is the breakage rate for the male condoms. The largest study to date reported breakage rates at over six times that of latex condoms. How much this is due to faulty application rather than the material itself is debatable. Although polyurethane is technically stronger than latex, the plastic is much less elastic, which can result in a higher breakage rate. If you're allergic to latex, but don't want to fret about your condom breaking, try layering a latex condom over the polyurethane one.

Other complaints that have surfaced about the Avanti involve its larger than standard size. Since polyurethane won't stretch as much as latex, the Avanti is made a bit wider than latex condoms—this

can result in a slippage problem. As well, Avanti condoms are considerably more expensive than latex condoms.

As for the female condom, the Reality may be harder to warm up to than its male counterpart. The Reality is a six-inch-long tube (as long as a condom, but wider), with one sealed end and a flexible, plastic ring at each end. The woman inserts one ring into her vagina, much like a diaphragm, while the ring around the opening remains anchored outside, resting flat against the labia.

There are several advantages to the female condom: It's great for those with latex allergies; women can take responsibility for its use; the condom can be inserted ahead of time; a man may find the loose fit of the female condom gives him increased sensation; and the coverage provided by the outer por-tion may help prevent transmission of STDs such as genital herpes or warts. The female condom is also suitable for anal use: Just make sure the outer ring doesn't slip inside the anus (it's helpful to leave about one inch of the condom hanging outside the anus). The insertive partner should be careful to use shallow thrusts—since the Reality condom is not as long as the rectum, longer thrusts may stress the condom.

The reported disadvantages of the Reality condom concern how difficult it is to use correctly. Because it is somewhat cumbersome and bulky, its effectiveness is diminished unless it is used correctly. One study of women using the female condom, which included those women who used it inconsistently or incorrectly, reported a pregnancy rate of 26 percent. With correct use, the female condom should have a failure rate of only five percent.

Here are some helpful hints: Position the inner ring carefully or the condom may twist; use enough lube or the condom will stick to the penis; make sure not to insert the penis or dildo between the condom and the vaginal wall; hold the outer ring in place to keep it from slipping into the vagina; and remove it very carefully to prevent ejaculate from leaking out. In addition, the outer ring may irritate the external genitalia, while the internal "one size fits most" ring may not fit *you*. Finally, don't use the Reality condom in combination with a latex condom—they will stick together.

I felt like we were having sex with a grocery bag, and the crinkly noise was a bit of a turn off.

We're not trying to rain on your parade if you're a polyurethane fan, we just want to tell you what we know about these products. If you're allergic to latex, polyurethane is definitely your best bet.

Lambskin Condoms

Made from the appendix of sheep, lambskin condoms should never be used for safer-sex purposes, as viruses may permeate small imperfections in the membrane's surface. Use latex condoms only, or wear a latex condom over a lambskin one if you're allergic to latex.

Condom Shopping Checklist

Some things to consider before buying your condoms:

✓ *Material:* Latex condoms are the most effective barriers against the transmission of disease, but some people are allergic to latex. If you have latex allergies, consider trying a polyurethane condom. Never use lambskin condoms for safer sex.

✓ *Size:* Large condoms are just over two inches wide while the "snug" variety are just under two inches. The minimum length for condoms is six and a half inches, though longer ones can exceed eight inches. The polyurethane condom is wider and shorter than standard latex.

✓ *Thickness:* Thinner condoms may feel great but aren't necessarily as strong as their thicker brethren. They do pass the basic air-inflation tests, yet have a tendency to break more often than other condoms. If you're new to condom use, start out with the thicker variety.

✓ *Flavor:* Condoms come in a variety of flavors, from mint to chocolate to tutti-frutti. If you're planning an evening of oral sex, we guarantee these'll spice up the occasion.

✓ *Lubrication:* Many people don't like the taste of lubricated condoms, and there are plenty of

unlubricated ones available. If you're allergic to nonoxynol-9, avoid condom lubes with this ingredient. Use lubed condoms for intercourse, especially if you don't have any additional lube on hand.

✓ *Texture:* Some condoms (Kimono Sensation) come with little nubs on the inside designed to stimulate the wearer's penis and some with ribbing on the outside, ostensibly to stimulate the receptive partner's vagina or anus. You may or may not be able to distinguish these subtle sensations.

✓ *Color:* Most condoms are available in a clear or semiclear color, but you can find condoms in every color of the rainbow as well as glow-in-the-dark.

✓ *Special features:* Do you want it to stick to the base of the penis? Cover the testicles? Massage the tip of the penis? Read the condom's package to determine whether it has any special feature.

✓ *FDA approval:* If you're not sure whether the condom has been approved by the FDA for use in prevention of disease or pregnancy, check the label.

Condom Care

In addition to learning how to put a condom on correctly, you also need to make sure that they are taken care of properly. To ensure your success:

- Check the expiration date on a condom before you use it. Some condoms also note a manufacturer's date, which is not the same as the expiration date.
- Make sure your condom is approved by the FDA if you'll be using it for contraception or disease prevention. It should say on the label.
- When opening the wrapper, tear along the dotted line or the seal. Don't use your teeth or scissors.
- Store condoms in a cool, dry place. Forget wallets and glove compartments. If you carry one in a pocket or purse, do so for a short time.
- If the condom looks gummy or brittle, throw it away.
- Don't reuse condoms.

The Cream of the Condom Crop

CROWN SKINLESS SKIN. Thin and strong. Good Vibration's bestselling condom.

TROJAN MAGNUM. Marketed as slightly bigger than regular condoms, they're wider at the head, which makes them good for uncircumcised men or men with thick penises.

KIMONOS. Thin and strong.

KIMONO SENSATION. Little nubs along the inside of the condom are designed to increase sensation for the wearer.

DUREX. Strong, fairly thin, lubed, and inexpensive. Also available in colors.

PLEASURE PLUS. Features a baggy pouch at the tip (more comfortable for uncircumcised men) that massages the penis with each stroke.

INSPIRAL. Similar to the Pleasure Plus, but the baggy tip spirals, increasing sensitivity. Also good for men with larger penises.

KISS OF MINT. Flavored and unlubricated.

Dental Dams

These six-inch squares of latex are used by dentists during oral surgery and have been co-opted for safer oral sex purposes. Dental dams offer an adequate—if somewhat thick—barrier between your tongue and your lover's labia or anus. Fortunately, a few thinner and larger dams are being manufactured (such as Glyde and Lixx) in a variety of flavors. An equally effective and easier-to-obtain alternative is a condom. Snip off the tip and then cut along one side of the condom. Open it up and voilà—you've got a very thin dam. You can do the same thing with a latex glove by snipping off the fingers and cutting open the side with the thumb. Plastic wrap is another option—though it hasn't received the testing that latex has, at least one study has determined that Saran Wrap is impermeable to virus-sized particles.

I love having dental dams when I am on my period, because that way my lover can still go down on me and not worry about making a mess.

How to Use Dental Dams

- Rinse off the dam before use. It's covered in a fine powder that can irritate the genitals.
- The lickee or the licker holds the dam in place over the genitals while the licker performs. A little lube on the side next to the genitals will increase sensation. Try sucking in little air bubbles with your mouth and snapping the bubble back against the skin for a unique sensation.
- Don't inadvertently reverse the dam—only one side of the dam should come into contact with the genitals. Use a pen to mark a nonreversible letter (like K or B, don't use A or X) on the dam. This will help you find the right side if the dam is dropped.
- We've seen an ingenious use of plastic wrap that frees up the pair of hands normally required to hold the dam in place. You can fashion yourself some plastic wrap underwear by first unrolling the sheet around your hips, then dipping it down between the thighs so that it covers the labia and anus, and back up around the hips. Plastic wrap is so clingy that it sticks together nicely.
- Throw away dams when finished. They are not reusable.

If you want your hands free, the alternative to plastic wrap undies is a dam harness or latex panties. The harness has two leg straps with snaps to secure the dam in place over the vulva. The latex panties look like men's briefs and are a one-time-use only garment.

Gloves

Latex gloves feel like a second skin when worn, and once you've lubed them up, they can be a slippery-smooth delight sliding over skin or in and out of orifices. Use gloves for any situation in which your finger or hand will be contacting mucous membranes, from fingering your partner's clit, to giving a hand job, to fisting (use plenty of lube for the latter). Make sure your nails are trimmed, your hands free of any rings or items that might pierce the glove, and your glove long enough to cover the part of your hand or arm that will come in contact with mucous membranes. Do not reuse gloves.

Gloves are another medical tool co-opted as an exotic safe-sex toy. Rinse the powder off the gloves before using them, as it can irritate. Standard latex examination gloves can be found at most drugstores.

Nitrile gloves offer those with latex allergies a synthetic alternative to rubber. They are stronger and thinner, can be used with oil-based lubes, come in a powder-free version, and are available in different sizes. These can be harder to find than latex gloves, so check with sex boutiques or condom retailers.

I like gloves for penetrating my female partner. It is so nice to take them off and instantly have a clean hand to touch again.

I think gloves make the fingers/hand slicker and keep lube wetter longer.

Finger Cots

Cots are like miniature latex condoms for your finger. If you plan on stimulating or penetrating someone with one finger only, this would do the trick. It's also a perfect size for smaller toys—butt plugs, minivibrators, or small dildos, though you'll need to tie something around the base of the cot to make sure it doesn't roll off.

My partner uses finger cots when his fingers are all messed up and cut from work, so that we don't need to worry about spreading infections or irritating anything on him or in me.

Gloves are great because your hands don't get pruney and your fingernails aren't as sharp. I've used these on women. I don't see the point of finger cots. Gloves are just as easy and give you more options.

Erotic Safer Sex

Safer sex is great! There are so many things you can do with a condom or a dental dam! Safer sex can also be great even for those in long-term monogamous relationships. If you are with a partner who is squeamish about oral sex or about rimming, you can do it with a barrier. Condoms also make for easier cleanup of sex toys or of sex during menstruation.

We wish everyone shared this woman's attitude about safer sex, but the truth is the majority of people today are not what you'd call enthusiastic about safer sex. Many are resigned to the practice, yet they approach it with about as much enthusiasm as they would a trip to the dentist. Some folks resent being told what they "should" be doing in the bedroom; some feel a certain sense of immunity; some just write off safer sex as a big nuisance.

And despite the likelihood that you or someone you know has an STD, broaching the subject can be made especially difficult by ignorance, denial, or stereotyping.

When I was 18, I contracted human papilloma virus from a partner. Although I was treated and have had no recurrences, this has been a difficult subject to approach with a new partner. I find it hard to just blurt out, "By the way, I had some irregular cells on my cervix that I had treated with liquid nitrogen" while we're standing in line at the movies or whatever.

"Umm…before this goes any farther…umm…I have to tell you something…I have this icky STD, nothing that could kill you, but one of those things that doesn't go away." People are usually very understanding, but it sucks to have to talk about it. So far, I haven't had anyone run away screaming.

You are responsible for your own and your partners' sexual health. We can tell you how to try to make sex safer as well as easy, fun, interesting, exciting, and erotic, but only you can make the words a reality. One good place to start is with your own attitude about safer sex. It's easy to complain about the taste or feel of condoms, but with a little creative research and imagination, you might change your opinions. You might learn something from today's youth, who came of age using condoms:

When I was first sexually active, condoms themselves turned me on—I would sometimes use them masturbating; just owning some was a sign that I might be having sex someday.

I've been using condoms since day one, except when I was on the pill and only sleeping with one person. I don't love 'em, but they do make some things easier (anal sex, for example), and at this point I've almost forgotten what it's like to have sex without one.

From almost the beginning I've learned the importance of using a condom to prevent disease and pregnancy. It's always been common sense to me, like wearing a seatbelt and not smoking.

You're probably reading this book searching for a few good ideas or a fresh approach. So why not embrace safe sex like you would any other toy or technique—with a playful spirit and a willingness to experiment?

I'm lucky that I've always liked latex—I used gloves long before most people ever heard of them.

Black, shiny rubbers on my white skin fetishize my dick as if it were a much larger dildo.

To illustrate our point, and to give you a place to start, we've listed some common complaints about latex, along with our suggestions for turning a potential problem into a playful activity.

Find me a condom that tastes like café mocha and then we'll talk! Thanks to the growing number of flavored latex supplies, your next oral sex adventure can be as tasty as a good café mocha. Mint condoms are perfect for an after-dinner blow job, while bubble gum dams might bring out the naughty schoolgirl in you. This is

great news for folks who find the actual taste and smell of latex less palatable. If you don't like the taste of lubricated condoms, buy them unlubricated and apply your own favorite lube. Think about how many tastes you've acquired in your life—perhaps coffee, beer, your lover's juices—latex too can be an acquired taste. After you've played with safer-sex accessories for a while, you may develop a Pavlovian response!

Even the smell of some types of condoms turns me on.

With the right condom/flavored lube it's kinda neat to give a blow job with a condom, though latex does still taste yucky alone.

I could never understand what people meant by "eroticizing" latex until I bought a latex dress. I got so turned on by the snug, supportive feel of rubber on my body that now just about any kind of latex turns me on.

Condoms reduce sensitivity. Certainly nothing will feel exactly the same as naked skin, but you can learn to enjoy the new and different sensations offered by a condom. You may discover that condoms reduce friction and thereby make your erection last longer. If you're having trouble maintaining an erection with a condom, try masturbating with different kinds to find the ones that feel the best—eventually your body will become conditioned to respond to this different kind of stimulus. And remember, not all condoms are identical—they vary in size, shape, texture, color, and taste—so there's bound to be at least one out there with your name on it! Japanese condoms tend to be thinner than American brands, so you may want to start with these to maximize sensation. You might enjoy condoms that fit more snugly because they keep your penis harder longer. Or maybe you find that contoured condoms—those that balloon a bit at the top and then become narrow below the head—increase sensation. The Kimono Sensation condom with nubs on the inside may provide just the extra stimulation you need. And we have to relay the comeback of one woman whose partner complained about the condom being *too* small: "If this condom can hold a gallon of water, it can hold your dick."

When you're with a partner and you're worried about not getting enough stimulation with a condom, you can always have him or her manually stimulate you until you're close to coming, then apply the condom for the duration of your sex play. Or you can see if your partner is interested in trying the Reality female condom, which can be used vaginally or anally.

Women should experiment too. The more comfortable and competent you are with applying condoms, the better it will feel to your partner.

Condoms become "unlubed" quickly and rub painfully during intercourse. This is nothing that a spare bottle of lube and a spray bottle with water in it won't fix. Having extra lubricant on hand is essential. And many people don't realize that water will reactivate the lube as it starts to dry up. A spray bottle or a bowl of water by the bed will do the trick.

It's so awkward to stop what we're doing and whip out the latex. Try not to think of it as stopping, but rather as expanding what you're doing. Don't you already pause once in a while to dim the lights, find the vibrator, or put in a diaphragm? You don't have to think of it as a chore, but as part of the fun.

> *I've always used condoms. I don't find those thirty seconds "awkward" or too "mood-ruining" like some people say. It's just a part of the dance, and it always has been.*

Try fantasizing when you're alone about using latex with your partner, imagining different ways you'd like to try the condom, dam, or glove. That way, when the time comes you'll have a few tricks up your sleeve. Have your safer-sex supplies at the ready so that you don't spend time searching around. We heard tell of one woman who liked to keep a glove stashed under the top of her stocking so that a hand traveling up her thigh would encounter it before going any further. Play with your toys together—your partner can put a condom on himself or herself, acting the exhibitionist, or you can put it on for him or her as part of your foreplay, teasing as you go. You could practice different ways of applying the condom. When using your mouth, for example:

- You'll probably want to use an unlubricated condom.
- Open the condom and unroll it slightly.
- Form your lips into an O and place the condom between your upper and lower lips, in front of your teeth. Make sure the condom is facing the right direction so that it unrolls correctly.

- Hold onto the penis or dildo with one hand, then place your mouth on the penis or dildo, tightening your lips and pushing down on the rim.
- Push from your neck to unroll the condom down the shaft.

As with many of the toys or activities we suggest in this book, part of the difficulty of incorporating safer-sex accessories into your sex life stems from embarrassment or awkwardness when trying something new. A sense of humor is crucial, and can help you ease into a new activity (as long as you're not laughing at someone else's unwitting expense). Colored condoms or the glow-in-the-dark variety might underscore the playfulness and fun of the activity.

Some of my lovers are reluctant to use condoms. At the risk of sounding preachy, if a sexual partner refuses to use a condom—or any other kind of safer-sex accouterments—at your request, ultimately it shows a lack of regard for sexual health. Being sexually assertive is something that doesn't come naturally to many of us, so it's important to be prepared for situations like this. There are several good books and websites that teach sexual assertiveness and specify how to ask for safe sex. Most of these stress the value of coming to terms with your wants and needs beforehand and school you on how to avoid common pitfalls like over-aggressiveness or defensiveness. And as this mom points out, standing up for your sexual rights is our greatest gift to the next generation:

> *I have always said that I am not willing to die for sex, and no one is worth my life when it comes to sex. I can only hope that my daughter, when she is old enough, has the common sense NOT to take her partner's word that he is "clean."*

Here are some of our customers' approaches to discussing safer sex:

> *My one rule is: no condom, no sex.*

> *When I start getting close to someone, I initiate a safe-sex talk. I state my sex history and that I have herpes.*

One very simple tactic is to reassess your approach, making the proposition as appealing as possible. For example, instead of the cold, direct approach:

Now it's time for you to put on the condom.

We can't have sex without condoms.

Try a nasty, yet equally direct approach:

I know exactly which condom will feel great on you.

There's a condom with your name on it itching to get out of my pocket.

Safe sex with you is something I've fantasized about.

It might help for you to make a list of what your specific personal rules are when it comes to safer sex, so that you'll be ready when the time comes. For example, you might list something like, "I don't want to go down on someone without a barrier," or "I will only perform fellatio with a condom." If your partner is unwilling, be empathetic and suggest that you compromise with some alternatives that are acceptable to both of you. She may not want to use a dam, so you'll both masturbate instead. He may refuse to use a condom, but you feel okay about giving him a hand job. It might be awkward at first, but confidence and comfort will come with practice.

Try to raise the subject of safer sex in conversations outside the bedroom. This way you can feel each other out before your judgment gets blurred during a lip-locked passionate embrace. If you're finding yourself tongue-tied when it comes to asserting your intention to use dental dams, pull one out and show it to your partner. Talk about how you feel; maybe you're nervous, shy, embarrassed, or intimidated—if you feel silly, say so. Find out how your partner feels as well. Maybe gloves remind her of a bad root canal, but the promise of a slow, smooth, and slippery genital massage will undoubtedly give her something much better to think about. Often just being honest about the situation can ease the tension. It provides an opportunity to air your concerns or fears, clear up any misconceptions, and reassure the person that you're doing this out of concern for both of you! Not to mention it gives you something new and different to look forward to.

Keep in mind that STDs are simply a fact of life for all of us. They don't target any one demographic, and they don't conform to stereotypes about who's most likely to be infected. The sooner we accept their presence in our everyday lives, the sooner we can get on with the business of enjoying sex—accessories and all.

I grew up in a time when STDs were mostly curable. Even herpes wasn't as prevalent. When our society finally admitted that AIDS was not "the gay disease," safer-sex practice was no longer just for intellectual discussion. AIDS awareness has also opened my eyes to other STDs, the curable as well as the incurable. I am from the Mexican-American community (Roman Catholic too), where the good wife stays home and is faithful. How many little women have been infected with STDs by roving husbands? Disease isn't just in the whorehouses, or the bathhouses, or for any one type of person in the population. Anyone can get infected at any time by even the most trusted person. I have come to accept that safer sex must be considered normal and part of our everyday health. For me it is not a taboo subject, I will discuss it as freely as polio or flu vaccinations.

Risk Management

Since the onset of AIDS, "risk reduction guidelines" were established to help people understand which activities presented a greater risk of transmitting those bodily fluids that contain HIV. The guidelines also help gauge the risk of transmitting STDs other than HIV, as most STDs are passed along through vaginal, oral, or anal sex.

Behaviors in the "unsafe" category generally involve semen or blood coming into direct contact with mucous membranes in the rectum, vagina, or mouth. Activities in the "possibly unsafe" category are less likely to transmit viruses. Activities in the "possibly safe" category either involve contact with low-risk fluids, such as saliva and urine, or will not transmit the virus unless your latex barrier breaks. The "safe" category reflects activities that involve no exchange of bodily fluids and are completely safe. For example, using a condom during intercourse reduces the chance of transmission, but the possibility that the condom may break means that intercourse is not entirely safe. Vaginal secretions may be infectious under certain conditions, which is why contact with vaginal secretions is considered possibly safe. For example, if the secretions come into contact with open sores or cuts, there's a risk of viral transmission. Or if you're experiencing a vaginal infection there is a higher concentration of the virus in your secretions.

Bacterial STDs such as chlamydia, gonorrhea, or syphilis can all be treated with antibiotics, but you should not have unprotected sex until the infection is resolved. While safer-sex education focuses on condom use as the key to reducing disease transmission, STDs that can be transmitted via skin-to-skin contact, such as genital warts or genital herpes, aren't necessarily covered by a condom. During an outbreak, therefore, it's safest to postpone intercourse or oral sex if you notice sores in areas not easily covered by condoms or dams. Given that it's possible to transmit herpes asymptomatically—that is, even when you aren't experiencing an active outbreak—folks with herpes may want to use barriers during every sexual encounter. However, it's up to you and your partners to make your own decisions regarding risk management.

For more detailed information, we suggest you contact STD hotlines (see our resource listings) or peruse one of the many excellent books available on the subject. Ultimately, it's up to *you* to assess your individual risk factors and to choose activities to suit your needs.

My spouse and I used to have very strict rules against body-fluid-exchange with other partners. In the last few years we have relaxed those somewhat for friends that we feel close to already (i.e. close friends with whom we later become sexual). The reasoning is this: We do not find oral sex (our preferred play act) to be a high-risk activity for HIV, but high-to-medium for other STDs. However, most other STDs have more prominent and early symptoms than HIV. When we are with a friend who is close enough that we trust to be honest about any STD symptoms, then we're willing to forgo barriers.

If I'm not in a long-term relationship, I don't do anything but mutual masturbation without protection. I know some people won't even touch without gloves, but I think that's the point at which it's no longer worth it to me. I do use protection for oral sex, although I know the risk is pretty low. I've often been the first one to ever insist on using a condom or Saran Wrap with a partner, but when I'm firm they've always accepted it.

Guidelines for Risk Management

Safe

Massage
Hugging
Mutual masturbation (touching your own
    genitals)
Dry kissing
Tribadism, dry humping, frottage
Fantasy
Voyeurism, exhibitionism
Phone/computer sex
Sex toys (provided condoms are used if toys are
    shared)
Bathing together

Possibly Safe

French kissing
Anal intercourse with condom
Vaginal intercourse with condom
Fisting with glove
Cunnilingus with latex barrier
Fellatio with condom
Rimming/analingus with latex barrier
Finger fucking vaginally or anally with latex
    glove or cot
Watersports (urine on unbroken skin)

Possibly Unsafe

Cunnilingus without a barrier
Finger fucking without a barrier
Fellatio without a condom
Sharing sex toys without cleaning or changing
    condoms in between uses
Fisting without a glove
Rimming/analingus without a latex barrier

Unsafe

Anal intercourse without condom
Vaginal intercourse without condom
Blood contact
Unprotected cunnilingus during menstruation

Beyond the Guidelines

One of the fundamental limitations of many safer-sex raps is their focus on how to avoid contracting a disease, rather than how to avoid transmitting one. "Learn how to stay squeaky clean," the underlying message goes, "so that you don't have to join the ranks of the untouchables." It's understandable that the focus of STD education would be on restricting the spread of disease, but where does this leave those of us who already have sexually transmitted diseases, yet have no desire to embrace celibacy?

It's quite common for the average sexually active adult to take this us/them perspective to heart, and to divide the world of potential partners into those people they judge to be at risk for disease and those they judge not to be at risk. We were quite depressed at the number of our survey respondents who, when asked about their experience with safer-sex accessories, answered something to the effect of "I know my partners, so we don't have to bother with the precautions that other people have to follow." Countless health professionals have explained that it's not who you have sex with, but what sexual activities you engage in that separates risky behavior from safe behavior. Is anybody listening?

People are listening, all right, but they're listening selectively. After all, media reports frequently aggravate the misconception that a wide gulf exists between a tragic caste of disease-ridden adults and "the rest of us clean folks." Take the infamous 1982 *Time* magazine cover story on herpes, entitled "The Scarlet Letter." Similarly, HIV has been labeled in a variety of ways over time—from a gay virus, to an intravenous drug-user's virus, to a low-income woman of color's virus. People seem to believe that the virus itself is selective about the sexuality and socioeconomic status of the body it invades, rather than recognizing that infection rates rise more rapidly in different populations at different times during the course of an epidemic. What's going on here? Massive denial, that's what. Sexually transmitted diseases of all kinds are rampant in the American population, and the notion that anyone belongs to a "safe" stratum of society is ridiculous.

For instance, one in five Americans is currently infected with genital herpes. Some 80 percent of these people are estimated to be unaware that they are infected with the virus, or that they have the potential to transmit it asymptomatically, that is, without actually experiencing an outbreak. Chlamydia is the most common STD in America, spreading particularly fast among people under 25. AIDS, still widely viewed as a gay white man's disease, is rampantly on the rise among African Americans, Latinos, and young people.

Acknowledging the prevalence of STDs in all classes and communities and setting up effective prevention methods is going to require a major overhauling of our social attitudes and proscriptions around sex. Our sex-negative culture is one of the prime culprits in the spread of disease. Sex is seen as shameful, and having an STD identifies you as a sexually active individual, which is even more shameful. Telling a partner you have an STD identifies you not only as sexually active (shameful), but also as someone who's sick. Being sick is also shameful in our society, where the punishing viewpoint "If you're sick, it's your own fault" still holds sway. All this shame results in secretiveness, and secretiveness results in further transmission.

The AIDS epidemic provides a distressing example of the inherent limits of public health campaigns to impose behavioral changes in the context of a sex-negative society. Despite the ubiquity of AIDS-prevention campaigns within the gay community and a decreasing rate of new infections throughout the late eighties, more and more gay men are reporting "falling off the safe-sex wagon," with optimism about the efficacy of new AIDS treatment drugs resulting in backsliding to unsafe-sex practices (such as "barebacking," having anal sex without a condom).

Societal unwillingness to be explicit about sexual activities often results in public health warnings being painted with such a broad brush that people wind up just throwing up their hands and taking no precautions whatsoever. Individuals with genital herpes may be advised to use latex barriers every time they have sex, owing to the outside chance of asymptomatic transmission. The "use condoms every time" injunction is the cornerstone of AIDS-prevention efforts, accompanied by laudable campaigns to eroticize latex. But blanket regulations can backfire. Just as teenagers who are urged to choose abstinence over sex are more likely to wind up pregnant than those who are provided with a more comprehensive range of options, adults who are urged to use latex barriers for every sexual encounter are likely to cheat. It's the American Way to seesaw wildly between extremes of abstinence and abandon: One more box of cookies tonight and I'll give up all fat and sugar tomorrow.

Individuals who weigh the specific risks of each encounter, and modify accordingly the safer-sex approach they choose to take, stand a much better chance of sustaining a safer-sex lifestyle over the long haul. For instance, you might decide that since you always know when a herpes outbreak is coming on, the risk of asymptomatic transmission is low enough that you'll forgo using a dental dam for oral sex. You might decide that you're willing to perform fellatio without a condom as long as you haven't flossed in the past few hours. And we hope that you'll insist on using a condom for vaginal intercourse with someone you've just met. We intentionally use the terms "risk management" and "risk reduction," rather than "risk elimination," to encourage you to take an active, dynamic approach to protecting your own sexual health.

Before I started having sex, I thought the point of safer sex was that you just have to do it all the time, no matter what. Now I think that it's really important to be able to communicate with a partner and determine risk and make informed choices. Meaning that sometimes it's okay not to have safer sex.

STDs and Your Self-Image

Because of our culture's sex-negativity, contracting an STD can really do a number on both your general and your sexual self-esteem. Common mental tapes include: "It's all my fault, I'm being punished for being sexual"; "If only I hadn't (fill in the blank) this would never have happened"; "I'm ruined, violated, no longer whole"; "No one will want me now that I'm a vector of disease." Compare the dramatic negativity of these thoughts with how you'd feel if you'd simply caught the flu from a coworker, and you'll have a sense of how extraordinarily vulnerable we all are around our sexuality.

It's common for people to experience a decrease in sexual desire immediately after contracting a disease. Some people stop masturbating, let alone engaging in partner sex.

One of the hardest things for me about my chronic herpes outbreaks was that I went from feeling very positive about my labia to viewing them as a painful,

sore, disgusting part of my body. It seemed to me that all my genitals did was let me down, and the less I had to think about or touch them, the better.

What's sad about this attitude is that you are effectively denying yourself access to one of your greatest sources of healing. While it's natural to feel a decrease in sexual energy when you're physically debilitated, you should try not to let this extend into a total shutdown of sexual activity. Honoring your right to be sexually active can be physically healing: Sex reduces stress, provides a cardiovascular workout, strengthens your pelvic muscles, and otherwise creates an all-over glow. Exercise is frequently recommended for people suffering from any kind of disease, so what better therapy for an STD than sexual exercise? Honoring your right to be sexually active can also be emotionally healing. Negative sexual feelings easily segue into an overall negative self-image. If you can keep the perspective that you have an unalienable right to sexual pleasure, then your health and self-esteem will benefit directly.

While it may seem flagrantly Pollyanna-ish to speak of the positive ramifications of contracting an STD, it's true that certain silver linings can emerge if you let them. Many people find that STDs have taught them to be more open and communicative with sexual partners, as they can no longer simply initiate sex with new partners without some sort of preliminary discussion. While honesty entails risking rejection, it's also one surefire way to separate creative, compassionate women and men from narrow-minded, fearful girls and boys.

Chronic, incurable diseases, such as herpes or HIV-infection, also force you to take a healthier approach to your entire life, to do what you can to reduce stress, and to build up your immune system.

Finally—we saved the best for last!—an STD can pull you out of a behavioral rut like nobody's business. Suddenly, you're forced to appreciate the fact that sex can be oh-so-much-more than commingling body fluids and sticking one body part into another orifice. A whole new world of toys, fantasy play, and full-body sensation can be yours…if only you'll let it.

I used to love fucking up the ass and getting fucked, because of the intimacy and sometimes roughness of the gesture. After I got anal herpes, from my days of unprotected sex, it became painful to get fucked and was a turn-off. Now I'm mostly a top (I wear a condom) or I delicately perform ass play on myself. Sometimes I squat on my partner's finger, gently jiggling against my prostate, so I can control the depth of the action. This is the hardest load I shoot. Being witnessed and having my partner's help in bringing me off makes me feel a rush of sexual appetite.

I first started making my partners use rubber gloves just so I wouldn't have to be distracted by worrying about cuts in their fingers and infecting them and all that. The unexpected bonus was that I love the way gloves turn a human hand into a slick, smooth little creature— sometimes I pretend I'm getting fucked by a seal.

If you're receptive to the possibility, a heightened consciousness around STDs can even inspire a unique level of sexual self-awareness. Whether you have an STD, your partner has one, or you have no idea what the true status of your partner's health is, it's up to you to make the call as to how to behave. Coming to terms with and identifying your personal safer-sex

guidelines is a golden opportunity—a chance for you to appreciate the myriad possibilities of your entire body, to face your fears, to name your desires, and to celebrate the triumph of sexual energy over ignorance and shame.

Sex for Fun

We thought about calling this book *Sex for Fun* because it expressed so simply and concisely the message we wanted to impart to our readers. By now you're probably tired of hearing us tell you that sex should be playful, experimental, communicative, and celebratory. But nowhere is this more worth repeating than in the conclusion to this chapter on safer sex. We've given you the information, the tools, and (we hope) the motivation to go out and play safely—but only you can take those latex products out of your medicine cabinet and treat them like the real sex-enhancing, communication-building, confidence-inspiring, turn-on toys they were meant to be!

Benefits of Safer Sex

People rarely stop to think about these benefits of practicing safer sex:

- It's a show of respect for both your own and your partner's sexual health.
- It gives you peace of mind.
- Condoms can help erections last longer (thereby prolonging intercourse or masturbation).
- Condoms can be effective contraceptives if used properly.
- Safer sex curbs the spread of sexually transmitted diseases.
- It keeps your sex toys clean.
- Latex barriers are ideal for those who might find sexual fluids unappealing.

- Latex barriers offer a unique tactile sensation, especially when used with lubricant.
- Safer sex frees you from having to rely exclusively on your partners knowing or telling the truth about their sexual histories.
- Condoms make for quick clean-up.
- Safer sex facilitates communication about sex.
- It allows you to be creative in your sex play.
- It can introduce an element of humor into the bedroom.
- It has resulted in phrases like "anal sex" and "intercourse" becoming commonplace in the media.

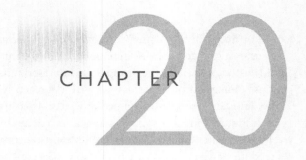

CHAPTER 20

Censorship

Just as reliable as the natural urge to express our sexuality is the societal urge to censor these expressions. In this chapter, we'll take a look at recent American trends in sexual censorship and give you tips on what you can do to stand up for freedom of expression.

"Unnatural" Acts

In the United States, a surprising number of consensual sexual activities are simply against the law. Until 1961, all fifty states prohibited various forms of consensual sex between unmarried adults. While many of these statutes were repealed during the seventies, well over a dozen states still have laws on their books criminalizing unmarried cohabitation; "fornication," which refers to sex between unmarried couples; and consensual "sodomy," which refers to oral or anal intercourse or both.

In other words, depending on where you live, your sex life may be literally felonious—and you *can* be prosecuted. In the late 1980s, a North Carolina man spent over two years in prison on a felony conviction for having oral sex with his ex-girlfriend. As of 2001, anal sex with a same-sex partner in Oklahoma carries a ten-year sentence, while anal sex with an opposite-sex partner in Idaho could get you five years to life.

These antiquated statutes are slowly being dismantled thanks to local legislative and court challenges—but no thanks to the federal government. You may recall the Supreme Court's *Bowers v. Hardwick* ruling of 1986. In a five-to-four decision, the Court ruled that same-sex couples don't have a constitutional right to privacy to "engage in sodomy" and upheld the existing Georgia state laws, in which consensual oral or anal sex between same-sex couples was a felony offense. The good news is that Georgia's sodomy laws were struck down by a lower court in 1998, but as the following letter suggests, attitudes die hard:

> After teaching human sexuality courses at the technical school and university levels for many years, I quit because I cannot discuss in open and honest ways all of the wonderful ways of pleasuring oneself and one another without incurring the wrath of the Georgia state legislature and the school system in which I work.

Most frequently, "sodomy" laws are used to discriminate against gays and lesbians in housing, employment, or child custody cases, but they can be used to discriminate against unmarried heterosexuals as well. As recently as 1996, an Idaho prosecutor charged unwed mothers with violating state fornication laws as a means to deny them welfare benefits. Check out our resource listings under "Freedom of Expression" to learn how you can help decriminalize the pursuit of sexual pleasure in your state.

Obscenity and the Law

Sexual expression becomes a crime when the materials that are produced, whether writings or images, are legally classified as "obscene." Obscene materials are exempt from the First Amendment guarantees of free speech. The legal definition of obscenity, and the inevitably subjective interpretations of this definition, determine what sexual materials we have access to and what materials we can create.

The Supreme Court definition of obscenity, which has been in effect since its 1973 *Miller v. California* ruling, allows states to regulate sexual materials according to their own community standards, provided the regulations be restricted to works that, "taken as a whole, appeal to the prurient interest in sex," that portray sexual conduct in "a patently offensive way," and that, "taken as a whole, do not have serious literary, artistic, political or scientific value." Only materials that are found by judges or jurors to meet all "three prongs" of this definition of obscenity may be deemed obscene.

You'll notice that these criteria are imprecise at best—in fact, some First Amendment lawyers feel *Miller* is so vague that if it concerned any topic other than sex, it would be considered unconstitutional. The dictionary defines "prurience" as "an inordinate interest in matters of sex," while the Supreme Court has helpfully added that prurient interests are those that are "sick and morbid," as opposed to "normal and healthy." Needless to say, it's as difficult to define "patently offensive" as it is to determine whether a photograph has *serious* artistic value or not.

The Golden Age

During the seventies, the flowering sexual revolution and women's movement created something of a Golden Age of sexual freedom of expression. In 1970,

the President's Commission on Obscenity and Pornography, which had been appointed by President Lyndon B. Johnson, submitted a report to President Richard M. Nixon stating that pornography had no discernible negative effects. The Commission recommended the repeal of most obscenity laws and called for improved sex education programs across the nation. While Nixon vigorously condemned these recommendations, the seventies were a boom time for books and magazines that satisfied the public desire for sexual information and depictions of sexual behavior. Early X-rated movies included work by directors and producers who were committed to pushing the envelope of sexual expression with serious dramas, and the success of sexually explicit mainstream films such as *Last Tango in Paris* and *Midnight Cowboy* suggested that Americans were finally "grown up" enough to embrace a popular culture that addressed sex in thoughtful and provocative ways.

The Reagan–Bush Years

The pendulum swung in the eighties with the dawn of the Reagan–Bush era (that is, the first President Bush) and the rise of the so-called Religious Right. President Ronald Reagan convened the U.S. Attorney General's Commission on Pornography, aka the Meese Commission, and charged it with a mandate to find the causal link between pornography and social ills that President Johnson's Commission had refuted over a decade earlier. The Meese Commission, an eleven-member panel of whom six were antipornography activists, obediently came to the conclusion that porn was a very bad, harmful thing indeed (but not before publishing its voluminous 1986 report, which was chock-full of excerpts from pornographic writings and plot summaries from adult videos).

The Commission's report concluded that pornography inspires sexual violence and abuse, a finding that was immediately disputed both by several of the sociologists whose research the report misrepresented and by two of the Commission's female members. These women—psychiatrist Judith Becker, whose career was devoted to studying and treating victims and perpetrators of sex crimes, and Ellen Levine, editor of *Women's Day* magazine—formally dissented from the Commission's report. They pointed out that the Commission suffered from limited funds, took no time to do independent research, and held heavily biased hearings—the majority of their "witnesses" being self-described "victims of pornography." In a public statement, Becker and Levine noted, "To say that exposure to pornography in and of itself causes an individual to commit a sexual crime is simplistic, [is] not supported by the social-science data, and overlooks many of the other variables that may be contributing causes."

Yet the Commission's detractors were ignored and the Justice Department, duly inspired by a mission to crack down on porn, created the National Obscenity Enforcement Unit. Under Presidents Reagan and George Bush, this unit developed a sophisticated strategy to take on the heavyweights of the adult industry. They targeted a handful of video manufacturers and distributors and harassed them with obscenity indictments in multiple jurisdictions. Since obscenity is defined according to community standards, the Justice Department set up sting operations to ensure jury trials in conservative communities: For example, FBI agents would pose as consumers and place mail orders for videos to be delivered to Oklahoma City, Dallas, or Salt Lake City.

These multiple jurisdiction lawsuits were a double whammy. First, most distributors couldn't afford the expense of mounting legal defense in several different states simultaneously, and the Justice Department counted on the fact that either the companies would agree to stop distributing videos, or they would drain all their financial resources on legal bills and simply go out of business. Second, if obscenity charges did stick in more conservative jurisdictions, companies could then face possible federal racketeering charges for interstate trafficking in obscene materials. While state obscenity convictions are usually misdemeanor charges, racketeering is a federal felony charge, which can result in large fines, long prison sentences, and the seizure of business assets.

One company that survived a staggering degree of federal harassment is PHE, the parent company of one of the nation's largest adult mail-order catalogs, the Adam and Eve catalog. PHE, located in North Carolina, was established in 1970 by two graduate students in family planning who saw the need for a mail-order condom catalog. Over the years, the company added novelties, lingerie, magazines, and videos, and grew large enough to attract the attention of the federal government. Between 1986 and 1993, the Justice Department waged a campaign to put Adam and Eve out of business, indicting the company on criminal obscenity charges in North Carolina, Utah, Kentucky, and Alabama.

Fortunately, PHE had the resources and the commitment to fight back and win. Unlike many video distributors who have no particular investment in the products they produce, and whose defense frequently boils down to "I know this video is a tasteless piece of crap, but dammit, I've got a First Amendment right to sell it," PHE's founder, Phil Harvey, stands behind his product line. He employs a panel of sex therapists and psychotherapists who screen every product under consideration for the Adam and Eve catalog. PHE not only successfully defended itself against every obscenity indictment, but went on to file a civil suit against the Justice Department for harassment and selective prosecution. This suit was settled in 1993 when the Justice Department agreed to cease further prosecution. (You can read the whole sordid tale in Phil Harvey's book *The Government vs. Erotica: The Siege of Adam and Eve*.)

Growing public awareness of these bullying tactics—exposed in the 1991 ACLU publication *Above the Law: The Justice Department's War Against the First Amendment*—together with the advent of a new administration led the Justice Department to shift its focus. Federal raids on adult businesses were shelved in favor of a new legal strategy: "protecting" helpless women and innocent children from the "degrading" effects of sexually explicit materials.

Protecting Women

In 1992, the Senate Judiciary Committee approved the Pornography Victims' Compensation Act, a bill that would have entitled the victim of a sex crime to sue producers, distributors, and retailers of books, magazines, and videos purported to have inspired the crime. In other words, manufacturers and retailers would be held liable for crimes committed by their customers. Although this Act never reached a vote in the full Senate, similar bills claiming a causal link between enjoying sexually explicit materials and performing criminal acts have been widely championed by antiporn activists Catharine MacKinnon and Andrea Dworkin and considered by a number of state and local legislatures.

The positive legacy of the aborted Pornography Victims' Compensation Act was the forging of alliances between publishers, distributors, retailers, media people, and First Amendment groups. Anticensorship organizations such as Feminists for Free Expression sprang up in response to this threat to freedom of speech, and numerous mainstream journalists and editors took a stand in defense of the constitutionality of sexually explicit materials.

The Canadian Supreme Court's *Butler v. the Queen* decision of 1992 provides a textbook example of what can go wrong when governments step in to "protect" their citizenry from "obscene" materials. Inspired by U.S. ordinances drafted by MacKinnon and Dworkin, which linked pornography to sexual discrimination against women, *Butler* mandates that Canadian customs seize all materials that officials deem to be "degrading" or "dehumanizing" to women. Canadian customs officials have taken the ruling as carte blanche to seize feminist, gay, and lesbian writings crossing the border and to target gay and lesbian bookstores for ongoing harassment. The lesbian erotic magazine *Bad Attitude* was one of the first publications to be seized, and has been followed by countless other volumes from *Hot, Hotter, Hottest* (detained before it proved to be a chili pepper cookbook!) to safer-sex handbooks to, you guessed it, two of Andrea Dworkin's own books.

Protecting Children

The specter of a vast commercial empire of child pornography helps to keep the wheels of the federal antiporn bureaucracy turning; however, there's no substantive proof that this empire exists. Lawrence A. Stanley convincingly argues in "The Child Porn Myth," his 1989 article in the *Cardozo Arts and Entertainment Law Journal,* that there's no commercial production or distribution of child pornography in the United States—kiddie porn exists only as a cottage industry of images shared among a small group of pedophiles. While it may be possible to find images online of minors engaged in sexual activity (hailing from overseas websites), these make up an exceedingly tiny fraction of all the sexual material on the Internet. Yet few in the Religious Right—or in government agencies, for that matter—distinguish between the production of sexually explicit materials for adults and the sexual exploitation of children. In fact, during the height of the Justice Department's war on the adult industry, the National Obscenity Enforcement Unit was renamed the Child Exploitation and Obscenity Section.

In 1996 Congress passed the Child Pornography Prevention Act, which expanded the definition of child pornography by making it a felony to produce, distribute, sell, or possess any visual depiction that "appears to be" or "conveys the impression" of a minor engaging in sexual activity. In other words, images of people *implied* or *simulated* to be under the age of 18 engaged in *implied* or *simulated* sexual activity would be defined as child pornography. As written, the law would have had major implications not only for the adult industry, but also for mainstream publishers, Hollywood filmmakers, museum curators, and advertisers—fortunately, it was overturned by the Supreme Court in 2002.

Politicians construct a moral high ground for their efforts to suppress the free exchange of sexually explicit materials by claiming that "we need to protect our children." The real target of these so-called Child Protection Acts, however, is the adult industry—yet pornographers are the first to agree that child pornography is criminally abusive. As sex educators, we'd be thrilled if the government went to the mat for children's civil rights, but it's difficult to see how pouring millions of tax dollars into preventing a married couple in Utah from receiving a mail-order porn video or trying to outlaw a Calvin Klein ad campaign truly combats the physical, emotional, and sexual abuse of the nation's children.

Censorship Online

The Internet, with its accessible, uncensored exchange of sex information and entertainment, is a natural lightning rod for free speech issues. It's a lot trickier to define "community standards," and therefore obscene materials, in a global medium. Congress's first pass at legislating sexual content on the Web was the Communications Decency Act (CDA) of 1995, which outlawed "indecent" online materials. The language of the CDA was so vague that it would have criminalized a huge range of sites—everything from the Breastfeeding Home Page to images of the Sistine Chapel. Free speech advocates successfully challenged the CDA, and it too was overturned by the Supreme Court in 1997.

The latest First Amendment skirmish involves access to online materials. Subsequent to the CDA's defeat, Congress passed the Child Online Protection Act (COPA), which would have criminalized sites containing material deemed "harmful to minors" if the sites were accessible to minors. COPA has never taken effect—it was promptly blocked by a Federal District Court on the grounds that it violates the First Amendment. As of this writing, the American Library Association and the American Civil Liberties Union are challenging the COPA requirement that public libraries install filtering software on their computers or risk losing federal funding. (See the World Wide Web chapter for more on filtering software.) It seems likely that the Supreme Court will ultimately find COPA unconstitutional—and equally likely that yet another online censorship law will rise from its ashes. The decentralized, democratic nature of the Web may confound regulation, but that hasn't deterred legislators nationwide from ongoing efforts to restrict online content and accessibility. You can expect the Internet to be a free-speech battleground for years to come.

Self-Censorship

Censorship efforts don't merely limit access to sexually explicit materials, they also limit what materials get produced.

Books

How do obscenity prosecutions affect what gets produced? Publishers of mainstream sex manuals err on the side of caution and avoid explicit photos in their books, even if the results—such as a sexual-positions guide in which all the images are carefully framed to keep genitals out of sight—are somewhat absurd.

Given our national obsession with "protecting" children from sex, it's not surprising that both adult and mainstream publishers are reluctant to accept stories related to child or adolescent sexuality—even though many of us had our adult eroticism forged during our youth. Most regrettably, the first casualties of laws ostensibly designed to protect children are often children's sex-education materials themselves. Nude photos of children have been deemed obscene in a range of court cases, and sex-ed resources such as the European classic photography book *Show Me* have been withdrawn from U.S. distribution.

Videos

Mainstream producers of porn are resistant to abandoning a formulaic approach to plot and content for fear of creating works that could be deemed "obscene" in another state. In a Catch-22 scenario, the censorship of sexually explicit materials limits the extent to which these materials can evolve into a more artistic genre that fewer people might consider worthy of censoring.

The Justice Department's single-minded pursuit of major adult video distributors in the early eighties produced a firestorm of preemptive self-censoring throughout the industry. If a plot device or sexual activity led to a video's conviction on obscenity charges somewhere in the country, the device or activity was added to the informal, yet rigid, set of boundaries beyond which porn producers would not venture. The no-no list includes fairly predictable activities such as bestiality, urination, and defecation. It also includes vaginal or anal fisting—the placement of any more than three fingers in the vagina is considered an "unnatural" act. Even female ejaculation is sometimes suspect.

Any hint of nonconsensual activities is similarly avoided, so bondage and genital-sex scenes are rarely, if ever, combined in the same film. Profanity is also scrupulously avoided, to the point where ejaculations such as "Oh God, I'm coming!" are edited out. Drugs and violence have all been white-washed out of modern porn, while images of brand-name products are edited out as well (brand-name sex toys are a welcome exception to the rule!).

Needless to say, the return of Republicans to the White House has put porn producers on high alert. Since the late nineties, when the threat of federal prosecution eased and sales of adult videos skyrocketed, the porn industry has developed something of a split personality. Large companies that release bigger-budget videos and produce soft-core, cable-ready versions of their films have more to lose and are naturally more prone to self-censoring. Smaller, maverick companies that release "wall-to-wall" hardcore videos push the envelope in terms of content. It remains to be seen how this split will play out under the current and subsequent administrations.

During the Golden Age of porn, it was possible to view adult videos that framed explicit sex scenes within the context of dramatic, passionate plots. Rape and murder were tackled head on in videos such as *Anna Obsessed* and *Midnight Heat*, videos with all the moody complexity of Hollywood film noir. Yet these classic films were among the first to go under the editor's knife in the early nineties when distributors were fleeing the threat of prison or bankruptcy. Other, far more light-hearted classics, such as *Opening of Misty Beethoven* and *Private Afternoons of Pamela Mann*, were also vigorously edited to remove any potentially controversial chunks of plot or dialogue. As an analogy, try to imagine taking classic films of American cinema, such as *Chinatown* or *The Godfather*, and excising all the scenes in which sex and violence are linked. The resulting erotic videos were a shadow of their former selves, rendered practically incomprehensible due to lack of continuity. The fate of porn's Golden Oldies is a sad reminder that adult video will never have a chance to grow up as long as censorship restricts it to the perpetual adolescence of lowest-common-denominator conformity.

Toys

While sex toys don't fall under any constitutional protection and have been ignored by federal legislators, several states have their own laws prohibiting the sale of "obscene devices." Obscene devices are usually defined as those "designed or marketed primarily for the stimulation of human genitals." Yup, in several states, including Texas and Georgia, sex toys are currently commercial contraband (though Texas does allow the sale of sex toys for therapeutic and medical reasons). While most of these laws are decades old, Alabama made headlines by outlawing sex toys in the year 1998, with the argument that there is "no fundamental right to purchase a product to use in pursuit of having an orgasm." Upon challenge by the ACLU and a group of six female sex toy consumers and retailers, this deeply silly law was promptly overturned by a District Court.

Adult bookstores in states such as Texas work around the laws by labeling their dildos "condom demonstration models" and their vibrators "novelties." In other words, folks selling and buying sex toys agree to pretend that they're being purchased either as a public health service or as gag gifts.

Zoning

Most of the statutes criminalizing the purchase of "obscene devices" date back to the seventies, when the increasing number of adult bookstores and massage parlors opening in major cities inspired opponents to devise whatever legislation they could dream up to limit the success of these businesses. Later, zoning laws became the method of choice for controlling adult retailers. Many cities and towns have zoning ordinances that restrict the location of adult-oriented businesses—specifying that they must be a certain number of feet from schools, churches, residential neighborhoods, etc.

At Good Vibrations, we ran afoul of similar zoning restrictions when we opened our second store in Berkeley in 1994. We had applied for a permit as a "book and gift store," as this is how our San Francisco store is zoned. A local resident complained that our store more closely resembled the zoning ordinance description of an adult-oriented business, namely one "which predominantly engage[s] in the sale of products or materials which appeal to a prurient interest or sexual appetite of the purchaser or user."

When we went before the zoning administrators, we were informed that any business with more than 25 percent of its inventory in sexual products was considered an adult business but that, given our educational mission, they'd allow us to carry up to 50 percent of sexually related inventory. We learned that a condom shop that had opened near Berkeley's college campus had been forced to limit condoms to less than 25 percent of its inventory…and promptly went out of business. So we went to work measuring the square footage of our fixtures and splitting hairs over which of our products qualified as "adult" versus "educational" materials.

In Good Vibrations' case, we were able to rally community support, which tipped the scales in our favor. Customers, friends, and colleagues deluged the Berkeley city council with faxes, phone calls, email, and letters of support. The local media had a field day, and five days later, city officials bowed to community pressure and reinstated our permit.

Other adult-oriented businesses in less tolerant communities aren't always so fortunate. Many people instinctively approve of zoning laws; after all, they're regarded as keeping adult businesses away from schoolchildren, rather than as violating First Amendment rights. Those who sprang to Good Vibrations' defense did so because they considered us to be "different" from "sleazy" adult bookstores with video viewing booths. In the eyes of most citizens, however, these fine distinctions would be purely academic, and any outfit distributing sexually explicit materials should be forced to hit the road. It's important to bear in mind that zoning laws are frequently the thin end of the wedge in attempts to legislate adult businesses right out of town. Whether zoning laws are being invoked to clean up Manhattan's Times Square, to remove X-rated videos from a mall's video store, or to keep a Good Vibrations from opening in your home town, we urge you to look beyond the antiporn hysteria to make reasoned judgments of your own.

What You Can Do

You can participate in the fight against censorship both on a national and local level. Check out the organizations listed under "Freedom of Expression" in our resource listings. These national organizations can keep you updated on upcoming federal legislation; it's crucial that you let your congressperson or senator know how you feel on all censorship-related bills. Don't assume that challenges to First Amendment rights fall along party lines—Democrats and Republicans are equally capable of trampling over your privacy rights, especially during an election year.

Working for change on the local level can take a bit more courage, since this may entail contacting friends and neighbors to let them know you support access to sexual materials. Since definitions of obscenity and zoning ordinances are influenced by community standards, it's particularly important that you speak out on the local level.

You can also combat censorship by flexing your consumer dollar. If you enjoy a certain adult director's work, ask your local video store to order more of his or her videos, and tell all your friends to consider renting them as well. If you crave porn with greater diversity in performers and body types, you may need to spend more to purchase independent videos. If one bookstore in your town carries sex books but another doesn't, patronize the sex-positive establishment and let its proprietors know you appreciate the range of their selection. Seek out the retailers who present the products and information you crave.

In your defense of sexually explicit materials, you're bound to grapple with your own preconceptions and subjective interpretations. One man's porn is another man's erotica, and one woman's utterly irredeemable filth is another woman's entertaining night on the town. You're certainly entitled to your own responses and opinions, and in fact we urge you to tease out and identify what does and doesn't give you pleasure in the videos, books, magazines, and toys you encounter. We hope, however, you'll maintain the point of view that it's better for there to be a wide-ranging variety of sexual materials than it is to shut down or ban any one genre. The mainstream adult industry suffers from a certain "outlaw" complex—folks who are producing commercial porn are definitely the lowest in the pecking order of First Amendment defense. The hypocrisy of having their work publicly scorned and politically persecuted, yet privately consumed in mass quantities, has resulted in an understandable amount of cynicism. As a result, adult-industry people have an incentive to circle their wagons and reject change rather than to expand the possibilities of their genre. Change will only come slowly and in direct response to consumer demand.

We recognize that it's much easier to say nothing than to stand up and identify yourself as someone who doesn't think that anal sex is a "crime against nature," who is happy that the town bookstore carries sex manuals, or who enjoys renting porn from the neighborhood video store. Yet as long as individuals remain silent about the books we read, the videos we watch, and the toys we enjoy, our rights to privacy and the pursuit of pleasure will continue to be threatened.

Kat Sunlove

"People fear what they don't understand, and so I put myself out there as best I can. When I get on TV and they have to look at me and I look like the grandma next door, they have to redefine who they think a pornographer is."

Kat Sunlove's career recapitulates every anticensorship battle of the past twenty years. A funny, feisty woman who still has the gentle Texas drawl and the energetic idealism of her youth, she's worked to defend sexual freedoms as an educator, writer, publisher, and most recently as lobbyist for the adult industry's Free Speech Coalition. Although she's long since given up her teenage ambition to serve as a Baptist missionary to Russia, we thank the Lord that Kat has channeled her missionary zeal into building a more sexually open and free society.

As Mistress Kat, the author of a column on erotic dominance and submission that ran in California's *Spectator* magazine, Kat made her first foray into the public arena in the early eighties. At the time, she and her partner, Layne Winklebleck, were teaching some of the first public S/M workshops ever held in this country: "S&M was totally and completely in the closet at that point. I knew from the letters I got that there were hundreds of thousands of people with these interests, yet scared to do anything about them—so sexual choice was one of the early censorship battlefields for me."

In 1992, Kat became publisher of *Spectator,* a weekly magazine that has been in constant publication since its origins in the sixties as the *Berkeley Barb. Spectator* features sex-related news, reviews, and pictorials, along with classified ads from sex professionals, and is distributed in coin-operated public news racks. In 1996, *Spectator* ran afoul of a new California law that banned adult newspapers from such news racks. Although the *Spectator* staff fought the law all the way up to the U.S. Supreme Court, ultimately they have had to self-censor content to stay in public news racks.

Kat has been active in adult industry trade organizations since the early eighties, and when she decided to leave *Spectator* in 1997, she was quickly hired as a lobbyist for the Free Speech Coalition (FSC). The mandate of the FSC is to provide resources, advocacy, and legal analysis on legislation that would impact the adult entertainment industry as a whole. The FSC was successful in challenging portions of the Child Pornography Protection Act.

If anyone has the energy and enthusiasm to change the world one constituent and one legislator at a time, it's Kat. "When I'm training budding citizen lobbyists, I often tell them, 'We have truth on our side, all we have to do is tell it!' I'm a well-educated woman who got into the adult industry in my mid-thirties, very self-consciously. I'm not a victim, okay? I used to be a union organizer for the Hotel, Restaurant and Bartenders International Union—you want to talk to me about oppressed women, let's talk about hotel maids!" She has taken her message to political events, through the corridors of the state house, and even into "the lion's den" of televangelist Pat Robertson's *700 Club:* "People fear what they don't understand, and so I put myself out there as best I can. When I get on TV and they have to look at me and I look like the grandma next door, they have to redefine who they think a pornographer is."

To find out more about the Free Speech Coalition, visit www.freespeechcoalition.com.

Endnote

We hope you've enjoyed reading this book, that it made you laugh and turned you on. Most of all, we hope it inspired you to expand your own sexual boundaries. By this, we don't mean we'll feel like failures if you don't want to tackle at least four new sexual positions or try at least six new sex toys as soon as you finish the last page. We would be happy if you simply felt encouraged to communicate more about sex.

The most revolutionary aspect of our work is not the nature of the products we sell or the way we sell them—it's the fact that we talk about sex. Enthusiastic, forthright, frank talk about sex is in desperately short supply in our society, and our customers tell us they're grateful for the opportunity we provide to speak freely about a subject that is shrouded in mystification. If you've felt similarly gratified by what you've read, we'd like to ask a favor of you in return.

You can help advance sexual expression on a grassroots level if you're willing to take some personal risks. It takes courage to identify your sexual feelings, fantasies, and fears without apologies or rationalizations or excuses. One of the biggest contributors to sexual shame and ignorance is people's reluctance to stand up and name what brings them pleasure. It's easier to fall silent than to ask a lover to touch you in specific ways. It's easier to dismiss activities as immature, dangerous, or politically incorrect than to examine the source of your preconceptions. It's easier to make assumptions about somebody else's sexual preferences than to acknowledge what fuels your own fantasies. It's easier to critique that "tedious" X-rated movie or that "trite" porn magazine than it is to identify the moment during viewing when your pulse speeded up or to point to the photo that made your juices start flowing. It's easier to pretend that your siblings don't have sex than it is to compare notes on how you've been influenced by the cultural messages you all received while growing up. Yet if you take the risk of speaking up about sex, a whole new world of perceptions and possibilities will open before you.

Why not try talking to a lover, a friend, a coworker, or a relative about sex in a way you never have before? Tell your lover the plot of your most powerful fantasy. Ask your best friend to take your kids to the movies so that you can stay home and masturbate. Interview your mother and your father about how they learned about sex. Present a vibrator at your sister's baby shower. Swap condom recommendations with a coworker. You may be surprised at how exhilarating it is to acknowledge yourself as a sexual person, and at how eagerly those around you respond to any encouragement to express sexual feelings and opinions.

We understand that many people feel that sex is a private matter, and that public discourse threatens to devalue it. The truth is, our society's tacit agreement to keep silent about where and how we get pleasure has created a situation in which the individual right to privacy is under siege and the right to free expression is subject to constant legislative threats.

The enjoyment of sex is a basic human right that we'd like to see guaranteed to all. When we were first working on this book, we used to joke that the final chapter should be entitled "We'd Like to Teach the World to Come," but perhaps a more accurate title would be "We'd Like to Teach the World to Communicate." Better communication leads to increased sexual pleasure, which, in turn, promotes health, self-esteem, intimacy, creativity, and joy. The world would unquestionably be a better place if sexual pleasure were more abundant. While we can't necessarily realize our dream of putting a vibrator into the hands of every U.N. representative or penetrating the nation's corridors of power with dildos and lubes, we can offer you encouragement, praise, and our heartfelt wishes for a lifetime full of all the sexual pleasure you desire.

Let's Talk About Sex—
Take Our Survey!

We're inviting all our readers to fill out as much of the following survey as they wish. Feel free to skip any questions that don't inspire you. We hope these questions will encourage you to identify what gives you pleasure. We're not looking for statistics—we simply want to get a sense of what sexual activities you're enjoying, so that we can best represent your experience in future editions of this book. We want to know what kind of sex you like and why you like it! If you're willing to share your responses (anonymously, of course), send your completed survey to: comments@anneandcathy.com.

We may choose to quote anonymously from portions of these surveys. If you do not wish to be quoted, even anonymously, please tell us.

Age   _____
Sex   _____
Sexual orientation   _____

Sexual Arousal and Response

1. Please describe your experience of any or all of the following:
    women: orgasm, multiple orgasm, ejaculation, G-spot stimulation
    men: orgasm, multiple orgasm, orgasm without ejaculation, prostate stimulation

2. Please describe how your experiences of desire, arousal, and orgasm have (or haven't) changed over the course of your lifetime. For instance, how have your experiences changed with age, during pregnancy, upon becoming a parent, while on medication, after surgery, etc.

Self-Image

3. What factors have had the biggest influence on your sexual self-esteem?

4. How has your sexual self-image changed over your lifetime?

Masturbation

5. What's your earliest memory of masturbating (consciously engaging in sexual self-stimulation)?

6. Describe your single most powerful masturbation experience.

Coming of Age

7. When did you start having sex with a partner, and what were these early experiences like?

8. What specific resources did you find most useful in learning about sex and sexual technique (books, partners, sex-ed class)?

9. What were the most positive and most negative messages you received when learning about sex?

Sex Play

10. What are your favorite sexual activities that don't involve intercourse (massage, oral sex, mutual masturbation, etc.)?

11. What types of online sexual entertainment or communication do you enjoy (cybersex, chatrooms, reading/writing erotica, etc.)?

12. Please describe your experiences with sexual power play.

Penetration

13. Please describe what types of vaginal and/or anal penetration (fingers, fist, penis, dildo, plug, vibrator, anal beads, etc.) you particularly enjoy.

14. What are your favorite positions for penetration?

15. Do you use lubricant; why or why not? If you do, what type do you prefer?

Sex Toys

16. Please describe your most enjoyable, amusing and/or disappointing experience with a sex toy.

17. What sex toys do you wish existed?

Fantasies

18. Please describe your (current) favorite fantasy.

19. Have you identified certain recurring themes in your fantasies, or have your fantasies changed over your lifetime?

20. What specific books, magazines, or videos reliably fuel your fantasies?

Communication

21. What have been some of the most difficult subjects to raise with a sexual partner?

22. What techniques have you found to be most (and least) successful in discussing sex with a partner?

Safer Sex

23. Please describe your experience with safer-sex accessories (condoms, dams, gloves, Saran Wrap, etc.)? If you do not practice safer sex, why not?

24. How has your attitude about safer sex changed (or not) over your lifetime?

Feedback

25. Are there any other specific questions or issues you'd like us to address in future editions of this book?

26. What comments and/or feedback do you have for us?

Resources

Shopping Guide

Adam and Eve
Catalog of toys, videos, and lingerie

> PO Box 800
> Carrboro, NC 27510
> (919) 644-1212 *or* (800) 274-0333
> www.adameve.com

Adam and Gillian's Sensual Whips and Toys
Catalog of bondage gear and whips

> 40 Grant Avenue
> Copiague, NY 11726
> (631) 842-1711 *or* (888) 476-8697
> www.aswgt.com

Aslan Leather
Online catalog of harnesses, bondage gear, and whips

> Box 102, Station B
> Toronto, Ontario
> Canada M5T 2T3
> (416) 306-0462 *or* (877) 467-1526
> www.aslanleather.com

Blowfish
Catalog of toys, books, and videos

> PO Box 411290
> San Francisco, CA 94141
> (415) 252-4340 *or* (800) 325-2569
> www.blowfish.com

Come as You Are
Retail store and online catalog of toys, books, and videos

> 701 Queen Street West
> Toronto, Ontario
> Canada M6J 1E6
> (416) 504-7934 *or* (877) 858-3160
> www.comeasyouare.com

Condomania
Retail stores and catalog of safer-sex supplies

> 647 N. Poinsettia Place
> Los Angeles, CA 90036
> (323) 930-5330 *or* (800) 926-6366
> www.condomania.com

> 351 Bleecker Street
> New York, NY 10014
> (212) 691-9442

Betty Dodson Productions
Online catalog of Betty's books, videos, and select toys

> PO Box 1933
> Murray Hill Station
> New York, NY 10156
> (866) 877-9676
> www.bettydodson.com

Dream Dresser
Retail stores and online catalog of fetish clothing, shoes, and toys

> 8444-50 Santa Monica Boulevard
> West Hollywood, CA 90069
> (323) 848-3480 *or* (800) 963-7326
> www.dreamdresser.com

> 1042 Wisconsin Avenue, NW
> Washington, DC 20007
> (202) 625-0373

EroSpirit New School of Erotic Touch
Catalog of erotic massage videos by educators, including Joseph Kramer and Annie Sprinkle

> PO Box 3893
> Oakland, CA 94609
> (510) 428-9063 *or* (800) 432-3767
> www.erospirit.org

E-Sensuals
Catalog of books and videos related to sex and
spirituality; national directory of Tantra teachers and
workshops

> PO Box 1818
> Sebastopol, CA 95472
> (707) 823-3063 *or* (800) 982-6872
> www.tantra.com

Eve's Garden
Retail store (woman-oriented) and catalog of toys,
books, and videos

> 119 West 57th Street, #1201
> New York, NY 10019
> (212) 757-8651 *or* (800) 848-3837
> www.evesgarden.com

Femme Productions, Inc.
Candida Royalle's erotic videos from a woman's
perspective

> (800) 456-5683
> www.royalle.com

Forbidden Fruit
Retail store and online catalog of toys and fetish
clothing

> 512 Neches Street
> Austin, TX 78701
> (512) 478-8358 *or* (800) 315-2029
> www.forbiddenfruit.com

Glyde Dams
Online catalog of safer sex supplies

> PO Box 9783
> Seattle, WA 98109
> (206) 283-7664
> www.sheerglydedams.com

Good For Her
Retail store and online catalog of toys, books, and
videos

> 175 Harbord Street
> Toronto, Ontario
> Canada M5S 1H3
> (416) 588-0900 *or* (877) 588-0900
> www.goodforher.com

Good Vibrations
Retail stores of toys, books, and videos

> 1210 Valencia Street
> San Francisco, CA 94110
> (415) 974-8980

> 1620 Polk Street
> San Francisco, CA 94109
> (415) 974-8985

> 2504 San Pablo Avenue
> Berkeley, CA 94702
> (510) 841-8987

Catalog of toys, books, and videos

> 938 Howard Street, #101-GB
> San Francisco, CA 94103
> (415) 974-8990 *or* (800) 289-8423
> www.goodvibes.com

Publishing/Production

> Down There Press: sexual self-help and erotic books
> Passion Press: erotic audio tapes
> Sexpositive Productions: erotic and educational
> videos

Grand Opening!
Retail store and online catalog of toys, books, and videos

> 318 Harvard Street, #32
> Brookline, MA 02146
> (617) 731-2626 *or* (877-731-2626
> www.grandopening.com

Heartwood Whips of Passion
Catalog of hand-crafted whips

> PO Box 490
> Herndon, VA 20172
> (703) 834-0757
> www.heartwoodwhips.com

House O' Chicks and Vulva University
Online sex education classes and video sales

> 2215-R Market Street, #813
> San Francisco, CA 94114
> www.houseochicks.com

JT's Stockroom
Catalog of S/M toys

> 2140 Hyperion Avenue
> Los Angeles, CA 90027
> (323) 666-2121 *or* (800) 755-8697
> www.stockroom.com

Libida
Online catalog of toys, books, and videos

www.libida.com

Lovecraft
Retail stores and online catalog of toys, books, videos, and lingerie

27 Yorkville Avenue
Toronto, Ontario
Canada M5R 1B7
(416) 923-7331 *or* (877) 923-7331
www. lovecraftsexshop.com

2200 Dundas Street, East
Mississauga, Ontario
Canada L4X 2V3
(905) 276-5772

Loveseason
Retail stores and catalog of toys, books, videos, and lingerie

4001 198th Street SW, #7
Lynnwood, WA 98036
(425) 775-4502 *or* (800) 500-8843

12001 NE 12th Street, #85
Bellevue, WA 98005
(425) 455-0533

724 Meridian Avenue E
Milton, WA 98354
(253) 952-0224

10607 SE 240th Street
Kent, WA 98031
(253) 859-0748

Pleasure Chest
Retail store and catalog of toys and clothing

7733 Santa Monica Boulevard
West Hollywood, CA 90046
(323) 650-1022 (retail)
(800) 753-4536 (mail order)
www.thepleasurechest.com

Purple Passion
Retail store and online catalog of toys, books, videos, and fetish clothing

211 West 20th Street
New York, NY 10011
(212) 807-0486
www.purplepassion.com

Romantasy
Catalog of custom corsets

2912 Diamond Street, #239
San Francisco, CA 94131
(415) 585-0760
www.romantasy.com

Rubber Tree
Nonprofit organization's catalog of safer-sex supplies

PO Box 8179
Santa Fe, NM 87504
(505) 988-5261 *or* (888) 792-8733
www.rubbertree.org

Safe Sense
Online catalog of safer-sex supplies

2015 Polk Street
San Francisco, CA 94109
(415) 351-1903 *or* (888) 702-6636
www.condoms.net

SIR Video Productions
Online catalog of lesbian-made erotic and educational videos

3288 21st Street, #94
San Francisco, CA 94110
www.sirvideo.com

Stormy Leather
Retail store and catalog of fetish clothing and toys

1158 Howard Street
San Francisco, CA 94103
(415) 626-1672 *or* (877) 975-5577
www.stormyleather.com

Toys in Babeland
Retail stores and catalog of toys, books, and videos

711 E. Pike Street
Seattle, WA 98112
(206) 328-2914 *or* (800) 658-9119
www.babeland.com

94 Rivington Street
New York, NY 10002
(212) 375-1701

Venus Book Club
Online catalog of erotic books and videos.

w ww.venusbookclub.com

Vixen Creations
Catalog of handcrafted silicone toys

1004 Revere, #B-49
San Francisco, CA 94124
(415) 822-0403
www.vixencreations.com

A Woman's Touch
Retail store and catalog of toys, books, and videos

600 Williamson Street
Madison, WI 53703
(608) 250-1928 *or* (888) 621-8880
www.a-womans-touch.com

Womyn's Ware
Retail store and catalog of toys and books

896 Commercial Drive
Vancouver, British Columbia
Canada V5L 3Y5
(604) 254-2543 *or* (888) 996-9273
www.womynsware.com

Xandria Collection
Lawrence Research Group
Catalog of toys, books, and videos

165 Valley Drive
Brisbane, CA 94005
(415) 468-3812 *or* (800) 242-2823
www.xandria.com

Magazines and Online Erotica

Adult Video News
Monthly trade magazine of the adult film industry:
news, reviews, and gossip

AVN Publications
(818) 718-5788
www.adultvideonews.com

Anything That Moves
Nonprofit quarterly bisexual magazine

2261 Market Street, #496
San Francisco, CA 94114
(415) 626-5069
www.anythingthatmoves.com

Clean Sheets
Online weekly magazine with erotica and
commentary

www.cleansheets.com

Dimensions Magazine
Bimonthly magazine celebrating BBWs (big, beautiful
women) and their admirers

PO Box 640
Folsom, CA 95763
(916) 984-9947
www.dimensionsmagazine.com

Erotica Readers and Writers Association
A forum for women and men interested in writing,
reading, or talking about erotica

www.erotica-readers.com

Good Vibes Magazine
Articles on sex and erotica published by Good
Vibrations and updated weekly.

www.goodvibes.com

Jane's Net Sex Guide
Jane is the Ralph Nader of online adult commerce:
she reviews hundreds of adult sites and provides
consumer tips.

www.janesguide.com

Libido: The Journal of Sex and Sensibility
Online literary sex magazine

PO Box 146721
Chicago, IL 60614
(773) 275-0842 *or* (800) 495-1988
www.libidomag.com

Loving More
Quarterly magazine on responsible polyamory

PO Box 4358
Boulder, CO 80306
(305) 543-7540 *or* (800) 424-9561
www.lovemore.com

Nerve
Online magazine of erotica, articles, and personals

www.nerve.com

On Our Backs
Bimonthly lesbian magazine

3415 Cesar Chavez Street, #101
San Francisco, CA 94110
(877) 999-6627
www.onourbacksmag.com

Scarlet Letters: The Journal of Femmerotica
Online magazine of erotica, articles, and advice

www.scarletletters.com

Spectator Magazine
Weekly sex news, reviews, and pictorials

PO Box 1984
Berkeley, CA 94701
(510) 849-1615 *or* (800) 624-8433
www.spectator.net

Sex Information and Organizations

Hotlines

Sexual Health

American Social Health Association hotline, (800) 971-8500

Centers for Disease Control national AIDS hotline, (800) 342-AIDS
Spanish, (800) 344-7432
Hearing impaired, (800) 243-7889

Centers for Disease Control national STD hotline, (800) 227-8922

Emergency Contraception hotline, (800) 584-9911

HIV/AIDS Teen hotline, (800) 440-TEEN

National Abortion Federation hotline, (800) 772-9100

National Herpes hotline, (919) 361-8488

Sexual Abuse and Domestic Violence

Domestic Violence hotline, (800) 799-SAFE

National Child Abuse hotline, (800) 4-A-CHILD

RAINN (Rape Abuse and Incest National Network), (800) 656-HOPE

Information

San Francisco Sex Information, www.sfsi.org
(877) 472-7374 *or* (415) 989-7374

Seattle Sex Information, (206) 328-7711

Sexual Health Resources

Circumcision Information and Resource Pages
Medical and historical articles, as well as information for parents and educators

www.cirp.org

FSD (Female Sexual Dysfunction) Alert
Feminist educational campaign challenging the medical myth of female sexual dysfunction and promoting a more holistic approach to women's sexual empowerment

www.fsd-alert.org

Safer Sex Page
A friendly, comprehensive, multimedia site

www.safersex.org

Isadora Alman's Sexuality Forum
An online community discussing sex and relationships

www.askisadora.com

Society for Human Sexuality
The largest online archive of sexuality materials

www.sexuality.org

Resources for Children, Teens, and Parents

Advocates for Youth
Promotes policies to help youth make informed and responsible decisions about sexual health

1025 Vermont Avenue, NW, #200
Washington, DC 20005
(202) 347-5700
www.advocatesforyouth.org

Coalition for Positive Sexuality
A sex education site run by teens for teens

www.positive.org

Go Ask Alice!
A site serving a student population and boasting an extensive archive of sex Q&A

www.alice.columbia.edu

Our Whole Lives (OWL)
A comprehensive, lifespan sexuality education series for grades K–12

Unitarian Universalist Association Bookstore
25 Beacon Street
Boston, MA 02108
(800) 215-9076
www.uua.org

Scarleteen: Sex Education That's for Real
Accurate sex advice for youth delivered in a friendly, nonjudgmental manner

www.scarleteen.com

Sex Etc.
A sex education site run by teens for teens

www.sxetc.com

Professional Organizations

American Association of Sex Educators, Counselors, and Therapists (AASECT)
Can provide list of AASECT-certified therapists and counselors; publishes *Journal of Sex Education and Therapy*

PO Box 238
Mount Vernon, IA 52314
(319) 895-8407
www.aasect.org

Sexuality Information and Education Council of the United States (SIECUS)
Annotated bibliographies on dozens of sex-related topics online or by mail

130 West 42nd Street, #350
New York, NY 10036
(212) 819-9770
www.siecus.org

The Society for the Scientific Study of Sex (SSSS)
Publishes *Journal of Sex Research*

Address and phone same as AASECT (above)
www.ssc.wisc.edu/ssss

Freedom of Expression Organizations

American Civil Liberties Union
Nonprofit organization offering educational and legal services to defend First Amendment rights

125 Broad Street, 18th Floor
New York, NY 10004
(212) 944-9800
www.aclu.org

Electronic Frontier Foundation
Nonprofit organization protecting civil liberties online

454 Shotwell Street
San Francisco, CA 94110
(415) 436 9333
www.eff.org

Feminists for Free Expression
Nonprofit anticensorship organization

PO Box 2525
Times Square Station
New York, NY 10108
(212) 702-6292
www.ffeusa.org

Free Speech Coalition
Trade organization providing resources and advocacy on legislation affecting the adult entertainment industry

www.freespeechcoalition.com

National Coalition Against Censorship
Nonprofit organization; publishes *Censorship News* four times per year

275 Seventh Avenue
New York, NY 10001
(212) 807-6222
www.ncac.org

National Coalition for Sexual Freedom
Nonprofit organization advocating for individual rights to consensual alternative sexual expression and working to change antiquated sex laws

1312 18th Street, NW, #102
Washington, DC 20036
(202) 955-1023
www.NCSFreedom.org

Peacefire
Youth alliance against Internet censorship; provides information on Internet filters and blocking software

www.peacefire.org

Sex and Disability Resources

Come as You Are
Online catalog site also features information on sex and disability

www.comeasyouare.com

Committee on Sexuality
Committee of professionals, parents, and people with developmental disabilities advocating for sexual rights

21450 Bear Creek Road
Los Gatos, CA 95030
www.w3ddesign.com/committee

Diverse City Press
Publishes sex resources for peoplewith developmental disabilities and their caregivers

460 Oak Street
Newmarket, Ontario
Canada L3Y 3X6
(877) 246 5226
www.diverse-city.com

Gimp Girl Community: Sex and Disability
An excellent resource site featuring articles, links, and discussion boards

www.gimpgirl.com/sex.html

Good Vibrations Shopping Guide for People with Disabilities
Advice and recommended products

www.goodvibes.com

Ragged Edge
Bimonthly magazine on disability rights that sometimes covers sexual issues

PO Box 145
Louisville, KY 40201
(502) 894-9492
www.ragged-edge-mag.com

Sexual Health
Extensive information and resources for people with physical disabilities, illnesses, or other health-related problems

www.sexualhealth.com

Transgender and Intersex Resources

CDS Bookstand
Online catalog of books, videos, and magazines about transgender issues

PO Box 491
Lionville, PA 19353
(610) 321-0858
www.cdspub.com

FTM
Information and peer support for female-to-male transsexuals. Publishes quarterly newsletter.

1360 Mission Street, #200
San Francisco, CA 94103
(415) 553-5987
www.ftm-intl.org

Gender Education and Advocacy (formerly AEGIS)
National nonprofit organization advocating for gender-variant people; publishes quarterly journal *Chrysalis* and newsletter

PO Box 33724
Decatur, GA 30033
www.gender.org

Gender Issues
A directory site with extensive links to transgender resources

www.songweaver.com/gender

GenderPAC (Public Advocacy Coalition)
National organization working to end discrimination and violence caused by gender stereotypes

1743 Connecticut Avenue, NW, 4th Floor
Washington, DC 20009
(202) 462-6610
www.gpac.org

International Foundation for Gender Education
Publishes quarterly *Transgender Tapestry* magazine

PO Box 540229
Waltham, MA 02454
781) 899-2212
www.ifge.org

Intersex Society of North America
National educational and advocacy organization

PO Box 301
Petaluma CA 94953
707) 636-0420
www.isna.org

S/M Resources

Dr. Gloria Brame
Informational site on BDSM "for literate adults"

www.gloriabrame.com

Eulenspiegel Society
Publishes quarterly magazine *Prometheus*

PO Box 2783
Grand Central Station
New York, NY 10163
(212) 388-7022
www.tes.org

National Leather Association, International
Provides referrals to local chapters; organizes annual "Living in Leather" event

4031 Wycliff Avenue, #958
Dallas, TX 75219
www.nla-i.com

QSM
Classes on S/M for all orientations; catalog of S/M books, magazines, and videos

PO Box 880154
San Francisco, CA 94188
(415) 550-7776
www.qualitysm.com

Society of Janus
Nonprofit, San Francisco–based education and support group

PO Box 411523
San Francisco, CA 94141
(415) 292-3222
www.soj.org

Bibliography

Nonfiction
Female Sexuality

The Black Women's Health Book edited by Evelyn White (Seal Press, 1994). A comprehensive health book with a good discussion of sexuality.

The Clitoral Truth by Rebecca Chalker (Seven Stories Press, 2000). Everything you ever wanted to know about the clitoris.

Cunt Coloring Book by Tee Corinne (Naiad Press, 1989). A coloring book of forty-two drawings of women's genitals (previously titled *LabiaFlowers*).

Femalia edited by Joani Blank (Down There Press, 1993). Thirty-two full-color photographs of women's genitals.

For Yourself: The Fulfillment of Female Sexuality by Lonnie Garfield Barbach (Penguin Group/Signet, 2001). A classic guide for women who have never had orgasms or who wish to enhance their sexual responsiveness. Revised.

The Good Vibrations Guide to the G-Spot by Cathy Winks (Down There Press, 1997). Encouraging and no-nonsense debunking of G-spot and female ejaculation myths, along with how-to advice.

The G-Spot and Other Recent Discoveries about Human Sexuality by Alice Kahn Ladas, Beverly Whipple, and John D. Perry (Bantam Doubleday Dell/Dell, 1982). A discussion of the G-spot, including first-person accounts of G-spot stimulation and female ejaculation.

The Mother's Guide to Sex by Anne Semans and Cathy Winks (Random House, 2001). Examines changes to a mother's sexuality, from pregnancy through postpartum and beyond. Includes a section on talking to kids about sex.

My Secret Garden by Nancy Friday (Simon & Schuster/Pocket Books, 1973). A groundbreaking collection of women's sexual fantasies.

New View of a Woman's Body by the Federation of Feminist Women's Health Centers (Feminist Health Press, 1991). A self-help classic, including an expanded definition of the clitoris and color photographs of women's genitals.

Our Bodies, Ourselves for the New Century by the Boston Women's Health Collective (Simon & Schuster/Touchstone, 1998). A wide-ranging sourcebook on all aspects of female sexuality and sexual health.

The Playbook for Women about Sex by Joani Blank (Down There Press, 1982). An interactive playbook/workbook designed to enhance sexual self-awareness.

The Survivor's Guide to Sex: How to Have an Empowered Sex Life After Child Sexual Abuse by Staci Haines (Cleis Press, 1999). How women survivors can rebuild a fulfilling sex life, identify dissociation, handle triggers, and cultivate sexual pleasure.

The Ultimate Guide to Anal Sex for Women by Tristan Taormino (Cleis Press, 1997). A thorough resource on anal sex for women of all orientations.

When the Earth Moves by Mikaya Heart (Celestial Arts, 1998). Exploration of female sexuality includes information about different types of orgasm, when and why women fake orgasm, multiple orgasms, and more.

The Whole Lesbian Sex Book by Felice Newman (Cleis Press, 1999). An all-questions-answered, savvy guide to lesbian, butch, bisexual, femme, androgynous, and transgendered sex.

Woman: An Intimate Geography by Natalie Angier (Anchor, 2000). Informative and wide-ranging tour of the biology of the female body.

Male Sexuality

Circumcision: What It Does by Billy Ray Boyd (Tatterhill Press, 1990). Facts about circumcision.

How to Make Love All Night: The Male Multiple Orgasm and Other Secrets of Prolonged Love by Barbara Keesling, Ph.D. (HarperCollins Publishers/Harper Perennial, 1994). Exercise regime teaching techniques to achieve and control the timing of orgasm without ejaculation.

Men Like Us by Daniel Wolfe and Gay Men's Health Crisis (Ballantine Books, 1999). The first comprehensive health resource book by and especially for gay men.

The Multi-Orgasmic Man by Mantak Chia and Douglas Abrams Arana (HarperCollins Publishers/ HarperSan Francisco, 1996). An illustrated guide to achieving multiple orgasms based on Taoist teachings.

New Male Sexuality: The Truth about Men, Sex and Pleasure by Bernie Zilbergeld (Bantam Doubleday Dell/Bantam Books, 1992). Encouragement and advice on concerns including performance anxieties, erection difficulties, and desire discrepancies (previously published as *Male Sexuality*, 1978).

The Playbook for Men about Sex by Joani Blank (Down There Press, 1981). An interactive playbook/workbook designed to enhance sexual self-awareness.

Sex: A Man's Guide by Stefan Bechtel and Laurence Roy Stains (Rodale Press, 1996). Engagingly written advice on 130 different sexual topics.

Sexual Male: Problems and Solutions by Richard Milsten, M.D., and Julian Slowinski (W. W. Norton & Co., 2001). Dedicated to erectile difficulties and other male sexual performance concerns.

Sexual Solutions: A Guide for Men and the Women Who Love Them by Michael Castleman (Simon & Schuster/Touchstone, 1983). An informative, down-to-earth guide aimed at men in heterosexual relationships.

The Ultimate Guide to Anal Sex for Men by Bill Brent (Cleis Press, 2001). Debunks myths and offers instruction.

Masturbation

First Person Sexual edited by Joani Blank (Down There Press, 1996). A collection of masturbation stories by men and women of all orientations.

I Am My Lover edited by Joani Blank (Down There Press, 1997). Photo-essay of twelve women masturbating before the camera.

Men Loving Themselves: Images of Male Self-Sexuality by Jack Morin (Down There Press, 1988). A photo-study of twelve diverse men expressing their feelings about masturbation.

Sex for One: The Joy of Selfloving by Betty Dodson (Crown Publishers/Harmony Press, 1987). A reassuring, entertaining guide to the techniques and pleasures of masturbation with erotic line drawings by the author (expanded from the previously self-published works *Liberating Masturbation* and *SelfLove and Orgasm*).

Solo Sex: Advanced Techniques by Dr. Harold Litten (Factor Press, 1992). A friendly, creative guide to the varieties of male masturbation.

Tickle Your Fancy by Sadie Allison (Tickle Kitty Press, 2001). A basic introduction to female masturbation.

Sex Manuals and Guides

Anal Pleasure and Health by Jack Morin (Down There Press, 1998). The classic guide to eliminating anal tension and enjoying anal stimulation, revised and updated.

Big, Big Love by Hanne Blank (Greenery Press, 1999). Tackles mainstream attitudes that render fat folks sexless, offering information on fat sex, love and romance, self-image, finding partners, adapting sexual positions, and sexual health.

The Big O by Lou Paget (Broadway Books, 2001). A concise guide to both male and female orgasm.

The Complete Guide to Safer Sex by staff of the Institute for the Advanced Study of Human Sexuality (Barricade Books, 1999). A valuable guide to learning healthy sexual behavior, with current information about the transmission and prevention of AIDS.

Enabling Romance: A Guide to Love, Sex and Relationships for the Disabled by Ken Kroll and Erica Levy Klein (No Limits Communications, 2001). A one-of-a-kind guide covering sexual concerns and techniques for people with a variety of disabilities. Features interviews and a thorough resource list.

Erotic Massage: The Touch of Love by Kenneth Ray Stubbs (Secret Garden, 1989). General techniques for massaging the entire body, presented in clear language and with excellent illustrations.

The Erotic Mind: Unlocking the Inner Sources of Sexual Passion and Fulfillment by Jack Morin, Ph.D. (HarperCollins Publishers/Harper Perennial, 1995). Explores the nature of arousal, the four cornerstones of eroticism, and how to develop a more fulfilling sex life. Also available in audiocassette.

The Ethical Slut by Dossie Easton and Catherine Liszt (Greenery Press, 1997). A frank and practical look at the logistics of open relationships.

Exhibitionism for the Shy by Carol Queen (Down There Press, 1995). Tips for dressing up, showing off, talking sexy, and communicating your desires with a partner.

For Each Other by Lonnie Barbach (Signet, 2001). An updated version of the classic guide to increasing intimacy and improving communication in long-term relationships.

The Good Vibrations Guide to Adult Videos by Cathy Winks (Down There Press, 1998). Reviews of selected videos, interviews with notable stars and directors, tips on watching with a lover, and a concise history of modern porn.

Good Vibrations: The New Complete Guide to Vibrators by Joani Blank and Ann Whidden (Down There Press, 2000). The ultimate guide to selecting, enjoying, and maintaining a vibrator and introducing your partner to one.

Guide to Getting It On: A New and Mostly Wonderful Book About Sex by Goofy Foot Press (Goofy Foot Press, 2000). An honest and humorous discussion of a variety of sexual interests and activities.

Hand in the Bush by Deborah Addington (Greenery Press, 1998). Thorough guide to vaginal fisting.

Health Care Without Shame by Charles Moser Ph.D., M.D. (Greenery Press, 1999). Geared primarily toward those with alternative sexual lifestyles, this book offers invaluable advice on talking to health care providers about sexuality.

Hot Monogamy: Essential Steps to More Passionate, Intimate Lovemaking by Dr. Patricia Love and Jo Robinson (Penguin/Plume, 1994). An exercise book for monogamous couples who want to improve sexual intimacy, communication, and technique.

Lesbian Sex Secrets for Men by Jamie Goddard and Kurt Brungardt (Plume, 2001). Tips for straight men on pleasing women.

101 Nights of Great Sex by Laura Corn (Park Avenue Press, 1995). A creative couple's book with different suggestions for exploring sexual intimacy on each sealed page.

Polyamory by Dr. Deborah M. Anapol (Intinet Resource Center, 1997). Information on negotiating relationships that include more than one lover.

Sex Tips for Straight Women from a Gay Man by Dan Anderson and Maggie Berman. (HarperCollins, 1997). The authors (a gay man and his straight female best friend) provide insight on hand jobs, blow–jobs, and a wealth of sexual techniques designed to please men.

Soulmates by Eric Copage (Plume, 2001). A beautifully illustrated and comprehensive sex guide for African-Americans.

Talk Sexy to the One You Love by Barbara Keesling, Ph.D. (HarperCollins, 1996). Learn to create and enjoy an erotic vocabulary.

Trust: The Hand Book by Bert Hermann (Alamo Square Press, 1991). The definitive guide to anal fisting.

The Ultimate Guide to Cunnilingus by Violet Blue (Cleis Press, 2002). Extensive guide to oral sex.

The Ultimate Guide to Fellatio by Violet Blue (Cleis Press, 2002). Extensive guide to oral sex.

The Ultimate Guide to Strap On Sex by Karlyn Lotney (Cleis Press, 2000). Guide to anally or vaginally penetrating a partner with dildos and assorted toys.

The Woman's Guide to Sex on the Web by Anne Semans and Cathy Winks (HarperSanFrancisco, 1999). Entertaining tour of the steamy side of the Web, with tips for shopping, gathering information, finding quality sexual entertainment, and chatting, plus dozens of site reviews.

Eastern Sexual Techniques

The Art of Sexual Ecstasy: The Path of Sacred Sexuality for Western Lovers by Margo Anand (Jeremy P. Tarcher/Putnam, 1989). An exceptionally accessible guide to Tantric and Taoist techniques.

The Multi-Orgasmic Couple by Mantak Chia, Maneewan Chia, Douglas Abrams, and Rachel Carlton Abrams, M.D. (HarperSanFrancisco, 2000). Techniques for cultivating sexual energy, oral sex, positions, masturbation, and sexual synchronization with a partner.

Sacred Sex: Ecstatic Techniques for Empowering Relationships by Jwala (Mandala, 1993). A Tantric sex guide.

Sex with Spirit by Michelle Pauli (Red Wheel/Weiser, 2001). Covers Tantra, Kabbalah, Paganism, Yoga, and more, with information on how to tune your body to achieve heightened states of bliss within partnered sex. Beautiful erotic photographs.

Sexual Energy Ecstasy: A Practical Guide to Lovemaking Secrets of the East and West by David and Ellen Ramsdale (Bantam, 1993). An accessible, updated guide to Tantric sexual practices.

Women's Kama Sutra by Nitya Lacroix (Dunne Books, 2001). In this unique, nicely illustrated version of the Kama Sutra the focus is on women's pleasure.

S/M and Power Play

Come Hither by Gloria Brame (Fireside, 2000). An informative, friendly guide to turning your kinky fantasies into satisfying expressions of love and desire.

Consensual Sadomasochism: How to Talk About It and How to Do It Safely by Sybil Holiday and Bill Henkin, Ph.D. (Daedalus, 1996). An expert guide to S/M.

Leatherfolk: Radical Sex, People, Politics and Practice edited by Mark Thompson (Alyson Publications, 2001). A diverse and provocative collection of essays by some of the best writers in the gay and lesbian S/M community.

Leatherman's Handbook by Larry Townsend (LT Publication, 2000). Recently revised guide to S/M for gay men, including instructional information and erotic first-person accounts.

The Loving Dominant by John Warren, Ph.D. (Greenery Press, 2000). A comprehensive guide to dominance and submission from a male perspective.

The New Bottoming Book by Dossie Easton and Janet Hardy (Greenery Press, 2001). Revised, illustrated guide to submission.

The Seductive Art of Japanese Bondage by Mistress Midori (Greenery Press, 2001). Erotic color photographs illustrate the intricate art of Japanese rope bondage.

Sensuous Magic: A Guide for Adventurous Couples by Patrick Califia (Cleis Press, 2001). A revised, accessible guide to S/M for couples of all sexual orientations.

Sexual Magic: The S/M Photographs by Michael Rosen (Shaynew Press, 1986). More than fifty photographs of S/M play, accompanied by the subjects' personal reflections.

Sexual Portraits: Photographs of Radical Sexuality by Michael Rosen (Shaynew Press, 1990). Portraits of practitioners of body modification, bondage, and S/M, accompanied by the subjects' personal reflections.

The Sexually Dominant Woman: A Workbook for Nervous Beginners by Lady Green (Greenery Press,1992). A step-by-step guide to planning, negotiating, and carrying out a female dominant S/M scene (geared toward heterosexuals).

SM 101: A Realistic Introduction by Jay Wiseman (Greenery Press, 1992). A thorough guide to S/M equipment and techniques, focusing on physical safety and geared toward heterosexuals.

The Topping Book by Catherine A. Liszt and Dossie Easton (Greenery Press, 1995). An illustrated guide to dominance.

Children, Teens, and Parents

Beyond the Big Talk by Debra Haffner (Newmarket Press, 2001). Advice for parents of preteens and teens on talking about sex.

Changing Bodies, Changing Lives edited by Ruth Bell (Random House/Vintage Books, 1987). A comprehensive guide to puberty and adolescence written for 14- to 19-year olds with quotes from teenagers.

Deal with It by Esther Drill, Heather McDonald, and Rebecca Odes (Pocket Books, 1999). From the founders of the popular website gURL.com, a hip guide for teen and preteen girls, with accurate information about bodies, feelings, and changing relationships.

The Eros of Parenthood by Noelle Oxenhandler (St. Martin's Press, 2001). An examination of the erotic aspect of the parent–child bond.

Harmful to Minors by Judith Levine (University of Minnesota Press, 2002). Provocative and intelligent discussion of how societal attempts to "protect" children from sex is ultimately harmful to the development of a healthy sexuality.

It's Perfectly Normal: Changing Bodies, Growing Up, Sex and Sexual Health by Robie H. Harris (Candlewick Press, 1996). Sex-education book for 10- to 14-year-olds, with cartoon illustrations.

It's So Amazing by Robie H. Harris and Michael Emberley (Candlewick Press, 1999). Well-illustrated, positive, informative, and fun guide for kids 7 to 10 about bodies, babies, and family love.

A Kid's First Book about Sex by Joani Blank (Down There Press, 1983). A lively presentation of sex information for young children—one of the few books that discusses sexuality as distinct from reproduction. Illustrated.

More Speaking of Sex by Meg Hickling (Northstone Publishing, 1999). A fantastic resource for parents needing help with age-appropriate responses to kids' sex questions.

The Period Book: Everything You Don't Want to Ask but Need to Know by Karen and Jennifer Gravelle (Walker Publishing Company, 1996). Information on the physical, emotional, and social changes that accompany puberty, cowritten by a teenager.

The Playbook for Kids about Sex by Joani Blank (Down There Press, 1982). An interactive playbook/workbook that encourages sexual awareness in children (text is the same as in *A Kid's First Book about Sex*).

Two Teenagers in Twenty: Writings by Gay and Lesbian Youth edited by Ann Heron (Alyson, 1994). A collection of essays (only some are about sex) by gay and lesbian teens.

What's Happening to My Body? Book for Boys; What's Happening to My Body? Book for Girls by Lynda Maderas (Newmarket Press, 1987). Written for preteens, these informative guides to the changes brought on by puberty are reassuring without being condescending.

Your Body Belongs to You by Cornelia Spelman and Teri Weidner (Albert Whitman and Co., 1997). In clear, simple statements, therapist Spelman explains to children what types of touch are okay, how they can decline being touched, and what to do when someone crosses their boundaries.

Older Adults

Menopause Naturally by Sadja Greenwood, M.D. (Down There Press, 1996). This informative common-sense guide balances a holistic with a medical approach, addressing cultural influences as well as physical facts.

Ourselves, Growing Older by Paula Brown Doress and Diana Laskin Siegal (Simon & Schuster/Touchstone, 1987). A source book on female sexuality and sexual health specific to the concerns of women over 35.

Sex Over 50 by Joel Block, Ph.D., with Susan Crain Bakos (Prentice Hall Press, 1999). Covers self-esteem, rekindling desire, sexual techniques, and a host of health issues.

Still Doing It edited by Joani Blank (Down There Press, 2000). A collection of first-person accounts about sex from women and men over 60.

Transgender

Body Alchemy: Transsexual Portraits by Loren Cameron (Cleis Press, 1996). Photographs of female-to-male transsexuals, with essays.

Gender Outlaw by Kate Bornstein (Vintage Books, 1994). First-person account of the author's transformation from heterosexual male to lesbian woman.

Lessons from the Intersexed by Suzanne Kessler (Rutgers University Press, 1998). Kessler interviews surgeons, endocrinologists, parents of intersex children, and adults who were treated for being intersexed at birth.

Pomosexuals edited by Carol Queen and Lawrence Schimel (Cleis Press, 1997). Features writing from all shades of the gender spectrum, focusing on the politics of gender roles and transsexuality.

Sex Changes: The Politics of Transgenderism by Patrick Califia (Cleis Press, 2002). An insightful analysis of the contemporary history of transsexuality.

Sublime Mutations by Del LaGrace Volcano (Janssen Verlag, 2000). Color photographs of people who are transgender and intersex.

True Selves: Understanding Transsexualism by Mildred L. Brown and Chloe Ann Rounsley (Jossey Bass, 1996). An ideal book for a family member, friend, or coworker who is struggling to understand a loved one's transition, with first-person accounts from both FTMs and MTFs.

Sex and Culture

Bi Any Other Name: Bisexual People Speak Out edited by Loraine Hutchins and Lani Kaahumanu (Alyson Publications, 1990). A collection of seventy bisexual coming-out stories.

Bi Lives edited by Kate Ondorff (See Sharp Press, 1999). Eighteen interviews with bisexual women.

Susie Bright's essay collections are funny, provocative, and inspirational:

> *Full Exposure: Opening Up to Your Sexual Creativity and Erotic Expression* (HarperSanFrancisco, 1999).
>
> *How to Read/Write a Dirty Story* (Venus Book Club, 2001).
>
> *Susie Bright's Sexual Reality: A Virtual Sex World Reader* (Cleis Press, 1992).
>
> *Susie Bright's Sexual State of the Union* (Simon & Schuster, 1997).
>
> *Susie Bright's Sexwise* (Cleis Press, 1995).
>
> *Susie Sexpert's Lesbian Sex World* (Cleis Press, 1990).

Defending Pornography: Free Speech, Sex and the Fight for Women's Rights by Nadine Strossen (Doubleday/Anchor, 1995). A feminist perspective on the dangers of censorship.

Erotic Impulse: Honoring the Sexual Self edited by David Steinberg (Putnam/Jeremy P. Tarcher/Perigee Books, 1992). A wide-ranging collection of writings on sexuality from noted novelists, poets, therapists, and sexperts.

Gender Shock: Exploding the Myths of Male and Female by Phyllis Burke (Anchor Books, 1996). A provocative and inspirational attack on our rigid gender system.

Intimate Matters: A History of Sexuality in America by John D'Emilio and Estelle B. Freedman (University of Chicago Press, 1997). Explores the evolution of American sexual attitudes over the past four centuries. Second edition.

A New View of Women's Sexual Problems edited by Ellyn Kaschak and Leonore Tiefer (Haworth Press, 2001). A collection of essays comprising a feminist critique of the medical approach to women's sexual health.

Post Porn Modernist by Annie Sprinkle (Cleis Press, 1998). Annie chronicles her career in massage parlors, adult films, and performance art in a book that is part autobiography, part photo album.

Public Sex: The Culture of Radical Sex by Pat Califia (Cleis Press, 1994). The noted sex writer's collected essays on pornography, S/M, sexual repression, and other topics.

Real Live Nude Girl by Carol Queen (Cleis Press, 2002). First-person chronicle of sex-positive culture.

Sex in History by Reay Tannahill (Scarborough House, 1992). An engaging exploration of sexual attitudes and practices in the major world civilizations from prehistoric times up to the present day.

Sex Is Not a Natural Act by Lenore Tiefer (Westview, 1995). A collection of short essays challenging the assumptions underlying cultural constructions of sexuality

Sex Work: Writings by Women in the Sex Industry edited by Frédérique Delacoste and Priscilla Alexander (Cleis Press, 1998). A candid and provocative collection of writings by women sex workers.

Sexual Politics and Disability by Tom Shakespeare, Kath Gillespe-Sells, and Dominic Davies (Continuum, 1996). First-hand accounts about sex and disability.

Speaking Sex to Power: The Politics of Queer Sex by Patrick Califia (Cleis Press, 2002).

The Technology of Orgasm: "Hysteria," the Vibrator, and Women's Sexual Satisfaction by Rachel P. Maines (Johns Hopkins University Press, 1999). The true history of the invention of the vibrator.

Fiction

Erotica Series

Best American Erotica edited by Susie Bright (Simon & Schuster/Touchstone).

Best Bisexual Women's Erotica edited by Cara Bruce (Cleis Press).

Best Black Women's Erotica edited by Blanche Richardson (Cleis Press).

Best Gay Erotica edited by Richard Labonté (Cleis Press).

Best Lesbian Erotica edited by Tristan Taormino (Cleis Press).

Best Women's Erotica edited by Marcy Sheiner (Cleis Press).

Herotica Series, Volumes 1-7, various editors (Penguin/Plume).

Noirotica edited by Thomas Roche (Black Books).

Wicked Words: Black Lace Short Story Collection edited by Kerri Sharp (Black Lace).

Anthologies

Best Transgender Erotica edited by Hanne Blank and Raven Kaldera (Circlet Press, 2002).

Black Silk: Collection of African American Erotica edited by Retha Powers (Warner Books, 2002).

Brown Sugar: A Collection of Erotic Black Fiction by Carol Taylor (Plume, 2001).

Caliente: Latin American Erotica edited by J. H. Blair (Berkeley Publishing Group, 2002).

Erotic Travel Tales edited by Mitzi Szereto (Cleis Press, 2001).

Mammoth Book of Best New Erotica edited by Maxim Jakubowski (Carrol & Graf, 2001).

Neurotica: Jewish Writers on Sex edited by Melvin Jules Bukiet (Bantam, 2000).

On Our Backs: The Best Erotic Fiction (Alyson Publications, 2001).

Oy of Sex: Jewish Women Write Erotica edited by Marcy Sheiner (Cleis Press, 1999).

Ripe Fruit: Erotica for Well-Seasoned Lovers edited by Marcy Sheiner (Cleis Press, 2001).

Sex Spoken Here edited by Carol Queen and Jack Davis (Down There Press, 1998).

Sex Toy Tales edited by Anne Semans and Cathy Winks (Down There Press, 1998).

Sweet Life: Erotic Fantasies for Couples edited by Violet Blue (Cleis Press, 2001).

Zaftig: Well-Rounded Erotica edited by Hanne Blank (Cleis Press, 2001).

Novels

Autobiography of a Flea by Anonymous (Carroll & Graf, 1983).

Fanny Hill by Anonymous (Carroll & Graf, 1990).

Marketplace Trilogy: *The Marketplace, The Slave, The Trainer* by Laura Antoniou writing as Sara Adamson (Mystic Rose Books, 2001).

Sleeping Beauty Trilogy: *Claiming of Sleeping Beauty, Beauty's Punishment, Beauty's Release* by Anne Rice writing as A. N. Roquelaure (New American Library/Plume, 1983, 1984, 1985, respectively).

Story of O by Pauline Reage (Ballantine, 1973).

Strictly Confidential by Alison Tyler (Virgin Publishing, 2001).

Vox by Nicholson Baker (Random House, 1992).

Audio Erotica

The Butcher by Alina Reyes (Passion Press, 1995).

Cinematique: Erotic Audio Screenplays (Passion Press, 1999).

Cyborgasm: Erotica in 3D Sound (Passion Press, 1998).

Cyborgasm 2: The Edge of the Bed (Passion Press, 1998).

Erotic Edge edited by Lonnie Barbach (Passion Press, 1995).

The Erotic Reader: Selected Excerpts from Banned Books (Passion Press, 1995).

Herotica, Volumes 1-6, various editors (Passion Press).

Libido's Best: Erotic Audio Sense and Sensibility by Libido, Inc. (Passion Press, 1999).

Art

Collections

Body and Soul: Black Erotica by Rundu Staggers (Crown Publishing, 1996).

Erotic by Nature edited by David Steinberg (Red Alder and Down There Press, 1988).

Erotica Universalis edited by Giles Neret (Taschen, 1995).

The Illustrated Kama Sutra translated by Sir Richard Burton (Inner Traditions, 1991).

Love Lust Desire edited by Michelle Olley (Thunder's Mouth Press, 2001).

Male Nudes edited by David Leddick (Taschen, 2001).

Male Nudes by Women edited by Peter Weiermair (DAP, 1995).

Mammoth Book of Illustrated Erotica edited by Maxim Jakubowski and Marilyn Lewis (Carroll & Graf, 2001).

Naked Libido by Eugene Zakusilo (Libido, Inc., 1999).

Nice Girls Don't edited by Laurence Jaugey-Paget (Janssen Verlag, 1999).

Nothing but the Girl: The Blatant Lesbian Image edited by Susie Bright and Jill Posener (Cassell, 1996).

One Thousand Nudes edited by Michael Koetzle (Taschen, 1995).

Voyeur edited by Charles Melcher and Steven Diamond (Harper Collins, 1999).

Women En Large: Images of Fat Nudes edited by Laurie Edison and Debbie Notkin (Focus Books, 1994).

Notable Erotic Photographers:

Carlos Batts
Phyllis Christopher
Tee Corinne
Charles Gatewood
Della Grace
Laurence Jaugey-Paget
Richard Kern
Eric Kroll
Robert Mapplethorpe
Jill Posener
Herb Ritts
Michael Rosen
Jan Saudek
Michele Serchuk
Eric Stanton
Roy Stuart
Trevor Watson

Videography

Thanks to Susie Bright for introducing us to many of the following videos.

Erotic Classics from the Golden Age of Porn

Autobiography of a Flea directed by Sharon McNight and the Mitchell Brothers (1976). A wonderfully naughty Victorian romp.

Behind the Green Door directed by the Mitchell Brothers (1972). Marilyn Chambers is spirited away from humdrum reality to live out her fantasies.

Devil in Miss Jones directed by Gerard Damiano (VCA, 1972). Thought-provoking and arousing, with excellent performances.

Every Woman Has a Fantasy directed by Edwin Brown (VCA, 1984). John Leslie portrays a husband who dresses in drag to eavesdrop on his wife and her friends as they recount their sexual fantasies.

Nightdreams directed by Rinse Dream (Caballero, 1981). A surreal presentation of one woman's erotic delusions.

Other Side of Julie directed by Anthony Riverton (Cal Vista, 1978). When Julie discovers that her husband (played by John Leslie) is earning their living as a gigolo, she decides to assert her own sexuality.

Outlaw Ladies directed by Henri Pachard (VCA, 1981). Five women aggressively pursue (and achieve) sexual satisfaction over the course of a day.

3 A.M. directed by Robert McCallum (Cal Vista, 1976). A great erotic tragedy with superior acting.

Notable Contemporary Directors

Brad Armstrong is a multiple *Adult Video News* Award winner. He is lauded for quality production and editing, great sets, and stories.

Maria Beatty (of Blue Productions) focuses on images of S/M and the powerful female, immersing them in contemporary film noir aesthetics.

Andrew Blake has won many fans with his glossy, stylized videos, all of which are notable for high production values, attractive performers, and minimal plots.

Ernest Greene directs erotic and educational fetish and S/M films. Explicit genital contact is not common in films that also depict bondage and discipline, due to potential legal repercussions, but Greene's stylish videos of erotic power play generate plenty of heat.

Veronica Hart's films focus on relationships and hot sex, while featuring high production values, great acting, compelling stories, and good chemistry.

John Leslie's films aren't for the hearts-and-flowers crowd, but they deliver strong plots, tight editing, and athletic, nasty sex between the hottest performers in the business.

Antonio Passolini, who has been directing since the Golden Age of Porn, is best known for his film *Bliss*, which features complex relationships and supercharged sex.

Candida Royalle, of Femme Productions, takes a feminist approach to creating heterosexual porn. Her films celebrate romance and foreplay, and are often less in-your-face than mainstream adult videos (i.e, no external come shots and fewer genital close-ups).

Jackie Strano and Shar Rednour are the lesbian filmmakers behind SIR Productions, specializing in real-lesbian adult videos as well as specialty how-to videos. Their dyke drama *Hard Love and How to Fuck in High Heels* won an *Adult Video News* award, while the anal sex how-to *Bend Over Boyfriend* has been a runaway best-seller since its release.

Paul Thomas delivers satisfying plots, elicits strong performances, and dedicates plenty of screen time to authentic female orgasms in some of the most compelling videos in the industry today.

Educational

Ageless Desire (Afterglow Productions, 2000). Under the expert direction of Juliet "Aunt Peg" Anderson, three truly loving, real-life couples enact playful scenarios that demonstrate their favorite recipes for sexual pleasure, complete with suggestions, information, and explicit imagery.

Bend Over Boyfriend, Volumes 1 & 2 (Fatale and SIR Videos, 1998, 1999). Skilled blow jobs, unrestrained anal penetration, and lots of dirty talk fill these guides to strapping on dildos and penetrating male partners. Directed by Shar Rednour and Jackie Strano.

Better Sex for Black Couples, Volume 1 & 2 (Sinclair, 1999). Romantic and explicit demonstrations by real couples blend with explanations by sex experts to shatter long-held cultural stereotypes and explore issues that shape African American sexuality.

Carol Queen's Great Vibrations directed by Joani Blank (Fatale, 1995). Author of *Exhibitionism for the Shy* and a Good Vibrations staffer, Carol Queen offers explicit vibrator demonstrations together with tips for women and men alike.

Celebrating Orgasm (Betty Dodson, 1996). Betty Dodson offers private coaching in masturbation techniques to five different women ages 26 to 63.

The Complete Guide to Sexual Positions (Pacific Media, 1995). Explicit demonstrations of 100 different sexual positions for heterosexual couples, along with tips for intensifying G-spot stimulation.

Fire in the Valley (EroSpirit, 2000). Famed sex educators/pleasurists Annie Sprinkle and Joseph Kramer team up to bring you the consummate guide to female genital massage.

Guide to Advanced Sexual Positions (Sinclair, 1996). Two real-life, loving couples thoroughly describe and demonstrate an extensive variety of positions for oral, anal, and genital sex.

How to Female Ejaculate (Fatale, 1992). A group of five women discuss their experiences of female ejaculation and then demonstrate in a very fluid circle-jerk.

The Joy of Erotic Massage (Sinclair, 2001). A beautifully shot, tasteful video that gives step-by-step instructions on erotic massage.

Nina Hartley's Guides
 ...to Anal Sex (Adam & Eve, 1996).
 ...to Couples Sexploration (Adam & Eve, 2001).
 ...to Cunnilingus (Adam & Eve, 1994).
 ...to Fellatio (Adam & Eve, 1994).
 ...to Making Love to Men (Adam & Eve, 2000).
 ...to Making Love to Women (Adam & Eve, 2000).
 Porn star Nina Hartley delivers accurate anatomical information and demonstrates techniques with male and female pals with her trademark humor, enthusiasm, and professionalism.

Selfloving (Betty Dodson, 1991). A filmed version of Betty's Dodson's Bodysex workshop, in which a group of ten women discuss sexual self-image and feelings, after which Betty leads them in a guided masturbation ritual.

Sexuality Reborn narrated by Ben Vereen (Kessler Institute for Rehabilitation, 1993). Five couples dealing with spinal cord injuries discuss and demonstrate their sexual techniques (available only through the Kessler Institute).

Sluts and Goddesses directed by Maria Beatty and Annie Sprinkle (EroSpirit, 1992). Annie's diverse female cast explores erotic energy from a New Age perspective, and the video culminates in Annie's five-minute orgasm.

The Tantric Guide to Better Sex (Sinclair, 1997). Tantric experts teach ancient techniques to improve partner orgasms, and several real-life couples explicitly demonstrate the practices.

The Ultimate Guide to Anal Sex for Women, Volumes 1 & 2 (Evil Angel Productions, 1999, 2001). A how-to featuring arousing anal sex scenes (straight and lesbian) mixed with funny, genuinely enlightening conversations about all things anal.

Unlocking the Secrets of the G Spot (Sinclair, 1999). Established sex experts dispel myths while real couples illustrate G-spot techniques and ways to achieve male multiple orgasm.

Viva la Vulva (Betty Dodson, 1998). Led by Betty Dodson, a group of twelve women trim and primp their pubic hair, pose for close-up photo shots, discuss how they learned to love their genitals, and practice full-body massage on each other.

Sex Positive Productions (Good Vibrations' own line
of videos)

Please Don't Stop (2001). Made by and for lesbians
of color, this video focuses on a workshop in
which African American women learn about
sex techniques and toys, which inspires several
of the couples to experiment further at home.

Slide Bi Me (2001). An insurance company's
playfully lusty employees set out to enjoy a
company picnic and wind up having
uninhibited bisexual sex in every possible
combination, and with lots of toys.

Whipsmart (2002). Professional dominatrix
Mistress Morgana instructs viewers on the how
to's of adding power, pleasure, and pain to their
sexual encounters.

Voluptuous Vixens (2002). A diverse group of big
beautiful women play solo and together with
toys.

Index

crura, 18

cunnilingus, 123–125

cybersex, 251, 253–254

cyberskin, 96, 139, 188, 277

D

D/S, 258. *See also* S/M

Deal With It, 43

deep throat, 127

Defending Pornography, 238

dental dams, 129, 130, 283, 288–289; flavored, 130

Depo-Provera, 32

depression, 60–61

desire discrepancy, 75–76

desire, 30–32, 52–54

DHEA, 31, 57

diabetes, 26, 59, 104

Diagnostic and Statistical Manual of Mental Disorders, 30

Dictionary of Sexual Slang, 217

dildos, 136, 139, 140, 150–151, 183–200; acrylic, 189; cleaning, 185–186, 193; cyberskin, 188; double, 150–151, 195; and G-spot stimulation, 21; and genderplay, 199; history of, 183; jelly, 188; latex, 189; and lesbians, 184; and prostate stimulation, 25; prosthetic penis attachments,187–188; realistics, 187; rubber, 186–187; silicone, 189; size, 192; use with partner, 193–194; vegetables, 191; vibrating, 150–151. *See also* butt plugs

Dirty Dice, 222

disability, 58–59, 74, 261–262, 279; and massage, 111; and oral sex, 121; and vibrators, 135

discipline, 213

dissociation, 62

Doc Johnson, 278, 279

Dodson, Betty, 83, 89, 90, 102, 132, 138, 155, 190, 207, 237

Doing It for Daddy, 13

dominance, 257

Down There Press, ix, 8, 228

drug use, 163,174, 263

dry humping, 181–182

DSL, 244

Duncan, Gosnell, 279

Durex, 288

Dworkin, Andrea, 299–300

E

E! Entertainment, 233

Ecker, M. J., 100

ejaculation, in men, 25, 27–28, 83; and oral sex, 122; retrograde, 27; as separate from orgasm, 27–28, 37–38; in women, 21–22, 122, 146, 236

ejaculatory inevitability, 27, 28

Elders, Jocelyn, 100

Ellen/Annie, 16

embodiment, 62

Embrace, 107

Emmanuelle, 232

encryption software, 249

enema, 171

erectile dysfunction, 26–27

erection, 26–27; in older men, 57

Eros Bodyglide, 106

Eros of Parenthood, 119

Eros, 277

Eroscillator, 144

erotic art, 231, 231

Erotic Mind, 77, 81, 223, 262

erotic photography, 231

erotica, 227, 228–232, 250–251

Erotica Readers and Writers Association, 224, 251

estradiol, 31, 56

estrogen, 31–32, 33, 56, 103

Every Woman Has a Fantasy, 234

excitement, 29–30

exhibitionism, 209, 219

Exhibitionism for the Shy, 67, 220

e-zines, 250

F

Faces of Ecstasy, 8

family-building, 51–56

Fanny Hill, 229, 246

Fantasex, 233

Fantasy Joystick, 133

fantasy, 74, 185, 208–224, 230; and S/M, 259, 263

Fat Girl, 249

Fatale Videos, 236, 242

FBI, 299

feces, 129, 170–171

Federal Communications Commission (FCC), 218.

fellatio, 125–127

female-to-male transsexuals (FTMs), 33, 35, 199

Femalia, 8, 11

feminist porn, 235

Feminists for Free Expression, 246, 300

Femme Productions, 159, 235

fetish, 262

Reality female condom, 286–287
rectum, 29, 170–173, 174, 202
Rednour, Shar, 236
refractory period, 37
rejection, 66–67
Religious Right, 44, 132, 276, 298
Replens, 56
reproductive technologies, 51
resolution, 29–30
restraints, 268–269
Rice, Anne, 228
rimming, 129
risk management, 292–294
Ritts, Herb, 231
Robertson, Pat, 304
role-playing, 216, 258–259, 265
Romeo and Juliet, 5
Rosen, Michael, 231
Rourke, Mickey, 272
Royalle, Candida, 145, 151, 159, 233, 235

S

S/M, 213, 257–274 ; community, 258; erotica, 230;
    equipment, 266–274
sadomasochism. *See* S/M
safer sex, 180, 281–296; and communication, 72,
    291–292; and lubricants, 108–109, 283; and
    masturbation, 90, 98; and oral sex, 122, 129–131;
    risk, 292–294
safety, 262–263, 266, 268, 274.
safeword, 266
San Francisco Sex Information, 8
Saran Wrap, 129–130, 283, 288
Saudek, Jan, 231
Scarlet Letters, 247
Scarleteen, 247
science fiction, 228, 229–230
Scorpio Products, 279
Screaming Orgasms, 236
Screw, 239
scrotum, 23–24
secondary sex characteristics, 33
selective serotonin reuptake inhibitors (SSRIs),
    60–61, 104
self-censorship, 391
self-esteem, 9–15; and masturbation, 12; and STDs,
    295–296
self-knowledge, 67–68
SelfLoving, 90, 102, 138, 237

Semans, Anne, ix
seminal vesicles, 27
seniors, 57–58
sensory deprivation, 271–272
Sensuous Woman, 5
sex boutiques, 153, 189, 227
sex education, 43–44, 301; abstinence-only, 44; lack
    of, 45, 66; online, 246–247; videos, 237
Sex Etc., 43, 247
Sex for One, 11, 102, 138
sex guides, xi, 3, , 230
sex reassignment surgery, 33
sex toys, 275–276, 302; cleaning, 153, 185, 193, 270;
    design, 277–278; and fantasy, 220–221;
    manufacturers, 2, 275–280; and massage, 117–118;
    and masturbation, 83, 92, 99; and sex manuals, xii,
    133
Sexpositive Productions, ix, 235
sexual abuse, 61–62
sexual assault, 61–62
sexual fluids, 122, 130. *See also* safer sex
sexual identity, 33, 34, 35
Sexual Magic, 231
sexual response cycle, 29–30
Sexuality Information and Education Council of the
    United States (SIECUS), 247
sexually transmitted disease (STD), 24, 72, 108,
    129–131, 281–296; bacterial, 282; symptoms,
    282–282; viral, 282
shaft, of clitoris, 18; of penis, 23
shame, 2, 11
Show Me, 301
Siffredi, Rocco, 233
Silverberg, Cory, 59
Simon & Schuster, 228
SIR Videos, 235, 236
sixty-nine, 127–128
slappers, 271
slash, 251
sleeves, 146; vibrating, 135, 149
Slide Bi Me, 235
Slip Not, 198
Slippery Stuff, 105, 106
Sluts and Goddesses, 16
smut, 226, 229
Society for Human Sexuality, 247, 256
sodomy, 120
spam, 255
Spectator, 304

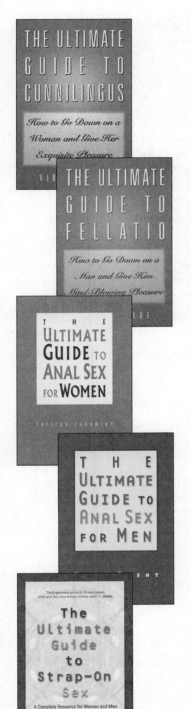

Classic Sex Guides

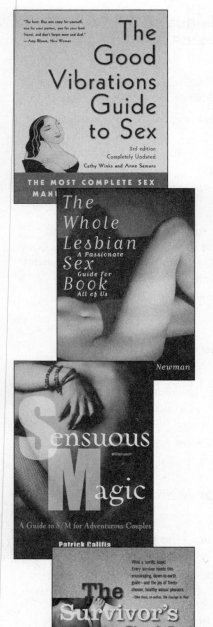

The Good Vibrations Guide To Sex
THE MOST COMPLETE SEX MANUAL EVER WRITTEN
THIRD EDITION

Cathy Winks and Anne Semans
Illustrated by Phoebe Gloeckner

"Nobody knows what's really going on in America's bedrooms like the gals at Good Vibrations." —Susie Bright

$24.95 • ISBN:1-57344-158-9 • Illustrations, bibliography, resources, index

The Whole Lesbian Sex Book
A PASSIONATE GUIDE FOR ALL OF US

Felice Newman

"The most complete, all-questions-answered, savvy guide to lesbian, butch, bisexual, femme, androgynous and transgendered sex! Keep it next to your bed!" —Good Vibrations

"Superb. Why can't more heterosexual sex manuals be this good?" —Library Journal

$24.95 • ISBN: 1-57344-088-4 • Illustrations, bibliography, resources, index

Sensuous Magic
A GUIDE FOR ADVENTUROUS COUPLES
2ND EDITION

Patrick Califia

Califia's much-loved beginner's guide to S/M for couples is for all readers who harbor fantasies of erotic dominance and submission. Completely revised and updated, featuring all-new erotic stories by Califia.

$14.95 • ISBN: 1-57344-130-9 • Bibliography, resources

The Survivor's Guide to Sex
HOW CREATE YOUR OWN EMPOWERED SEXUALITY
AFTER CHILDHOOD SEXUAL ABUSE

Staci Haines

The first encouraging, sex-positive guide for all women survivors of sexual assault. "What a terrific book! Every survivor needs this encouraging, down-to-earth guide—and the joy of freely-chosen, healthy sexual pleasure."—Ellen Bass

$21.95 • ISBN: 1-57344-079-5 • Illustrations, bibliography, index

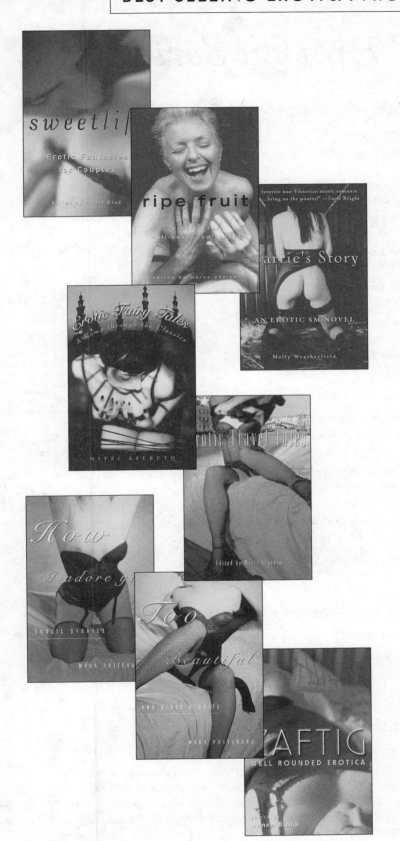

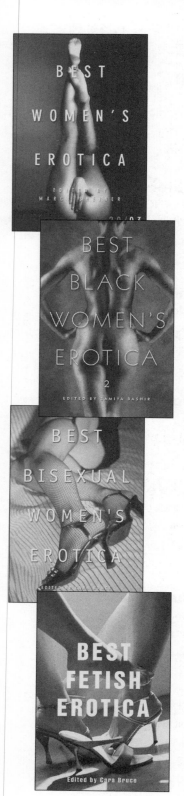